N.I. HEALTH AND SOCIAL SERVICES
QUEEN'S

4/73

CONGENITAL ABNORMALITIES
IN INFANCY

CONGENITAL ABNORMALITIES IN INFANCY

EDITED BY
A. P. NORMAN
M.D. F.R.C.P.

*Physician, The Hospital for Sick Children
Great Ormond Street
Paediatrician, Queen Charlotte's
Maternity Hospital*

SECOND EDITION

BLACKWELL SCIENTIFIC PUBLICATIONS
OXFORD AND EDINBURGH

© 1971 by Blackwell Scientific Publications
5 Alfred Street, Oxford, England, and
9 Forrest Road, Edinburgh, Scotland

All rights reserved. No part of this publication may be reproduced, stored in a retrieval system or transmitted, in any form or by any means, electronic, mechanical, photocopying, recording or otherwise without the prior permission of the copyright owner.

ISBN 0 632 05640 1

First published 1963
Second edition 1971

Distributed in the U.S.A. by
F.A.Davis Company, 1915 Arch Street,
Philadelphia, Pennsylvania

Printed in Great Britain by
Alden & Mowbray Ltd
at the Alden Press, Oxford
and bound by
The Kemp Hall Bindery

Contents

	List of Contributors	vii
	Preface	ix
	Acknowledgments	xi
1	Incidence and Aetiology *C.O.Carter*	1
2	Abnormalities of the Central Nervous System *K.M.Laurence and R.Weeks*	25
3	Abnormalities of the Cardiothoracic System *R.J.K.Brown*	87
4	Abnormalities of the Ear, Nose and Throat *H.S.Sharp*	131
5	Abnormalities of the Eyes and associated structures *C.A.Brown*	147
6	Abnormalities of the Genito-urinary System *D.I.Williams*	199
7	Abnormalities of the Gastro-intestinal System *H.H.Nixon and A.W.Wilkinson*	230
8	Orthopaedic Abnormalities *G.C.Lloyd-Roberts*	256
9	Abnormalities of the Skin *E.J.Moynahan*	289
10	Special Syndromes *A.White Franklin*	350
11	Syndromes due to Chromosomal Abnormalities *A. P. Norman*	392
	Index	416

List of Contributors

C.A.BROWN M.A. M.D. F.R.C.S. D.O.M.S.
Consultant Ophthalmic Surgeon, United Bristol Hospitals (Bristol Eye Hospital) and South Western Regional Hospital Board

R.J.K.BROWN M.B. M.R.C.P.
Consultant Paediatrician, Queen Elizabeth Hospital for Children, London and Middlesex Hospital

C.O.CARTER B.M. F.R.C.P.
Medical Research Council, Clinical Genetics Unit, The Hospital for Sick Children, Great Ormond Street

K.M.LAURENCE M.A. M.B.
Senior Lecturer in Paediatric Pathology, Welsh National School of Medicine, Llandough Hospital, Penarth; Consultant Pathologist, Cardiff United Hospitals

G.C.LLOYD-ROBERTS F.R.C.S.
Orthopaedic Surgeon, The Hospital for Sick Children, Great Ormond Street and St George's Hospital

E.J.MOYNAHAN F.R.C.P.
Physician-in-charge, Dermatological Department, The Hospital for Sick Children, Great Ormond Street; Physician, Dermatological Department, Guy's Hospital

H.H.NIXON M.B. F.R.C.S.
Paediatric Surgeon, The Hospital for Sick Children, Great Ormond Street and Children's Hospital, Paddington Green

A.P.NORMAN M.D. F.R.C.P.
Physician, The Hospital for Sick Children, Paediatrician, Queen Charlotte's Maternity Hospital

H.S.SHARP M.B. F.R.C.S.
Surgeon, E.N.T. Department, The Hospital for Sick Children, Great Ormond Street, and Charing Cross Hospital

A.WHITE FRANKLIN M.B. B.CH. F.R.C.P.
Hon. Consulting Paediatrician, Queen Charlotte's Maternity Hospital and St Bartholomew's Hospital

A.W.WILKINSON CH.M.EDIN. F.R.C.S.ED. F.R.C.S.
Nuffield Professor of Paediatric Surgery, Institute of Child Health, University of London; Surgeon, The Hospital for Sick Children, Great Ormond Street

D.INNES WILLIAMS M.D. M.CHIR. F.R.C.S.
Genito-urinary Surgeon, The Hospital for Sick Children, Great Ormond Street; Surgeon, St Peter and St Paul's Hospital

Preface

TO FIRST EDITION

I very much welcomed the suggestion that I might edit a book on Congenital Abnormalities. And I have often felt the lack of one. However, in planning it, it became evident that an attempt to cover the field of congenital abnormalities comprehensively, would either result in an excessively large volume or would be too cursory. It seemed best to limit the scope to anomalies apparent, by and large, in the first weeks of life. It has been by the side of the cot of a newborn baby that I have most often wished for some handy authority to which I could refer.

The contributors of the 10 chapters are all experts in their own fields and most have special knowledge of the newborn. In collecting this distinguished panel, it was interesting to find, however, how remote some specialities are from contact with the very young baby. On the other hand, reading some of the contributions shows that an almost new world of diagnosis may open to those who have been alerted to the possibilities and who have the knowledge and skill to recognize what they see.

I owe all the contributors a considerable debt of gratitude for permitting me to alter their text in places—in some instances to cut it very severely, and for allowing the interpolation or alteration of the genetic counselling sections in each of their chapters. This last has been carried out by Dr. Cedric Carter and in some cases the risks he gives are based on unpublished work of his own. Where there is no note on genetics, it may be assumed that there is no genetic cause or that the genetic effect is insignificant. I am, furthermore, most grateful to Cedric Carter for his advice and support throughout.

The name of certain syndromes gives rise to a little difficulty; for instance, there is pressure to alter terms such as mongolism and gargoylism. As alternative names are not yet generally accepted, I have used the term Down's syndrome (mongolism) at the first mention or where it forms a main item in each chapter and thereafter continued to use mongolism.

PREFACE

The use of illustrations also poses a problem as very high quality or numerous illustrations increase the cost of publication very considerably. In order, therefore, to keep down the cost of this book the number of illustrations has been limited to those which seem to show something not easily explained in the text or requiring emphasis.

A. P. NORMAN

January 1963

TO SECOND EDITION

Many of the chapters in the second edition have been extensively rewritten and R.D.Weeks has collaborated with Dr. Laurence to supply the clinical aspects of abnormalities of the Central Nervous System. The additional chapter on Chromosomal Abnormalities written by the Editor may require an apology on the grounds that it is both too brief and the writing too condensed, but in fact syndromes due to known chromosomal abnormalities and recognizable at birth are, with the exception of Down's syndrome, very rare; and form only a small though important section of congenital abnormalities as a whole.

A. P. NORMAN

March 1971

Acknowledgments

Dr. C.O.Carter for his constant advice and help, and for checking or inserting in each chapter the sections on incidence, genetic transmission, and empiric risks.

The consultant staff of The Hospital for Sick Children, Great Ormond Street, for permission to publish photographs of children in their care.

The Department of Medical Illustration, The Hospital for Sick Children, for supplying many of the illustrations; Mr. G.Lyth of this department for some of the diagrams; Mr. R.Lunnon, Director of the Department of Medical Illustration for allowing me to reproduce his ultraviolet photograph of palmar ridges and tri-radii in the normal hand.

Professor Paul Polani for his kindness in sending me the photographs and karyotypes of Patau's and Edwards's syndrome and of the hand and dermatoglyphics in Down's syndrome, taken by Dr. A. Boyers.

Dr. Beryl Corner, and Messrs. Cassells, for permission to reproduce illustrations from Dr. Corner's book *The Premature Baby*, in Chapter 5.

Miss Isabelle Forshall for supplying, and permission to publish, the illustrations in Chapter 3.

The Department of Medical Photography, University of Bristol, for supplying most of the illustrations in Chapter 5.

I

Incidence and Aetiology

C.O.CARTER

The Total Incidence of Congenital Malformations

Congenital malformations may be defined as abnormalities of structure present at birth and attributable to faulty development. Estimates of their total incidence are inevitably subjective. Such estimates will depend on the inclusion or exclusion of malformed stillbirths, the care with which children are examined, the period for which the children are followed, the number of minor malformations that are included and whether the estimates refer to hospital births or include domiciliary births as well. The incidence of children with at least one major malformation apparent at or soon after birth, stillbirths included, is, however, of the order of 15 per thousand total births. If the children are followed for a year and some minor malformations are included, the incidence rises to 4 or 5 per cent. The incidence of individual malformations differs widely in different races of man, but the total incidence appears to be similar in such varied races as European and North American Whites and Japanese, though probably lower in Negroes.

In Table 1.1 is summarized the incidence of the commoner major malformations, apparent at or soon after birth, in three large population series each of the order of 40,000 to 100,000 total births, from England (Birmingham), Sweden and Japan (Hiroshima and Nagasaki), together with one smaller series of just over 16,000 births from Nigeria (Lagos). In Table 1.2 are listed the incidence in the Birmingham series, after the children had been followed for 5 years; in the Japanese series after the children had been followed for 9 months; and in a relatively small, but exceptionally thoroughly investigated North American series, in which the children were followed for a year.

TABLE 1.1
Incidence of malformations (per 1000 total births). Estimates soon after birth (after McKeown & Record, 1960; Leck et al., 1968 and Lesi, 1968)

	Birmingham	Sweden	Japan	Nigeria
Total births	94,474	44,109	64,750	16,720
Anencephalus	2·0	0·5	0·6	0·8
Spina bifida	2·5	1·1–1·5	0·3	0·2
Hydrocephalus	0·9	1·0	0·3	0·3
Cardiac malformations	2·2	0·8	4·2	0·0
Cleft lip and palate	1·5	1·8	2·8	0·4
Dislocation of the hip	0·0	0·0	0·3	0·0
Talipes	4·2	2·8	1·1	1·1
Mongolism (Down's syndrome)	0·9	0·5	0·1	0·2
All individuals with major malformations	about 20·0	11·2	12·2	about 4·0

TABLE 1·2
Incidence of major malformations (per 1000 total births). Estimates based on observations beyond the neonatal period (after McKeown & Record, 1960)

	Birmingham	New York	Japan
Period of observation	(to 5 years)	(to 1 year)	(to 9 months)
Total births		5,749	16,144
Anencephalus	2·0	1·6	0·6
Spina bifida	2·6	1·6	0·3
Hydrocephalus	1·4	0·9	0·5
Cardiac malformations	4·2	8·5	7·0
Cleft lip and palate	2·0	1·6	3·0
Dislocation of the hip	0·7	1·2	7·1
Talipes	5·7	5·2	1·4
Mongolism (Down's syndrome)	1·6	1·9	0·9
All individuals with major malformations	about 25·0	Not given (total malformed 75·3)	24·5

The Contribution of Congenital Malformations to Death in Infancy

The death rate from congenital malformations has only recently begun to fall in technically advanced countries and any fall is attributable to better treatment rather than a decline in incidence. It would seem, therefore, that the influences responsible for congenital malformations are, in general, unaffected by a rise in the standard of living. In England and Wales the infant deaths certified as due to congenital malformations remained at 4 to 5 per thousand live births from the turn of the century until the last few years, while the total infant mortality has declined from 130 to under 20. In 1967 of 18·3 infant deaths 3·8 were ascribed to congenital malformations. In the year 1900 congenital malformations were responsible for only about 1 infant death in 30; they are now responsible for between 1 in 4 and 1 in 5. This is probably an underestimate since a malformation which is a major contributory cause of death, for example Down's syndrome (mongolism) in a child dying from bronchopneumonia, is not always entered on the death certificate.

The Frequency of Individual Malformations

Central Nervous System

In north-western Europeans it is the central nervous system and the heart which are most often malformed to a degree which constitutes a danger to life. The Birmingham series shown in Table 1·1, with an incidence of anencephaly of 2·0 per thousand total births and an incidence of spina bifida cystica of 2·5 per thousand, is representative of other English series. These two types of malformations are aetiologically related.

They occur with an even higher frequency in the north and west of the British Isles. Outside north-west Europe and areas inhabited by peoples of similar race the incidence in most instances is much lower. It will be seen in Table 1.1 that in Sweden the incidence was 0·5 per thousand for anencephaly and about 1·2 per thousand for spina bifida cystica, in Japan the figures were 0·6 and 0·3 per thousand, in Nigeria 0·8 and 0·2 respectively. It is noteworthy that in Japan and Nigeria the relative incidence of the two malformations is reversed, and anencephaly is commoner than spina bifida. Two new areas of high incidence in addition to north-west Europe are that of the Sikh community in the

Punjab and Alexandria in Egypt. It is not yet known how widely these high-incidence areas extend.

Figures for the incidence of congenital hydrocephaly are less reliable; malformations may be listed as hydrocephaly where the essential abnormality is a spina bifida cystica with an associated Arnold–Chiari malformation. Also where the hydrocephaly develops after birth it is not always clear, even on autopsy, whether the lesion responsible was congenital or acquired. The true incidence is probably of the order of 0·5 per thousand total births in Europe.

The Heart and Great Vessels

The incidence of congenital heart malformations may only be ascertained by careful follow-up of cohorts of children at best up to the time of examination by the school medical service. Estimates of 4 to 7 per thousand total births have been reported from Birmingham, Liverpool, Gothenberg, British Columbia and San Francisco. The true incidence is probably somewhat higher as some cases will be missed among neonatal deaths and some will not be detected till school age. The small but carefully followed series of Richards *et al.* (1965) gave an incidence of 8 per thousand total births.

The approximate percentage subdivision into the commoner types are: ventricular septal defects 20 per cent; patent ductus arteriosus, atrial septal defect, coarctation of the aorta, pulmonary stenosis, Fallot's tetrology and transposition of the great vessels each 10 per cent; aortic stenosis 5 per cent; and a miscellaneous remainder 15 per cent.

Cleft Lip and Cleft Palate

Family studies show that cleft lip, with or without an associated cleft palate, is genetically distinct from midline cleft palate without malformation of the lip; but estimates of the incidence often refer to the combined incidence. Western European data show incidences of 1·2 to 1·9 per thousand total births, and of these about three-quarters have cleft lip with or without cleft palate, and one-quarter have cleft palate alone. Cleft lip with or without cleft palate, therefore, has an incidence in western Europe of about 1·2 per thousand and isolated cleft palate about 0·4 per thousand. The W.H.O. survey of maternity hospital and other data indicates that the highest incidence is in southern Mongolians (including Japanese) where cleft lip ($\pm$ cleft palate) reaches up to 2·0 per thousand, next in northern Mongolians and American Indians, next in western Europeans (about 1·5), next in eastern Europeans (about 0·7) and lowest in Negroes (about 0·3).

Congenital Dislocation of the Hip
The incidence of congenital dislocation of the hip is especially difficult to estimate because of varying standards of diagnosis. In Britain and Sweden the incidence when diagnosis is made late is about 1 per thousand total births. Diagnosis in the neonatal period appears to give an incidence of about 4 per thousand, and it is to be presumed that 3 out of 4 of these would recover spontaneously. High incidences in children after the neonatal period are associated with the practice of tight swaddling in hip extension and adduction, as among the Lapps and certain American Indian tribes. This practice may prevent spontaneous recovery. The incidence is probably lower in Indians, Chinese and Negroes than in Europeans. The high figure for Japanese shown in Table 1.2 may represent diagnostic error.

Talipes
Estimates of the incidence of talipes equinovarus and other forms of talipes will be much influenced by the inclusion, or not, of minor degrees of the malformation. The total incidence is of the order of 4 per thousand in Whites. The incidence of severe talipes equinovarus is about 1 per thousand in Britain. The highest incidences of talipes equinovarus occur in Polynesians; an estimate of 6 per thousand has been made for Maoris.

Pyloric stenosis
Pyloric stenosis is not listed in Table 1.1 and 1.2 since it is not certain that it is truly congenital or truly a malformation. It has an incidence of about 3 per thousand total births in Britain and Sweden. It is rather less common in North America and the mainland of Europe, and rarer still in African and Asian populations.

Ulnar Polydactyly and Pre-helicine Fistula
The incidence of these two minor malformations is of interest in that they are each particularly common in Negroes. For example, in a series of just over 2000 births from Kampala (Simpkiss and Lowe 1961), there were no less than twenty-eight examples of ulnar polydactyly, forty-six of pre-helicine fistula and five of accessory auricles. In Lagos

the incidence of polydactyly was 9 per thousand. Radial polydactyly is relatively common in Chinese. In Europe and Japan, the incidence of polydactyly is only about 1 per thousand.

The Special Senses
Only one congenital malformation of the eye is common, and that is congenital cataract. In the carefully examined New York series, the incidence was 2 per thousand total births. In the British national survey (Manson *et al.* 1960) of the effects of virus in pregnancy, in which only the severer forms would have been noted, the incidence was 0·4 per thousand live births.

In this British national survey the total incidence of hearing defects of probably congenital origin, at the age of 2 years, was 0·8 per thousand live births.

Down's Syndrome
Down's syndrome (mongolism) is usually classed among the congenital malformations. The incidence of Down's syndrome in North America, north-west Europe and Australia appears to be between 1·5 and 2·0 per thousand. The condition is known to occur in other races, for example Indians, Africans, Chinese and Japanese; no reliable incidence figures are available because of high infant mortality and the difficulties of early diagnosis, but there are no indications of any racial or geographical variation in incidence other than that due to maternal age variation.

AETIOLOGY

General Considerations
Embryonic and foetal development, like postnatal development, proceeds under the interaction of genetic and environmental factors. Abnormalities of embryonic and foetal development may be due to abnormalities of the genetic potential for development, or to abnormalities of the intra-uterine environment, or to both genetic and environmental factors. Twin and family studies suggest that it is the last situation, a genetically determined lack of resistance to an environmental insult, which is responsible for the majority of naturally occurring congenital malformations in man and animals.

Twin Studies
Twin studies, based on consecutive series of patients, are mostly on too

small a scale to be definitive, but for most malformations they indicate that the proportion of identical co-twins also affected is well below 100 per cent, but more than that for fraternal twins of like sex. For anencephaly and spina bifida cystica, the low concordance for like-sex twins suggests that the concordance for identical twins is low and may be little more than that for fraternal twins, although family studies suggest some degree of genetic determination. This is also the case with congenital malformations of the heart. A large twin study of talipes from southern Germany gave 25 per cent concordance for identical twins and only 2 per cent for fraternal twins. For cleft lip, with or without lateral cleft palate, and also for pyloric stenosis, the concordance of identical pairs appears to be of the order of 30 per cent, but only about 5 per cent for fraternal pairs. A large-scale twin study for congenital dislocation of the hip gave 40 per cent concordance for identical twin pairs, and about 2 per cent for fraternal pairs. Only in the case of Down's syndrome, among common congenital malformations, do twin studies suggest complete genetic determination, since identical twins of patients have almost always had Downs' syndrome.

It should be noted, however, that a rare case of discordance of identical pairs is not incompatible with complete genetic determination, since the genetic abnormality might result from a somatic mutation early in the development of the twin. An example is a case of an identical twin pair, one a normal boy, the other with Turner's syndrome. It should also be noted that where a condition may be caused in more than one way a concordance of below 100 per cent for identical twins is compatible with complete genetic determination of a proportion of cases. There is evidence, for example, with congenital dislocation of the hip, that in some cases genetic predisposition is an important factor, while in others an environmental factor, abnormality of intra-uterine posture, is more important.

The analysis of genetic–environmental interaction in causing malformations is inevitably complicated, and will lag behind that of malformations whose aetiology is, for practical purposes, purely genetic or purely environmental. But in general it is these malformations of complicated aetiology which are the common ones.

Purely Environmental Determination

The brilliant studies of the experimental embryologists, for example

Warkany and his colleagues, over the past two decades in inducing abnormalities by a wide variety of environmental means, naturally led to hopes that such agencies could be incriminated in man. The list of such agents which, affecting or administered to the pregnant maternal animal, may cause malformations in her offspring, is an ever-growing one.

1. Dietary deficiency: including deficiencies of protein, vitamin A, riboflavin, folic acid, thiamine, and those induced by vitamin antagonists such as galactoflavin and folic acid antagonists.
2. Dietary excess: e.g. hypervitaminosis A.
3. Hormones: pituitary, thyroid, pancreatic, adrenal and gonadal.
4. Chemical agents: nitrogen-mustard, some antibiotics, purine antagonists, nucleic acid antagonists, azo-dyes.
5. Physical agents: radiation, hypoxia, hypo- and hyperthermia.
6. Infection.

In fact, however, there is no evidence as yet that any of the first five groups of environmental agents cause any appreciable number of human malformations.

Malformation, especially microcephaly, has been induced by the treatment of pregnant women with radium for cervical cancer; but only seldom since the dangers were recognized in 1925. A number of microcephalic infants were born to mothers pregnant at the time they were exposed to radiation from the atomic explosions in Hiroshima and Nagasaki. A number of instances are known where the use of drugs, aminopterin and recently thalidomide, have resulted in malformed infants. Similarly a few instances are known of malformation following therapeutic dosage of the mother with cortisone. Some genetically female children have been born with varying degrees of masculinization of the genital tract following the administration of androgenic drugs, such as ethisterone, in the treatment of threatened abortion. It has been claimed but not fully established, that there is an increased malformations rate in infants born to mothers with diabetes.

The specific dietary defects and excesses used to induce malformations in animal experiments are greater in degree than those likely to be experienced by human beings, and there is as yet no clear demonstration of any association between maternal diet and malformations in man.

Rubella in Pregnancy

Infection is of greater practical importance. At least ten viruses are capable of producing intra-uterine infection and foetal damage. Two infective agents only, however, has been incriminated as a cause of congenital malformation in the strict sense; these are rubella and cytomegalovirus. Toxoplasmosis can cause inflammation and degeneration of the foetal brain and eye, but these are not true malformations.

Rubella, occurring in the first 3 months of pregnancy, is specifically associated with malformations of one or more of three organs, the eye (congenital cataract), the ear (congenital deafness), and the heart. The proportion of children who are found to be malformed, following maternal rubella in the first trimester, has varied in different prospective series, and perhaps in different epidemics. The highest proportion, 50 per cent, was found in Paris. Most series, however, show between 20 and 30 per cent affected with severe malformations which are apparent in the first 2 years of life. This proportion will be increased if the children are carefully examined later for minor degrees of deafness, and such minor degrees of deafness may follow infection up to the end of the fourth month of pregnancy.

Relatively few cases are recorded of rubella in the first 4 weeks of pregnancy, but there is an indication that the risk of major malformation is highest after such early infection; it is then about 50 per cent and falls to about 30 per cent for infection in the second 4 weeks and to about 15 per cent in the third 4 weeks.

There are, however, differences in the risk of malformation of individual organs according to the period of infection. The incidence of cataract is highest following infection in the first 4 weeks, and there is little or no risk after the twelfth week. The incidence of congenital malformations of the heart is highest following infection in the first and second month, and is still present, though much reduced, in the fourth month. The risk of congenital deafness is highest after infection in the second month and continues into the fourth month.

An additional association with maternal rubella is microcephaly with or without some degree of mental retardation. Severe mental retardation is however uncommon, the incidence is of the order of 1 to 2 per cent, and no good data are yet available on the incidence of minor degrees of mental retardation, or the total range of intelligence in children born after maternal rubella.

Cytomegalic Virus and Herpes Virus 2 in Pregnancy
The relationship of intra-uterine cytomegalic virus infection to malfor-

mation is less well documented than that of rubella virus. Microcephaly and hydrocephaly, microphthalmia and chorioretinitis may follow such infection. Similar damage to the nervous system has been reported in a few cases following herpes virus 2. More recently congenital malformation in the strict sense, first arch malformations, including deafness, cleft lip and palate have been reported with cytomegalovirus infection.

Congenital Heart Malformations
There is suggestive, but as yet not conclusive, evidence that infection of the foetus with coxsackie B viruses may cause congenital heart malformations. There is more tenuous evidence that infection by mumps may also cause such malformation.

Birth Order and Maternal Age Effects
A more indirect indication of environmental influences is shown by maternal age and birth order effects. The most striking maternal age effect is shown by Down's syndrome and other trisomies (trisomy 16 in abortuses appear to be an exception). These are genetically determined conditions, but it appears that the likelihood of chromosomal non-disjunction increases rapidly after a maternal, age of 30 years. Birth order has no influence independent of maternal age. Anencephaly and spina bifida show a U-shaped relationship to birth order and maternal age, the risks being highest in first-born and late birth orders, also at maternal age under 20 and over 35 years. The effects of maternal age are still seen after standardization for birth order and vice-versa. Talipes is also commonest at under 20 and over 40 years. Uncomplicated hydrocephalus shows a very marked late maternal age effect. Polydactyly in contrast shows a declining rate with increasing maternal age. Congenital dislocation of the hip is markedly more common in first-born, presumably due to the influence of the frank breech malformation.

Except in the case of congenital dislocation of the hip the mechanism by which maternal age and birth order affects these is not known.

A paternal age effect is seen with some severe dominant conditions in the sporadic instances where the patient is affected by a fresh mutation.

PURELY GENETIC DETERMINATION

It is useful to distinguish between two main classes of genetic abnormalities that are responsible for malformations in man. The first class, chromosome mutation, involves mutations of whole chromosomes or of fragments sufficiently large to be visible under the microscope. The second class, point or gene mutations, involves mutations at single gene loci on a chromosome, or of fragments of a chromosome too small to be recognized microscopically.

In chromosome mutations many gene loci are involved, many biochemical processes will be disturbed, and the effect will be to produce abnormalities affecting many systems of the body, as in Down's syndrome and Turner's syndrome. In gene mutations there will often be an abnormality of the production of only a single enzyme or other protein, and only a single biochemical process will be involved. This will sometimes affect the development of several bodily systems, as in Ellis–Van Creveld's syndrome; perhaps more often only one bodily system will be affected, as in achondroplasia or aniridia. This will depend on whether several, or only one, type of cell makes use in its metabolism of the particular gene product concerned.

Chromosome Mutation

It is now established that there are twenty-three pairs of chromosomes in man. There are twenty-two pairs of autosomes in which each member of the pair are alike, and one pair of sex chromosomes consisting of two like X chromosomes in women and an X chromosome and a small Y chromosome in men. The autosomes are classified by their total length and by the relative length of the long and short arms of the chromosome, as divided by the centromere. They are numbered in descending order of total length from 1, the largest, to 22, the smallest; though several are of much the same size, for example the two small pairs of 21 and 22 cannot reliably be distinguished from each other.

Two types of chromosome mutation are at present known to cause malformation in man. The first is *non-disjunction*, the second is *structural change leading to translocation or deletion*.

Autosomal Non-disjunction

In non-disjunction there is a failure of the two members of a chromosome pair to separate in germ cell formation. This will result in a germ cell with either one chromosome too many, both members of the pair having passed into the germ cell; or one chromosome too few, neither member of the pair having passed into the germ cell. After fertilization by a normal germ cell derived from the other parent, the zygote will have either one chromosome too many, that is three chromosomes of one type, and is said to be *trisomic* for that chromosome; or have only one member of the chromosome pair (that derived from the normal germ cell) and be *monosomic* for that chromosome. The non-disjunction may occur either at the first reduction division in germ cell formation

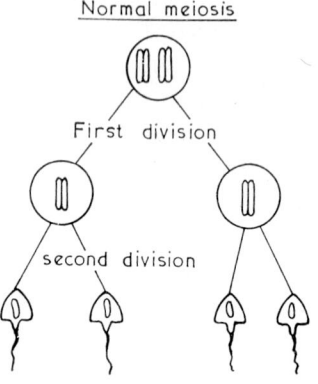

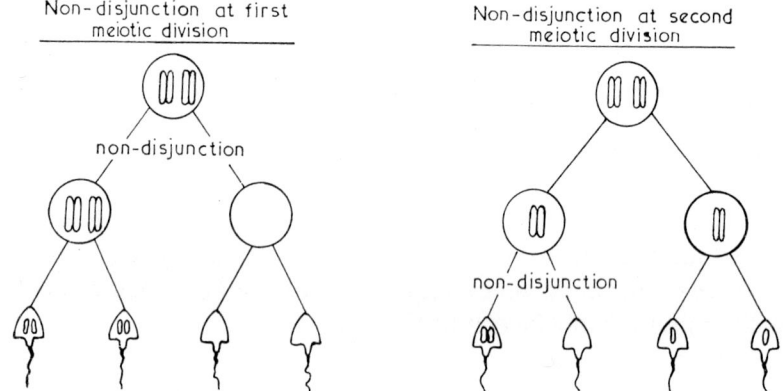

FIG. 1.1. Non-disjunction of chromosomes in germ cell formation.

or the second, and it is not yet known which is the more usual. The possibilities are shown diagrammatically in Fig. 1.1 for sperm cell formation. In non-disjunction at the first reduction division, the two chromosomes present in one parent will both be present in the germ cell that receives both members of the pair. In non-disjunction at the second cell division the two chromosomes in the cell receiving both members of the pair will both be derived from only one of the parental chromosomes.

The now classical example of autosomal *trisomy* caused by non-disjunction is Down's syndrome (mongolism). Here there is an extra small chromosome which it is conventional to call 21, but 21 and 22 cannot be distinguished and it may be that trisomy of either will cause Down's syndrome. Almost all children with Down's syndrome born to mothers over the age of 35 years have this genotype. However a minority of patients with Down's syndrome, especially those born to younger mothers, have the normal number of chromosomes, forty-six including a pair of chromosome 21; but they also have one chromosome which is unduly large, and incorporates the major part of a third chromosome 21. These anomalies are produced not by non-disjunction, but by translocation (*vide infra*). A few instances of partial Down's syndrome have been recognized, in which some of the cells show trisomy 21 and other cells have a normal chromosome complement (mosaicism—*vide infra*) or in which only part of an extra chromosome 21 is present.

Two other examples of autosomal trisomy are now associated with a characteristic syndrome of malformations, though neither of these appears compatible with survival beyond infancy. The first involves trisomy of a chromosome which is either 17 or 18. The syndrome includes mental defect, a malformed heart (usually interventricular septal defect), micrognathia, low-set malformed ears, webbed neck and ulnar deviation, with flexion deformity, of the fingers. The second example involves trisomy of a chromosome in the 13 to 15 group (probably 13), and the syndrome includes mental defect, microphthalmia and colobomata, interventricular septal defect, cleft lip and cleft palate, low-set ears and polydactyly.

Other types of autosomal trisomy are found only in first-trimester spontaneous abortions. The most common is trisomy 16. In addition 'triploidy', the presence of all the chromosomes in triplicate, is a common finding in early abortions. Trisomy of 21 is also common in abortions and probably more than half of all zygotes with trisomy 21 abort in the first trimester. Trisomies of the larger autosomes 1 to 12 are also found in abortions. It is likely that one zygote in about four has a major chromosomal anomaly and that over half of all spontaneous abortions in the first trimester are due to chromosome anomalies. No examples of autosomal monosomy are at present known, even in abortions. This is probably because such monosomy is lethal in early embryonic life, perhaps before the mother recognizes that she is pregnant. It is known from animal experiments that loss of chromosome material is more damaging than the presence of extra chromosome material.

Non-disjunction of the Sex Chromosomes
Non-disjunction of the sex chromosomes is responsible for Klinefelter's syndrome and Turner's syndrome. The recognition of these sex anomalies in recent years has been much simplified by the earlier discovery that in a cell with two X chromosomes there is a chromatin body visible at the edge of the nucleus in 20 to 60 per cent of cells. A normal female is therefore chromatin-positive and a normal male is chromatin-negative. The general rule is that the number of chromatin bodies to be seen is one less than the number of X chromosomes. One body appears when two X chromosomes are present, two bodies when three X chromosomes are present and so on. The probable explanation is that only one X chromosome in a cell is active; this does not take up stain, but any other X chromosomes present are condensed and appear as chromatin bodies.

The majority of patients with Klinefelter's syndrome, although they have male external and internal genitalia, are chromatin-positive. On chromosome examination they are found to be trisomic for the sex chromosomes and have the genotype XXY. The majority of children with Turner's syndrome, externally immature females, are chromatin-negative and are monosomic for the sex chromosomes, having one X chromosome and no second sex chromosome.

Klinefelter's syndrome is not likely to be recognized in the neonatal period unless routine nuclear sexing is carried out. In Turner's syndrome, the webbing of neck, the increased carrying angle at the elbow, the widely spaced nipples, oedema of the feet, and sometimes the presence of heart malformation may all be recognized neonatally. Some of the milder examples of Turner's syndrome are chromatin-positive and have no webbing of the neck; several of these have been found to be mosaics (*vide infra*), having some cells of genotype XO and others of genotype XX. The XO genotype is also one of the most common findings in abortuses.

Boys with an XYY genotype, the 'Extra Y' syndrome, are clinically normal in infancy and only detectable through their chromosomes. This genotype produces a tendency to develop increased stature, mild mental subnormality and impulsive (sometimes psychopathic) behaviour.

Chromosomal Translocation
The initial mutation in translocation does not involve a loss or addition of chromosome material, and usually produces no malformation. The

mechanism is a break of two chromosomes with a subsequent cross-union of the fragments, a process called reciprocal translocation. Thus if the breaks are in chromosomes 15 and 21, as in Fig. 1.2, the cross-union of the fragments will give a large composite 15/21 chromosome

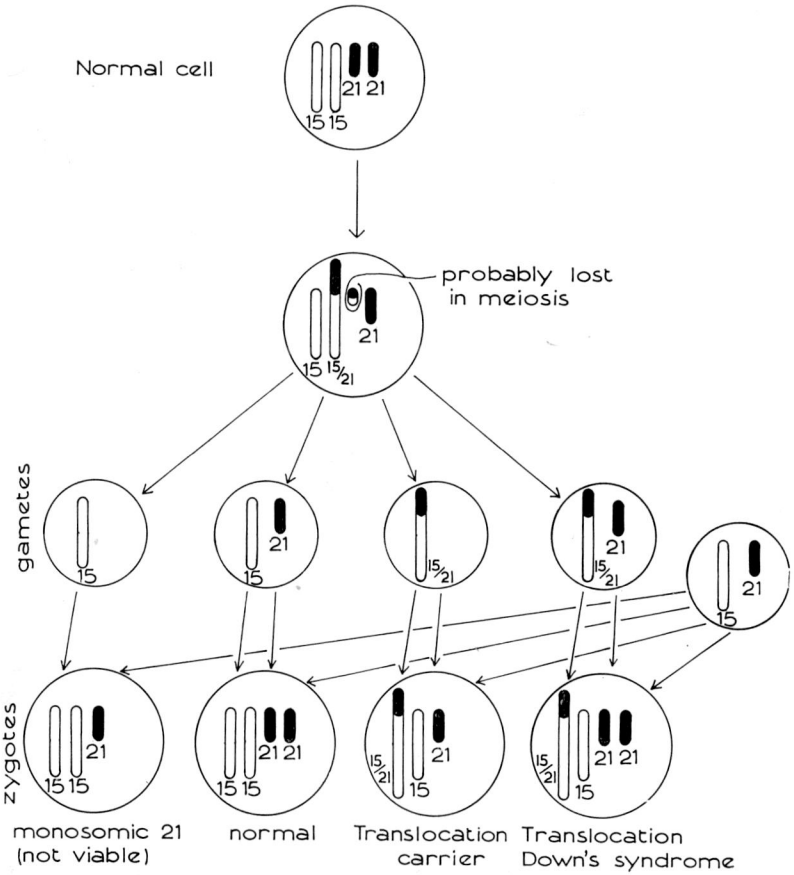

FIG. 1.2. Translocation of chromosomes 15 and 21 resulting in Down's syndrome.

comprising the major parts of both chromosomes and a small 15/21 fragment comprising the small residues of the two chromosomes. In subsequent cell division this small residue may be lost, leaving a genotype of forty-five, not forty-six, chromosomes, but a complete complement of chromosome material apart from the small lost fragments.

The translocated chromosome probably pairs preferentially with the larger normal 15 chromosome, and four types of germ cell may result: one containing a 15/21 and a 21 chromosome, one containing a 15/21 and no 21 chromosome, one containing a 15 and a 21 chromosome and one containing a 15 and no 21 chromosome. These germ cells can in turn produce four types of zygotes, though not necessarily with equal frequency; the first has forty-six chromosomes, but is in effect trisomic for chromosome 21 and develops into a child with Down's syndrome; the second is a clinically normal forty-five chromosome translocation carrier; the third is a normal child; and the fourth being monosomic for chromosome 21 is probably non-viable and has not been found. Chromosome translocations between 22 and 21 are also known in connection with Down's syndrome.

Another form of translocation involves a break at the centromere of a chromosome, with subsequent union end to end of two similar arms of a chromosome, producing what is called an *isochromosome*. If the two long arms of a chromosome are involved then a child who receives the isochromosome is in effect nearly trisomic for the chromosome involved. Isochromosomes of the X chromosome and of chromosome 21 are known in connection with Turner's syndrome and Down's syndrome.

Smaller mutations involving alterations in the structure of chromosomes are known in plants and animals. These include inversions of a chromosome, deletions and reduplications of parts of a chromosome. Two small deletions are now known regularly associated with clinical syndromes. In the 'cri-du-chat' syndrome there is a deletion of the short arm of chromosome 5, and a more serious group of anomalies is perhaps associated with a deletion of the short arm of chromosome 4, though the distinction between the two chromosomes is difficult. Recognizable syndromes are also associated with deletion of part of the long arm of chromosome 18, deletion of part of the short arm of chromosome 18, and deletion of part of chromosome 21. The latter has been called the 'anti-mongol' syndrome. With greater technical skill there is little doubt that many such smaller changes will, in the future, be recognized in man in association with malformations.

Mosaicism

In a proportion of instances of patients affected by chromosome anomalies there are two different cell lines present. Where such cell lines both arise from a single zygote this is called mosaicism. Where such cell lines arise from two different zygotes (from, for example, exchange of cells in the uterus between two dizygotic twins) the condition is called chimaerism. In the case of chromosome anomalies mosaicism usually arises from non-disjunction at an early metabolic division of the embryo.

Mosaicism is most commonly seen with sex chromosome anomalies and usually modifies the clinical picture in the way that one might expect. Examples of XO/XX or XO/XX/XXX mosaicism have partial Turner's syndrome; examples of XO/XY and XX/XXY mosaicism may have true hermaphroditism. Mosaicism is also occasionally seen in children with some, but not all, of the manifestations of Down's syndrome. Intellectual function in these trisomy 21/normal mosaics may be normal, but is very variable. Such a mosaicism in a mother may rarely account for the presence in a sibship of two regular trisomic children with Down's syndrome.

Point or Gene Mutations

Understanding of gene mutations, even more than that of chromosome mutations, is based on a mass of experiments on animals, plants and micro-organisms over the past half-century. There are a wide variety of types of human malformations which are essentially determined by gene mutations. Individually, however, if involving any considerable risk to life, they tend to be rare, because the frequency of gene mutations is much lower, for example, than that of non-disjunction of chromosome 21 or of the sex chromosomes.

It is useful to distinguish between two classes of mutant genes, those that affect development in *heterozygotes*, that is those who have the mutant gene on only one member of the chromosome pair, and those that affect development only in *homozygotes*, that is those who have the mutant gene on both members of the chromosome pair. The former genes are commonly called *dominant*, and the latter *recessive*. The distinction is somewhat artificial, as it is found that with sufficiently sensitive tests more and more mutant genes have some effect in heterozygotes, even though this leads to no obvious malformation or disability.

Some examples of malformations which are probably due to autosomal dominant mutant genes are listed below:

Skeletal system:
    Achondroplasia, classical variety
    Cleidocranial dysostosis
    Craniofacial dysostosis
    Brachydactyly: most varieties

Ectrodactyly of 'lobster-claw' type
Vascular and lymphatic system:
  Milroy's disease: many instances
Genito-urinary system:
  'Adult' form of polycystic kidneys
Skin:
  Congenital ectodermal dysplasia: many instances
Eyes:
  Congenital ptosis: many instances
  Congenital cataract: many instances
  Aniridia: many instances
Syndromes:
  Marfan's syndrome
  Holt–Oram syndrome
  Apert's syndrome
  Waardenburg's syndrome

By no means all patients with these conditions will have a parent affected, since many will be affected as a result of fresh mutations. This is particularly the case where the malformation considerably reduces the likelihood that the patient will have children.

A fresh mutation is hardly ever involved with malformations due to the patient being homozygote for an autosomal recessive gene. The patient is affected because both parents happen to be heterozygous carriers of the gene. Some malformations determined in this way are listed below:

Skeletal system:
  Diastrophic dwarfism
  Acrocephalopolysyndactyly
Central nervous system:
  Congenital deafness: most instances
Gastro-intestinal system:
  Apple-peel variety of jejunal atresia
Skin:
  Ichthyosis congenita
  Epidermolysis bullosa dystrophica (severe form)
Eyes:
  Buphthalmos: many instances
  Congenital subluxation of the lens with ectopic pupil
Genito-urinary system:
  Infantile form of polycystic kidneys with hepatic biliary ectasia

Ductless glands:
  Intersex due to congenital adrenal hyperplasia
Syndromes:
  Dandy–Walker syndrome with cystic kidneys
  Ellis–Van Creveld syndrome
  Fanconi's anaemia syndrome
  Marchesani's syndrome
  Laurence–Moon–Biedl syndrome
  Marinesco–Sjögren syndrome
  Conradi's syndrome
  Larsen's syndrome
  Pendred's syndrome

Mutant genes on the X chromosome show special features because most, perhaps all, of the gene loci on the chromosome have no corresponding gene locus on the little Y chromosome. A female may therefore be homozygous or heterozygous for such a mutant gene, whereas a male who has the mutant gene on his single X chromosome is said to be hemizygous for it. Such a male with a sex-linked 'recessive' mutant gene will tend to be as severely affected as a homozygous female and to be much more severely affected than heterozygous females. Some malformations determined in this way are listed below:

Central nervous system:
  Aqueduct stenosis: one form
Skin:
  Congenital dyskeratosis
Eyes:
  Megalocornea
Genito-urinary system:
  Testicular feminization
Syndromes:
  Reifenstein syndrome
  Oro-facio-digital syndrome (the oro-facio-digital syndrome may well be an X-linked 'dominant' lethal in males).

PART-GENETIC AND PART-ENVIRONMENTAL DETERMINATION

A feature of the experimental induction of malformations in animals by various teratogenic agents is that in one inbred strain of animal a particular agent is a potent source of malformations, while in a different inbred strain another agent is more damaging, Genetic factors are therefore important in potentiating or suppressing the action of these environmental agents.

Twin studies in man, as mentioned above, suggest that most of the common malformations in humans have a mixed genetic and environmental causation. For example, in the case of pyloric stenosis, and cleft lip and cleft palate, there are indications that the genetic predisposition is 'polygenic', that is to say it involves genes at several gene loci. In pyloric stenosis the primiparity effect in patients where the disease has a late onset, and the later onset of symptoms in children born in hospital than those born at home, suggest that maternal handling and feeding routines may play a part in producing symptoms. The major element in aetiology however is polygenic predisposition. In congenital dislocation of the hip the excess of first-born breech births suggests that the intra-uterine position of flexed hips and extended knees is an aetiological environmental factor, while two probably independent genetic predispositions, one for generalized joint laxity and one for a shallow acetabular socket, also play a part.

It will take time to disentangle these complex interactions, but in the long run this will be rewarding. It may well provide the opportunity for protecting those embryos which are genetically predisposed to develop malformations for the environmental triggers which are also required.

Genetic Counselling: General Principles

Knowledge of risks to the relatives, especially to the later sibs and the children of patients with congenital malformations, is useful in two ways. It helps the medical practitioner to make an early diagnosis and begin early any treatment that is required. For example, a newborn baby with signs of intestinal obstruction, who is a younger brother of a child with Hirschsprung's disease, probably also has Hirschsprung's disease; the son of a woman who had pyloric stenosis herself in infancy, must, if he should start vomiting in the first 4 months of life, be assumed to have pyloric stenosis until the contrary is proved. It also enables the practitioner to answer, as accurately as present knowledge permits, the parents' own questions on the risks to any children or any further children they may have. Any decision on whether to have children or not must rest with the parents, but they are entitled to any information which will help them to make the decision.

The estimation of genetic risks is not always straightforward. Two varieties of a condition, apparently very similar, may be determined by different genes with different patterns of inheritance. The patient's family history may be helpful in distinguishing the two varieties, and so may a knowledge of the frequency of the two varieties in the population. Therefore, while information on family risks is given in the later chapters of this book in connection with individual conditions it will, unless the situation is straightforward, often be wise to refer the patient for advice to one of the specialist genetic clinics now established in the main medical centres.

Genetic advice is most straightforward where there is reason to suppose that the condition is entirely environmentally determined. Later children born after a child who is malformed following maternal rubella or who have lesions following intra-uterine infection with toxoplasmosis run no risk of being affected in the same way.

Counselling in Conditions Due to Mutant Genes of Large Effect

Advice is also straightforward for dominant conditions determined by those autosomal mutant genes which always cause malformation in those heterozygous for them. When an affected child is born to normal parents it is probably that it is affected as a result of a fresh mutation. Such a mutation probably occurs late in the lineage of cells leading to the production of germ cells, and there is little risk of the parent having a second affected child. However, when the affected individual comes to have children, there is a 1 in 2 risk that any child of his will be affected in the same way. There is no risk to the children of individuals in the family who are unaffected.

Where a malformation is due to the patient being homozygous for an autosomal recessive gene, the risk of further children being affected is 1 in 4, that is 3 to 1 on an unaffected child. Any such unaffected brothers and sisters of the patient have a 2 in 3 chance of being heterozygous carriers of the mutant gene like the parents, but if they are carriers they will not have an affected child unless they are unlucky enough to marry a person heterozygous for the same mutant gene. Where it is not possible to detect the heterozygous carriers of such genes, parents at risk cannot be detected before they have had an affected child. With certain recessively determined conditions, for example sickle-cell anaemia and congenital microcytosis, carrier detection is possible and married couples, both heterozygous for the same recessive gene, may be warned of the 1 in 4 risk to their children.

Advice to parents who have had one boy with a malformation due to a mutant gene on the X chromosome is straightforward when there is evidence from the family that the mother is heterozygous for the gene concerned; if for example, her brother, father, mother's brother or sister's son is affected there is a 1 in 2 risk that any further boy will be affected and a 1 in 2 risk that any girl is a heterozygous carrier. Where no other member of the family is affected, it is possible that the boy's abnormality is a result of a fresh mutation; that the mother does not carry the gene and that there is no risk to later children. In the absence of any reliable test for the heterozygous state, however, it is more likely than not that the mother is a carrier, the odds being about 2 to 3 that she is a carrier even when affected boys die young and so do not contribute to the heterozygous carrier girls of the next generation. Where an affected male is considering having children, there is no risk of his transmitting the mutant gene to a son, since these inherit a Y chromosome and not an X chromosome from their father, but all daughters will be heterozygous carriers.

Counselling in Conditions Due to Chromosome Mutations
The general principles of genetic counselling for conditions due to chromosome mutations are not yet fully understood. For example, all the dozen or so children so far examined of women with trisomy for the X chromosome have been chromosomally normal. Again the offspring of translocation carriers, for example of 15/21 translocated chromosomes, may show significant departures from the expected proportion of affected, carrier and normal children even allowing for early abortions of some affected embryos. Empirical evidence at present suggests that where mother carries a 15/21 translocation the risk of Down's syndrome in a child surviving to term is between 1 in 5 and 1 in 10, but that it is less than 1 in 20 where father carries the translocation. Where either parent is a carrier aminocentesis and the culture of amniotic cells now offers the possibility of screening the foetus in the fourth month of pregnancy to see if the outcome of the pregnancy would be a child with Down's syndrome.

Counselling in Conditions of Mixed Aetiology
In many instances where a malformation has a mixed aetiology it is possible to give an empirical figure of the risk based on large-scale family studies. Examples are given later in the book, for example, for

anencephaly and spina bifida, cleft lip with or without lateral cleft palate, pyloric stenosis and congenital heart malformations.

There is inevitably some doubt, in giving empirical risk figures of this kind, whether they are appropriate to a particular family. For example, the risk to a woman, who has given birth to two children with anencephaly or spina bifida, of having a similarly affected child in a later pregnancy, is higher than the risk to a woman who has only had one such child. Some of this relatively high-risk group is included among women who have only had one such child, but at present there is no way of recognizing these women analogous to that now available in Down's syndrome from chromosome studies. Nevertheless these empirical risk figures are useful until they can be replaced by more exact methods.

Some Psychological Principles in Counselling
The ordinary skills that the medical practitioner uses in interviewing patients must be applied in giving advice on genetic risks. An attempt must be made to relieve anxieties, or feelings of guilt, and to put the situation in perspective for the couple concerned. For example, it is probable that most individuals are heterozygous for two or three autosomal recessive genes, which would cause severe malformation or disease in homozygotes. Unrelated parents of a child affected by such genes are the victims of bad luck in that both are heterozygotes for the same gene, and are in no way to blame.

Parents who have, for example, a 1 in 30 risk of a second child with a congenital heart malformation, should be encouraged to see this, admittedly additional and specific, risk in relation to the 1 in 50 risk that any pregnancy will result in a malformed child. The proportion of instances of malformation where there is a high risk of a second malformed child is fortunately low.

Many parents, though they do not raise the question, may have anxieties for the offspring of their other, healthy children and advice, which will usually be reassurance, will be helpful.

SELECTED REFERENCES

CARTER C.O. (1969) Genetics of common disorders. *Br. med. Bull.* **25**, 52
IDELBERGER K.I. (1939) Die Zwillingspatholigie der angeborenen Klumpfuss. *Zeit. f. Orthopäedie Suppl.* 69

IDELBERGER K.I. (1951) *Die Erbpathologie der sogennanten angeborenen Hüftverrenkung*. Munich: Urban & Schwarzenberg

JACKSON A.D.M. & FISCH L. (1959) Deafness following maternal rubella. *Lancet* **ii,** 1241

KALTER H. & WARKANY J. (1959) Experimental production of congenital malformations in mammals by metabolic procedure. *Physiol. Rev.* **39,** 69

LECK I., RECORD R.G., McKEOWN T. & EDWARDS J.H. (1968) The incidence of malformations in Birmingham, England, 1950–1959. *Teratology* **1,** 263

LESI F.E.A. (1968) 'A Study of Congenital Malformation in Newborn in Lagos'. Ph.D. thesis

MANSON MARGARET M., LOGAN W.P.D. & LOY RUTH M. (1960) 'Rubella and other virus infections during pregnancy'. *Ministry of Health Reports on Public Health and Medical Subjects, No.* **101.** H.M.S.O.

McINTOSH R., MERRITT KATHARINE K., RICHARDS MARY R., SAMUELS MARY H. & BELLOWS MARJORIE T. (1954) The incidence of congenital malformations: a study of 5964 pregnancies. *Pediatrics* **14,** 505

McKEOWN T. & RECORD R.G. (1960) 'Malformations in a population observed for five years after birth.' *Ciba Foundation Symposium on Congenital Malformations.* London: J. & A. Churchill

PENROSE L.S. (1957) Genetics of anencephaly. *J. ment. defic. Res.* **1,** 4

PITT D.B. (1961) Congenital malformations and maternal rubella: progress report. *Med. J. Aust.* **1,** 881

POLANI P.E. (1969) Autosomal imbalance and its syndromes, excluding Down's. *Br. med. Bull.* **25,** 81

RICHARDS MARY R., MERRITT KATHARINE K., SAMUELS MARY H. & LANGMANN A.G. (1955) Congenital malformations of the cardiovascular system in a series of 6053 infants. *Pediatrics* **15,** 12

SIMPKISS M. & LOWE ANNE (1961) Congenital anomalies in the African newborn. *Arch. Dis. Child.* **36,** 404

STEVENSON A.C., JOHNSTON H.A., STEWART M.I. PATRICIA & GOLDING D.R. (1966) *Congenital malformations: A report of a study of series of consecutive births in 24 centres.* Supplement to Vol. 34 of the *Bulletin of the World Health Organisation.*

2

Abnormalities of the Central Nervous System

K.M.LAURENCE AND R.WEEKS

The usual concept of malformations is not easy to apply to the central nervous system, as the development of the brain continues many years beyond the birth of the infant and as many developmental anomalies do not become apparent until postnatal life. On the other hand, the immature nervous system may react to injury by resorbing the injured portion without leaving a trace. In addition destructive processes may mimic developmental defects. It is thus clear that any discussion of 'malformations' found about the time of birth must include some acquired conditions and omit some developmental defects. In many instances the aetiology remains unknown and the morphogenesis poorly understood. Experimental teratology has helped greatly in the understanding of some of these malformations, but has also shown that the same end result may be obtained by a number of entirely different exogenous and endogenous processes.

The major dysraphic central nervous system malformations which include anencephaly and spina bifida cystica are among the commonest serious anomalies seen in the British Isles and are found in about 1 in 150 births. They cause much family distress and, where the child does survive, lead to a great deal of morbidity in addition. Other central nervous system abnormalities such as hydrocephalus, Down's syndrome (mongolism), agenesis of corpus callosum, microcephaly and so on, all less common, account for an appreciable proportion of the patients in our hospitals for the mentally subnormal.

DEFECTS OF CLOSURE OF THE NEURAL TUBE

Defects of closure of the neural tube account for the great majority of the central nervous system malformations. This group includes the gross anomalies such as anencephaly, and the most trivial, the dermal sinuses.

ANENCEPHALY

Anencephaly, with its great preponderance of females (about 4:1 females to males) accounts for almost half the severe neural tube malformations in Britain and is the commonest serious malformation seen in stillbirths. The term anencephaly is an unfortunate one as there always is, even in the severest forms, some brain tissue recognizable, while in the least severe cases there may only be an absence of both cerebral hemispheres. There is always acrania and often craniorachischisis. The facial features are grotesque with protruding eyes; abnormal ears and the relative absence of the neck add to this odd appearance.

Pathology
The congested haemorrhagic mass lying on top of the head consists of recognizable neural tissue pervaded by angiomatous spaces, often with choroid plexus and ependyma. In some cases the brain stem, and even the cerebellum, are quite well developed. The spinal cord, when formed, is small and congested, with absent pyramidal tracts; it is covered with congested meninges.

The cranial vault is completely absent, with the frontal bone missing above the orbital ridges, the parietal bones represented only by their most inferior parts and the squamous portion of the occipital bone represented only in the absence of a spinal defect. The basal bones are also grossly abnormal, with small orbits, and a small or absent anterior cranial and pituitary fossa. The eyes, although externally normal, show absence of the ganglion cells of retina, but the internal ear is usually normal. The pituitary gland can nearly always be found, if diligently sought; it is represented by anterior lobe only and is a small congested but otherwise normal structure. The thyroid is usually mature with abundant colloid; the thymus is often very large. In contrast the adrenals are very small due largely to virtual absence of the foetal zone, and are frequently described as being hypoplastic. However, the narrow zona medullaris is as well developed in the anencephalic as in the adult with acinar structures. The medulla is also better developed than in many normal newborns. That the gland is fully mature and shows precocious development rather than hypoplasia is confirmed by the high pressor amine content; in addition it contains small amounts of adrenaline and noradrenaline.

The lungs are frequently hypoplastic and poorly lobated. Other abnormalities may be present but are less often seen.

Management

Anencephaly should always be suspected when hydramnios develops, as it is the commonest foetal condition with which this is associated. Confirmation amply justifies an x-ray of the hydramniotic abdomen, for it helps the obstetrician to plan management of the pregnancy and delivery. Thought must be given to preparing the mother for the outcome and the pregnancy should probably be terminated. With hydramnios, artificial rupture of the membranes followed by an oxytocin drip is a standard method. More recently, amniocentesis followed by intra-amniotic injection of hypertonic saline has been proving most effective. As these foetuses are usually born prematurely they present no obstetric problem, but when they are delivered at term or postmaturely, difficulty may be experienced with the shoulders. In the knowledge that the foetus is malformed drastic measures such as the use of hooks or destructive operations may be used. Indeed in the absence of hydramnios, the anencephalic pregnancy may go well beyond term, probably because of the low foetal pituitary–adrenal activity, which is normally responsible for initiating labour in humans. Anencephalics are usually stillborn, or die within minutes. On occasion one will continue to live for hours or even days.

There is a considerable geographic variation, with the rates as high as 4 per thousand births in Ireland, 3·5 per thousand in South Wales and Liverpool, 2·8 in Birmingham and 1·8 in south-eastern England. The incidence is said to be low in eastern France and eastern Europe and the U.S.A. and very low amongst the Negroes and Chinese. Social class, seasonal, and secular variations in the incidence occur.

The empirical risk of another child with a central nervous system malformation being born to parents who have already had one child with either anencephaly or spina bifida cystica is about 1 in 25. However, if the mother has already had two children affected by one of the dysraphic malformations, the risk rises to about 1 in 8. In view of the considerable geographical variation in the incidence the recurrence risk is probably better expressed in terms of risk above the relevant population incidence. The risk of recurrence is about seven times the population incidence. The risk of recurrence is about seven times the population risk after one affected and about 30 times after two affected children.

Aetiology
Experimentally, anencephaly can be produced in the rat by subjecting the embryo to any of a large number of teratogenic agents only between the eighth and tenth day, i.e. just after gastrulation. The cephalic end of the neural tube remains open, but first the cerebral hemispheres, then the corpus striatum and finally the olfactory bulbs and the choroid plexus make their appearance. On the sixteenth day just as histogenesis of the cortex is proceeding the whole tissue begins to necrose. From abnormal early human embryos which have been studied it would appear that the process is similar in man, and that the causative factor has to act between the sixteenth and twenty-sixth day after conception. It is possible the developing embryo may be abnormal even before the sixteenth day.

The familial incidence suggests that the aetiology of the condition is in part genetic. Adequate twin studies are not yet available; in part because the patients mostly die before the type of twinning is established. There is little doubt however that most monozygotic co-twins of patients are not affected, and so there must be also a considerable environmental component in the aetiology. This is confirmed by the geographical and seasonal variations, and the increased frequency in the lower socio-economic groups. It is likely that one is dealing with a polygenically inherited predisposition interacting with as yet unidentified, but probably often quite minor, environmental trigger mechanisms.

Other Gross Brain Abnormalities

A number of other gross brain abnormalities, all incompatible with life, occasionally occur. In microcephaly acrania the skull bones may be present but abnormally small, completely enclosing a tiny degenerate brain, while in exencephaly the cranial vault is absent but scalp covers a sac containing fluid and degenerate brain tissue. Iniencephaly, where there is a confluence of the cranial and spinal cavities and a fusion of a large part of the cranial and vertebral skeleton with an uptilting of the face, is associated with a less degenerate brain. All grades of variation between these abnormalities and anencephaly, with which they are closely related, are seen. Cyclopia and cebocephaly, both very rare, though very occasionally seen with anencephaly, do not seem to be related to it. In the first condition more or less fused eyes are situated in a single midline orbit which is surmounted by a proboscis representing the nose. In the second, the eyes are paired. In both usually the brain shows some degree of arhinencephaly such as alobar holoprosencephaly with its grossly abnormal fused cerebral hemispheres and its single cerebral ventricle. Some of these cases are associated with trisomy of the 13–15 (D) chromosome.

Spina Bifida

Embryology, Anatomy and Pathology
The nervous system develops from a thickened area of ectoderm (medullary plate) which runs the length of the embryo in the midline dorsally. This plate infolds by the formation of medullary ridges on either side which then approximate and fuse to form a medullary tube, beginning in the mid-dorsal region and extending in both directions. It is almost complete by the end of the third week and the last points to close at either end, the neuropores, disappear by the end of the fourth week.

The neural tube then segments and supersegments at the cephalic end to form the various structures of the brain, while the cells of the tube proliferate to form ependyma, neurones, glial cells and pyramidal cells, etc. In the meanwhile the mesoderm surrounding the tube completely separates neuroectoderm and ectoderm and the mesenchyme segments into somites which develop into the vertebral column. The meninges, the pia arachnoid and dura are also formed from the mesenchyme at the time of separation of the neural tube from ectoderm. In all forms of spina bifida, i.e. spina bifida occulta and cystica, some part of this foregoing process is abnormal (Fig. 2.1).

Spina bifida occulta, the least serious, represents an abnormality of the mesodermal elements in the main, in that there is non-fusion of the laminae, with the spinal cord and its meninges remaining in their normal situation. In some cases both ectoderm and neuroectoderm may participate in the anomaly as evidenced by skin and cord abnormalities which are encountered.

Spina bifida cystica, the more serious abnormality, is conveniently subdivided into meningoceles and myeloceles. In the meningocele, in addition to spina bifida, the meninges, both dura and arachnoid, herniate out of the spinal canal while the cord remains in its normal position in the spinal canal. The meninges may be exposed on the surface or be covered by skin and the surrounding skin (as in spina bifida occulta) may be malformed. In this condition there may be associated anomalies of spinal cord and occasionally of the brain.

Myelomeningoceles, myelocytoceles, hydromyeloceles and syringomyeloceles, localized rachischisis and myeloceles are all essentially the

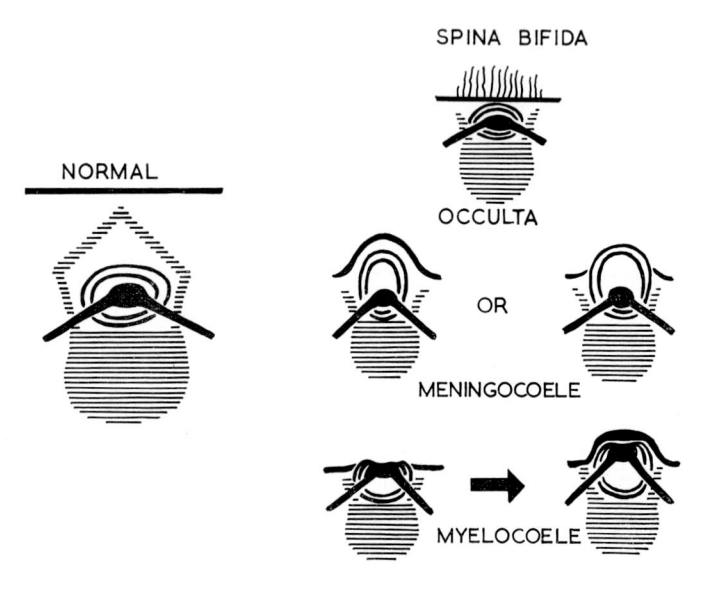

FIG. 2.1. Diagrammatic representation of the anatomy of the normal spinal column and spina bifida.

same lesion, and best regarded as myeloceles. In all these lesions the neural plate has locally failed to close over completely to form a tube; in most cases the cord tissue, with some degenerative changes, which are very much less severe than in anencephaly, lies exposed on the surface (Fig. 2.3). At birth this 'open' lesion is seen as the raw, apparently ulcerated, central zona vasculosa which is generally surrounded by a bluish semi-transparent membranous area representing the meninges and by skin which is often malformed; the latter may show a naevoid discolouration and abnormal pattern of hair-bearing skin. From the ventral surface of the 'neural plate', nerve roots, both sensory and motor, leave to traverse the 'subarachnoid' space and gain exit through the root canals. The spinal cord above the lesion often shows abnormalities such as cysts, syringomyelia, gliosis, but more frequently hydromyelia, and just proximal to the myelocele, diastematomyelia, with or without a fibrous, cartilaginous or bony spur arising from the affected vertebral body. Below the lesion, if situated high up on the spinal axis, the cord reforms into a recognizable structure. On occasion, even without active treatment, the myelocele may epithelialize over from the surrounding skin in about 2 weeks. More usually, however, unless very stringent measures are taken to prevent it, the zona vasculosa becomes infected with ensuing fibrosis, leading to the typical thick scarred fundus of the myelocele. Accumulation of fluid, usually cerebrospinal fluid, below the plate before or after birth, leads to its cystic nature. In a small number of cases the lesion is 'closed' with complete skin cover at birth. These do not run the same risks of infection, etc.

Nearly all myeloceles (some of those in the sacral region being the exception) are associated with the Arnold–Chiari malformation of the hind brain and many have aqueduct malformations in addition.

SPINA BIFIDA OCCULTA

The genetic relationship of spina bifida occulta to the major dysraphic syndromes is obscure. Its incidence in some series is as high as one in every ten patients on radiological examination.

Spina bifida is generally situated in the lumbar or sacral spine, and takes the form of defects of the lamina, though in some cases widening of the spinal canal, fusion or cleavage of vertebra and other defects may be present as well. In the great majority of instances there is no disability associated with this bony maldevelopment. In a number of cases the presence of the spina bifida is suggested by abnormal dark hair, angiomatous malformation of the skin, lipoma or dimples in the region of the defect.

Occasionally spina bifida occulta is associated with neurological or musculoskeletal disturbances. Most of these have spinal cord abnormalities as the underlying basis. The central canal of the spinal cord may be dilated (hydromyelia) or sometimes the spinal cord splits into two separate bundles around a bony or cartilaginous spur or a fibrous band (diastematomyelia). Occasionally there is a local meningeal abnormality or cord gliosis or cyst within the cord or an intraspinal mass such as a lipoma, dermoid, teratoma or a meningocele pressing upon it. These patients suffer from abnormalities of posture or muscle tone; muscle weakness may lead to deformities of the feet, legs and hips and sensory loss may lead to trophic ulceration. Sphincter disturbances are not uncommon. These disabilities are generally mild but may at times be disabling. They are not usually noticed before the age of 1 year when the patient begins to walk or when sphincter control is expected.

Surgical treatment should not be contemplated unless there is neurological deficit with progression. Then the case should be investigated. Surgical exploration should only be undertaken if a filling defect or a spinal block is found on myelography and then any cause of the cord pathology such as a dermoid or a bony spur or band in diastematomyelia should, if possible, be removed. Ingraham and Matson in forty-four cases of spina bifida occulta which came to surgery were able to find a removable cause in thirty-six instances, but unfortunately not all were improved by the surgical intervention. It is of interest that of the 105 patients of Ingraham and Matson who sought neurosurgical opinion thirty-nine did so because of cutaneous, forty-five because of musculo-skeletal, and nineteen because of sphincter manifestations.

Spina Bifida Cystica

Incidence and Aetiology

Like the closely related anencephaly, spina bifida cystica shows considerable geographical variation in the incidence. In the British Isles alone the incidence varies from 4·2 per thousand total live births in South Wales to 2·8 per thousand in Buckinghamshire and about 1·5 per thousand in south-eastern England. The condition is uncommon in the Mediterranean countries and rare amongst Negroes and Mongolians. There seems to be a greater incidence in the lower socio-economic groups and there are variable seasonal and secular variations as well. So far no geographical or dietary factors nor acute viral diseases or drugs in early pregnancy, have been shown to be causative. Whatever the cause it must have acted before the fourth week of gestation, i.e. before the neural tube has completely closed. The empirical risk of recurrence is similar to that in anencephaly (p. 27).

Meningocele

Meningoceles are much less common than myeloceles and the more carefully a 'meningocele' is investigated the more frequently it is found really to be a myelocele, accounting for the great variation in the figures quoted. The true incidence is probably not more than 1 in 20 cases of spina bifida cystica.

The meningocele appears as a cystic pedunculated or semi-sessile swelling of variable size usually in the midline anywhere along the spinal axis but most commonly in the lumbosacral region (Fig. 2.2). It is

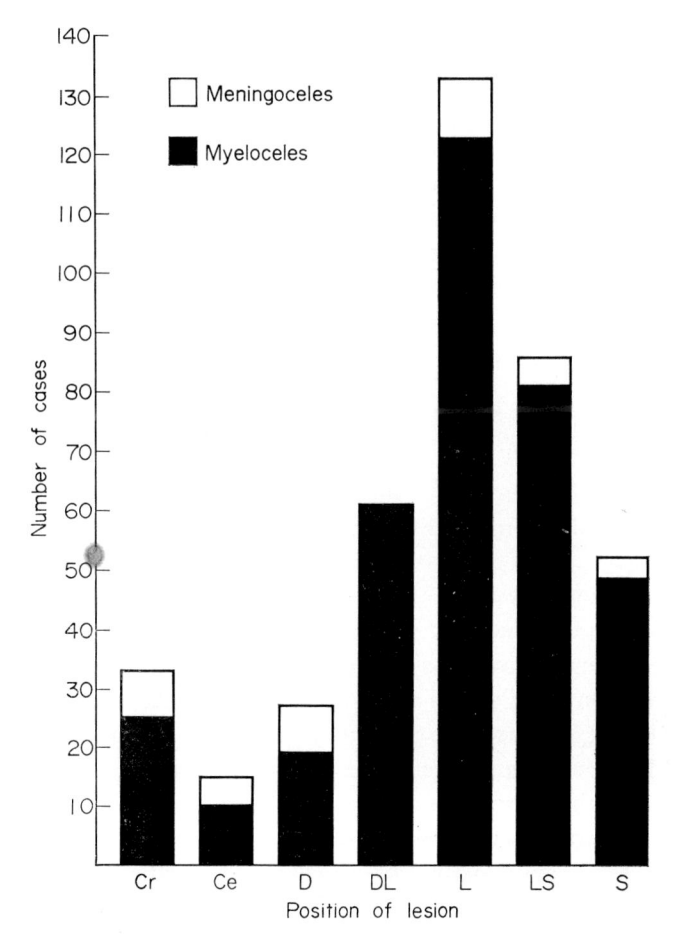

FIG. 2.2. The position of the lesion in 407 cases of spina bifida cystica. Cr = cranial; D = dorsal; D.L. = dorsilumbar; L = lumbar; L.S. = lumbosacral; S = sacral.
(Reprinted from *Arch. Dis. Childh.* (1964), **39**, 41, by permission of the Editor.)

covered either by a thin semi-transparent bluish membrane which represents the meninges, and in which blood vessels can be seen, or by full thickness of skin, which may show abnormalities such as hypertrichosis and angiomatosis. A lipomatous pad may be found at the base or overlying it, making the lesion appear very much larger. Sacs may have an impulse on coughing and may be compressible. Palpation and transillumination should not reveal any central nervous tissue in the wall of the sac, but it is generally not possible to be certain whether a lesion is a true meningocele until surgical exploration is carried out or until the sac itself has been examined histologically.

Although the spinal cord and its nerve roots are in their normal position, abnormalities of the cord similar to those sometimes seen in spina bifida occulta may be present, and account for the neurological deficit suffered by some of the patients. Occasionally malformations of the mid-brain, such as aqueduct stenosis and forking, or of the hind brain, such as the Chiari malformation, are found, accounting for the occasional development of hydrocephalus. The prognosis for survival and function of these cases is good.

MYELOCELE

The myelocele is a very much more serious lesion than the meningocele with regard both to morbidity and mortality.

(a) *Appearance*
The appearance as well as size of the sac at birth varies greatly, on occasions extending over the greater part of the back. It may be situated anywhere along the spinal axis, but most commonly in the lumbar region (Fig. 2.2). Those in the lumbar or sacral region are sometimes 'closed' lesions being covered over completely with skin, and are often associated with a lipomatous mass. More commonly the abnormality is 'open' and consists of a flat, more or less sac-like lesion with a central raw congested neural plate (zona vasculosa) situated at the fundus of the sac which is sometimes split into halves longitudinally. This is surrounded by a thin bluish semi-transparent parchment-like membrane (zona membranosa) representing the meninges, often containing blood vessels (Fig. 2.3).

When transilluminated the contents of the sac, nerve roots, blood vessels and spinal cord, may be seen. This can be important in deciding whether the lesion is actually a myelocele. The surrounding skin is frequently hair-bearing or naevoid. The myelocele contains cerebrospinal fluid which may ooze from the surface, either from the central canal of the cord, which occasionally opens into the surface near the upper end of the zona vasculosa, or from the neural plate or membrane damaged during or after delivery. A dermal sinus may be seen below the myelocele. Lipomata and rarely dermoid cysts or teratoma are sometimes part of the lesion.

After birth the sac may epithelialize over, but more usually the surface

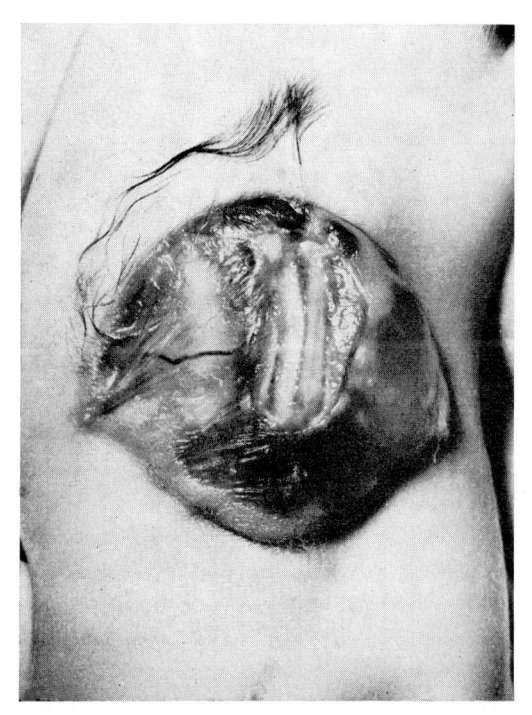

Fig. 2.3. Lumbar myelocoele at birth: the raw infected neural plate (zona vasculosa) is surrounded by a semi-transparent delicate membrane (zona membranosa) through which blood vessels and nerve roots can be seen. The surrounding skin shows hypertrichosis and angiomatosis.

becomes infected leading to an ascending meningitis, the most frequent and most serious complication. The sac wall sometimes becomes so infected that it bursts. This may also happen when the sac becomes very distended with cerebrospinal fluid. In either case ascending meningitis almost invariably ensues unless very stringent measures are taken.

If the infant survives, the spinal lesion will heal with more or less fibrosis and destruction of the cord tissue of the neural plate, and eventually epithelialize over. This results in the typical sac with the thick hard scarred fundus, and the whitish, rather parchment-like, opaque membrane surrounding it. Often the communication between the sac and the spinal subarachnoid space has been lost and the sac itself contains a series of loculations.

(b) *Neurological Involvement*

The great majority of myeloceles have a varying degree of nerve

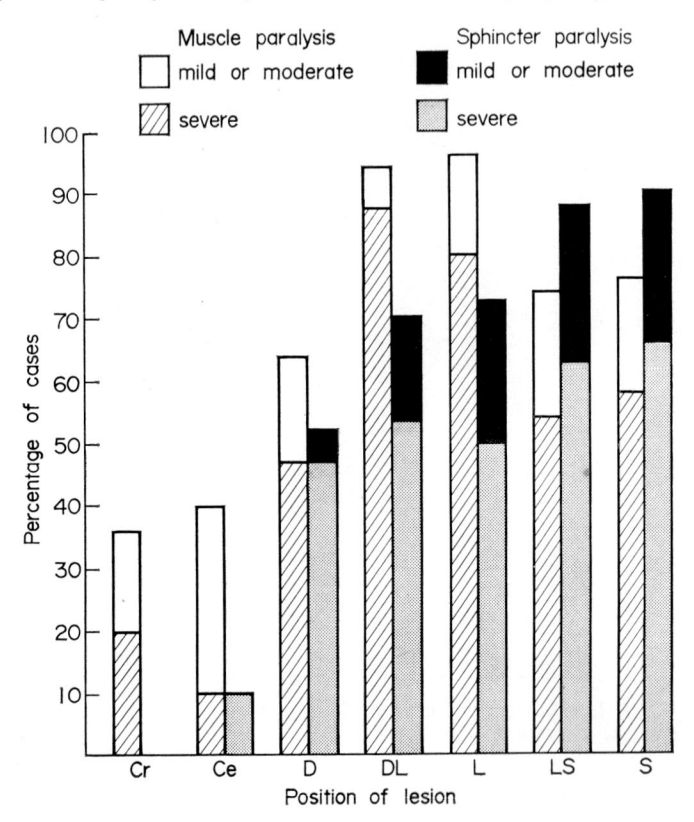

FIG. 2.4. The incidence and severity of muscular and sphincter paralysis in the 368 encephaloceles and myeloceles in the various positions along the cerebrospinal axis. Cr = cranial; Ce = cervical; D = dorsal; D.L. = dorsilumbar; L = lumbar; L.S. = lumbosacral; S = sacral.

(Reprinted from *Arch. Dis. Childh.* (1964), **39**, 41, by permission of the Editor.)

involvement, the distribution and amount depending not only upon the position and the extent of the lesion (Fig. 2.4) but also upon the secondary changes resulting from infection or trauma to the lesion.

Skeletal muscle involvement is the most frequent and obvious result of the spinal lesion and the level of the lesion determines which muscles are affected. Myeloceles in the cervical region often show no paralysis though some have involvement of the arm muscles. With lesions lower down, the abdominal and leg muscles may be involved; with extensive lumbar myeloceles both legs may be paralysed. Patients with sacral sacs may escape limb involvement altogether. Once a muscle is paralysed it will only rarely regain any appreciable amount of power. Contractures and joint abnormalities will ensue if the antagonistic muscles still functioning are allowed to act unchecked. Fractures may occur following trivial trauma.

Sphincter involvement is uncommon with cervical myeloceles and is seen increasingly as the lesion is situated lower down the spinal axis, until about 90 per cent of cases with sacral sacs suffer from at least some involvement of either the bladder or bowel sphincter, or both.

In the urinary system the bladder and the sphincter may be completely paralysed; the bladder is thin-walled and there is dilatation of the upper urinary tract as the ureteric sphincter may also be incompetent. These cases constantly dribble urine. In others the bladder is thick-walled and trabeculated often with diverticuli, and the bladder neck is spastic. These will develop reflux and later marked dilatation of the upper urinary tract. They tend to have intermittent but quite uncontrolled passage of urine. Recent intensive investigation of the urinary tract of these infants, using intravenous pyelography and micturating cystography, has shown that such changes, hydronephrosis, and ureteric reflux may be present at birth and progress more rapidly than has been supposed. With progressive dilatation of the urinary tract and the ascending urinary infection which so often accompanies it with its resulting pyelonephritis, increasing renal failure will develop, unless strenuous counter-measures are adopted.

When some anal function and sensation and an anal reflex are present, bowel control can generally be achieved with training. In these cases and where there is complete incontinence there is, however, a tendency for faecal overloading and acquired megacolon to develop.

Loss of sensation invariably accompanies paralysis, the distribution being strictly determined by the segments of cord involved. Lumbar and sacral lesions are most serious in this respect. Loss of sensation in the legs frequently leads to trophic ulceration and may cause pressure sores under any surgical appliances that may have to be worn to facilitate getting about. Saddle anaesthesia, almost constantly seen with sacral lesions, may allow severe excoriation around the penis, vulva or anus to occur, while ischial sores are seen in sitting patients. Chronic ulceration overlying bones may lead to osteomyelitis. Vasomotor disturbances in the affected limbs can also be troublesome.

(c) *Associated Malformations*
Of the true malformations outside the central nervous system, those of the skeletal system are the most frequently seen. Anomalies of the vertebral bodies, often at the site of the myelocele, may lead to severe kyphosis or scoliosis. Abnormalities of ribs (fused) are common especially with thoracic sacs. The skull is often small with a small posterior fossa, and frequently shows severe cranio-lacunia or even fenestra.

Talipes equinovarus is very frequent, while dislocation of the hip, arthrogryposis and genu recurvatum are often present. These are invariably associated with severe paralysis of the legs and can be accounted for on that basis in most cases. *In utero* the limbs take up their natural position only if the muscles are functioning normally. If, however, certain muscles are paralysed the limb is forced into unnatural positions by antagonists and the uterine compression. This after a time leads to any of those conditions listed. In only a few of these cases are dislocation of the hip or talipes equinovarus truly malformative.

Anomalies of the renal tract, such as double ureters, horseshoe kidneys and true congenital hydronephrosis, may be found in association. Cleft palate is a quite frequent concomitant while most other malformations are occasionally seen.

(d) *Hydrocephalus*
A very large proportion of myeloceles have concomitant hydrocephalus. In one investigation 83 per cent of cases were found to have ventricular dilatation of some degree at birth presumably due to malformations of the aqueduct or hind brain. Ascending meningitis from the myelocele then leads to post-inflammatory obstruction superimposed on the malformations, accounting for onset of hydrocephalus in some and rapid progression of the condition in others in whom the disease might otherwise have arrested spontaneously. Thus in a follow-up investigation on 407 cases of spina bifida cystica and cranium bifidum (including 368 myeloceles and encephaloceles), 82 per cent of cases had some hydrocephalus. In almost 80 per cent of these it was diagnosed by 3

months of age and in only a few cases was the onset after the age of 6 months, when the lesion is normally well epithelialized (Fig. 2.5).

Should hydrocephalus develop rapidly this must be treated expeditiously as otherwise the operation wound may leak cerebrospinal fluid, become infected and break down. The hydrocephalus that often develops after early surgery would probably have developed in any case, on

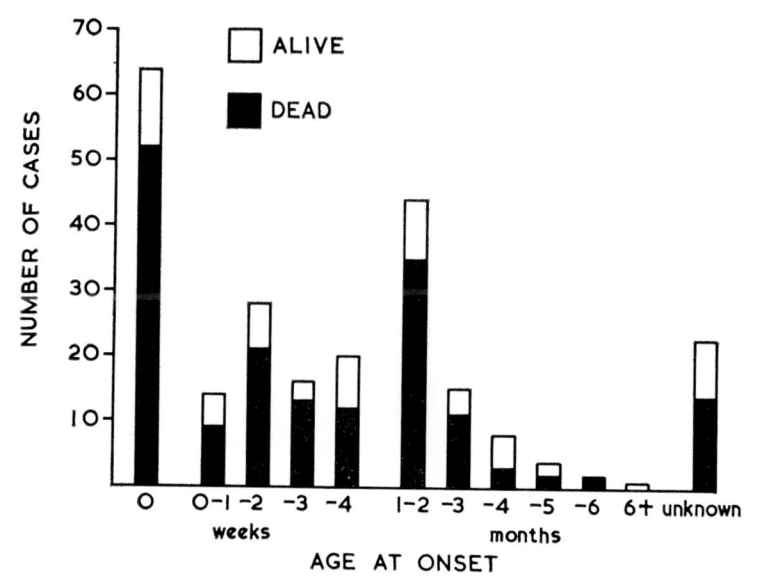

Fig. 2.5. Age of onset of hydrocephalus in 235 encephaloceles and myeloceles who had either moderate or severe hydrocephalus out of a total series of 368 cases. In twenty-three the age of onset was not known precisely.

account of the hind- and mid-brain malformation, though it is possible that in a few instances a mild reactive meningitis due to operative bleeding, damaged tissue or even infection might have accelerated its progress. There is no foundation to the theory that these sacs act as additional absorption surfaces and that their removal *per se* causes hydrocephalus.

Course and Prognosis

A large proportion of the cases of myelocele develop ascending meningitis from which many succumb. Many of those who survive this hazard then die of the effects of progressive hydrocephalus, often after a prolonged illness. A few of the older children suffer from renal infection and failure, recrudescence of an old meningitis or some sudden complication of hydrocephalus which had become arrested (Fig. 2.6). Trophic ulceration especially if neglected can be very debilitating.

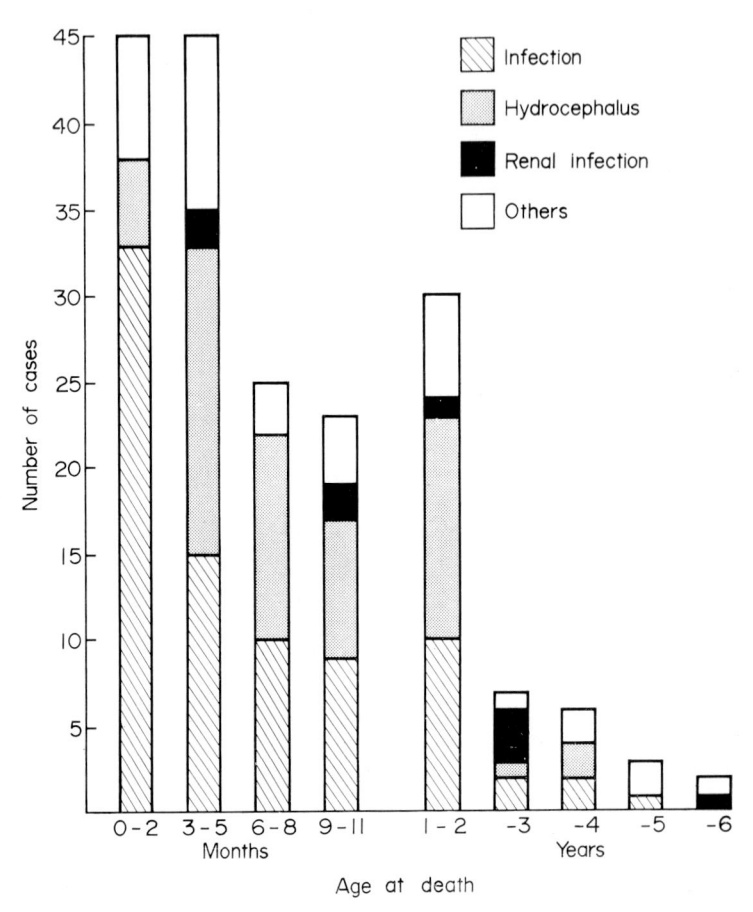

FIG. 2.6. A histogram showing the relation between cause of death and age at death in the 185 cases from a total series of 368 myeloceles and encephaloceles. Intracranial infection is responsible for most of the early and hydrocephalus for many of the later deaths.
(Reprinted from *Arch. Dis. Childh.* (1964), **39**, 41, by permission of the Editor.)

In the follow-up investigation referred to earlier, all of thirty-nine true meningoceles had survived the 10-year period, while 185 of 368 cases of myeloceles and encephaloceles (50 per cent) had died during the same time. This, however, gives a false prognosis as the series was not truly representative of the malformation in the community, both because many of the severest cases died before reaching the children's hospital where the investigation was carried out, and because this mode of computing prognosis takes no account of the actual number of cases at risk at any one time. When prognosis is computed on actuarial principles using a life table and chart as was done in a series of all the 425

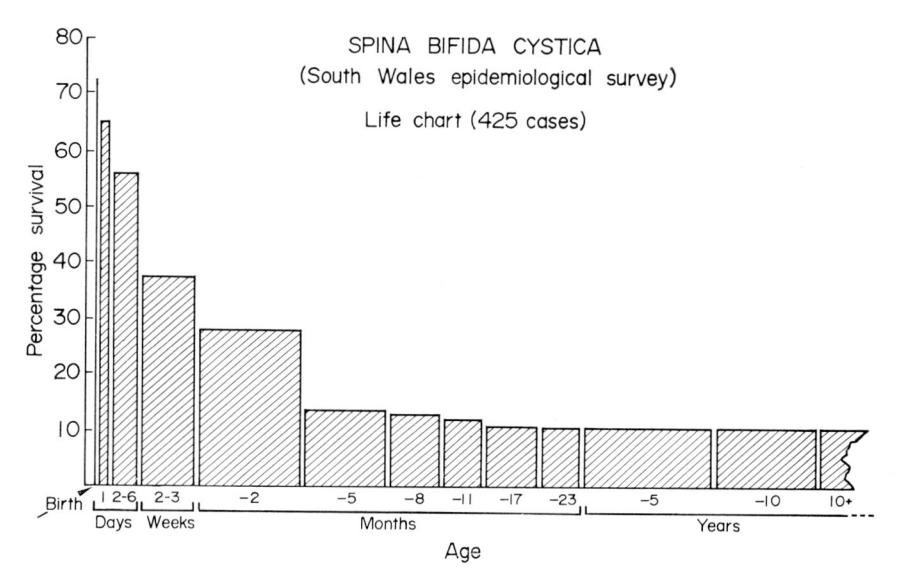

FIG. 2.7. Life chart of 425 cases of spina bifida cystica and encephaloceles born in a population of 850,000 over 7 years.
(By courtesy of the Editor of *Developmental Medicine & Child Neurology*.)

untreated cases in South Wales, born over a 7-year period, then it was found that only 16 per cent of all the total cases born reached their twelfth birthday (Fig. 2.7). Moderate or severe hydrocephalus associated with spina bifida appears to be a bad prognostic sign. Many of these eventually die while most of those without hydrocephalus, survive. The situation has now changed with more satisfactory methods of treating hydrocephalus. Though a large proportion of these children will grow up severely physically handicapped, intellectually they seem to be potentially normal. Intellectual impairment will, of course, result from repeated attacks of meningitis or severe hydrocephalus.

Treatment of the Spinal Lesion

Any surgeon who has attempted to carry out formal repair of fully epithelialized myeloceles is immediately aware of the inherent difficulties. Neural tissue (which may or may not be functional) is firmly fused to epidermis and nearly always has to be separated from it by sharp dissection. On the one hand, there is a risk of sacrificing neural tissue; on the other, of including epidermis within the reformed 'canal'. Such fragments of epidermis can provide a nidus for infection and may enlarge into epidermoid tumours. Electrical stimulation of the neural tissue is not much help because of the difficulty of interpreting physiological implications of muscle twitches produced in this way. Wide irradiation of the current gives one obvious source of error.

Separation of dura from epidermis is very difficult towards the fundus of the sac and consequently a cerebrospinal fluid fistula following repair is not uncommon. Surgeons were therefore receptive of the view first put forward in 1958 that the non-skin-covered meningoceles and myeloceles should be operated on as soon as possible after birth with the object of preventing meningitis and preserving such neural function as might be inherent within the exposed neural tissue. It is at this stage that the various elements composing the malformation can be most easily distinguished from each other and with experience even the largest defects can be closed with a single operation without recourse to skin grafting.

The essential steps in the closure of an extensive myelocele are:

(1) to gently free the nerves and zona vasculosa from the attached skin and zona membranosa;

(2) to refashion a dural tube to contain the neural tissue; the aim being to reduce the likelihood of a C.S.F. fistula but to avoid compression or strangulation of the neural plate;

(3) to obtain skin closure with full thickness viable skin flaps sutured without tension; for if there is tension then partial or total necrosis of the skin is unavoidable. It has been found that wide and long relieving incisions far out in the flanks are by far the most effective way of insuring primary healing of a big defect. These relieving incisions have secondary advantages in that they allow fluid to drain from beneath the skin flaps and they themselves heal rapidly without complications.

If the defect can be closed within 48 hours, or better, within 24 hours of birth without C.S.F. leak or skin necrosis, the incidence of meningitis and consequently the mortality falls dramatically, as was found in a retrospective study of the results in Cardiff.

Other advantages claimed for early closure are that it preserves and may actually improve the movement of the legs. It is generally agreed that if an infant born with an 'open' myelocele is examined frequently for the first 48 hours, movement present at birth may disappear after a few hours presumably due to drying out or exposure of the cord tissue.

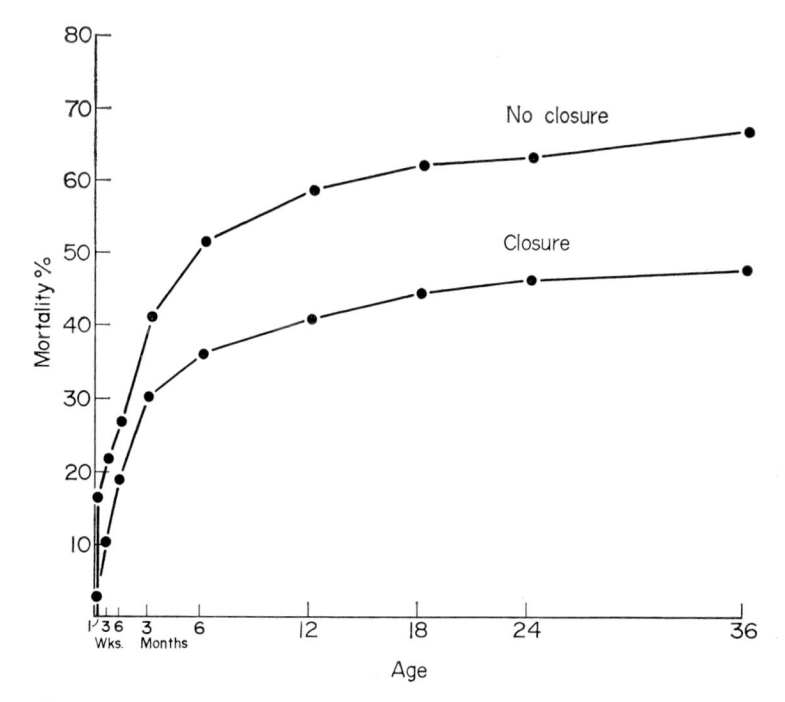

FIG. 2.8. Graph of mortality in patients treated operatively within the first 4 days of life compared with conservatively treated patients.
(Reprinted from Sharrard *et al.* (1967), *Develop. Med. Child Neurol.*, Suppl. **13**, 35, by courtesy of the Editor.)

In such cases movement may return to some extent after early closure of the defect but it is extremely doubtful if movement returns in limbs totally paralysed at the moment of birth.

Convincing evidence has now been obtained that early closure improves the mortality of this condition (Fig. 2.8) although the natural and the surgical mortality of a large thoracolumbar myelocele is still higher than the overall figure for myeloceles taken altogether.

Should early operation (i.e. within the first 48 hours) have been found to be impossible for one reason or another, such as late referral or severe surface infection, it is probably best to defer any surgical treatment until the area has fully epithelialized and can therefore be cleaned with antiseptic solutions prior to excision. If attempts are made to close the area before epithelialization, infected tissues are almost certain to be included within the lumbar subarachnoid space and local sepsis and meningitis follow inexorably. While waiting for epithelialization to occur, local wide-spectrum antibiotic can be used to keep down surface infection and the child should remain in hospital for the weeks necessary to achieve epithelialization.

It is generally accepted policy for these operations to be carried out only in special centres familiar with the problems involved. The transport of a child to such a centre should be arranged as soon as possible after birth and the lesion covered with damp sterile saline gauze to prevent infection or drying out of the lesion. On no account should caustic or irritant antiseptic solutions be used on the exposed neural tissue. The infants stand transportation quite well provided they are kept warm.

Faecal Incontinence
Faecal overloading which often results must be prevented by the judicious use of aperients and suppositories. When overloading is established it may be necessary to carry out manual evacuation. When there is some anal sphincter tone careful bowel training must be directed at regular defaecation in the absence of any rectal sensation. In this way full faecal continence can usually be achieved. Those cases with a completely patulous anus often do not achieve continence and it then may become necessary to carry out a colostomy as a last resort.

Urinary Incontinence
The aim of treatment is two-fold: to prevent renal damage resulting from retention and urinary infection and to relieve the socially unacceptable incontinence.

The urinary tract should be examined by means of intravenous pyelography and micturating cystography during the first month of life to assess its state, and the urine examined for infection. Whether the bladder is of the flaccid or of the trabeculated type it should be expressed regularly in order to keep residual urine to the minimum; some reflux which results together with the concomitant hydronephrosis cannot be avoided. The parents should be taught to be on the look-out for signs of urinary infection such as loss of appetite, general malaise and pallor. When any of these symptoms are reported the urine should be cultured and the appropriate antibiotic be given, if infected. The course is continued for at least 6 weeks regardless of whether the urine has become apparently sterile earlier.

A urinary diversion operation should be carried out as early as possible; and in any case should not be delayed beyond the third year. The ureters are transplanted into an artificial bladder (conduit) made from large or small intestine, connecting via stoma to a rubber bag into which the urine is collected. Once management is mastered the usual uriniferous smell is avoided. Other methods such as penile clamps, permanent urinals, in-dwelling catheters and the like are undesirable and have no place in the treatment of incontinence in spina bifida.

Orthopaedic Management
The efforts should be aimed at correcting existing deformities, and at preventing others from developing. A talipes equinovarus, whether paralytic or malformative, should be treated early, as the deformity of the feet will make walking very difficult. Other abnormalities of the joints, such as dislocation of the hip and arthrogryposis and the like, should also receive urgent attention. Many of the deformities seen later, that prevent locomotion and comfortable sitting in a chair, are, however, the result of the unopposed action of unaffected muscles. These may be prevented by means of judicious splintage and perhaps operative division of shortened muscles and tendon transplantation. The value of exercise and physiotherapy here is paramount. Walking calipers and aids, braces and supports are often of great benefit. In some instances it is better to amputate a severely deformed limb if thereby it becomes possible to sit in a chair or, with the aid of an artificial limb, to walk.

General Management
The general management falls into two parts: that of the parents and the family unit as a whole, and that of the child in question.

The parents, and especially the mother, must be told at once and sympathetically. An explanation of how the abnormality has come about will help to allay doubts and recriminations which may well arise. Tactful and candid discussion about the future is essential during the next weeks, but the paediatrician must avoid either too gloomy or too optimistic prognosis. Such explanations will help the parents to adopt a right attitude towards their malformed child. The mother should be helped to visit, handle, nurse and feed her child as soon as possible, which is often in a hospital some distance from where it was born. This will help to form a bond between them and lessen the risk of rejection. There should be frank explanations and discussions of plans of treatment and at some stage realistic genetic advice may be needed.

Parents may well require assistance, both moral and financial, during the all-too-frequent later hospital visits and admissions, and they may need to be enabled to have a holiday either with the child at a holiday centre with special provisions, or alone by arranging for the child to be admitted to a hospital, home or an institution for a short while. The parents should be advised to join the Association for Spina Bifida and Hydrocephalus (the Parents' Association) from which they derive much help and support.

Every effort should be made to enable the child to have contact with other children as early as possible in play centres or nursery schools to help to socialize these potentially isolated children. Later they should attend school, if possible a normal school; the education of these children, which is likely to be interrupted by repeated hospital admissions for the correction of deformity, must be as complete as possible as they, more than other children, are dependent on it for any form of separate existence.

Cranium Bifidum

Cranium bifidum is 'spina bifida' situated about the head. It warrants a special section as both features and prognosis are different.

Cranium Bifidum Occultum

Cranium bifidum occultum, a small midline occipital bone deficiency, usually found incidentally on x-ray examination of the skull. It is of no great clinical significance because remaining structures, such as dura and scalp, are sufficiently strong to prevent herniation of the skull content.

Cranial Meningocele and Encephalocele

Clinical Features

These lesions are less common than those along the vertebral column. Ingraham and Matson's and other series suggest that they account for about 1 in 5 of all the cases seen. This is rather a high figure, possibly because many such patients survive and tend to be referred to the larger centres for treatment.

The great majority of sacs are situated in the occipital area, diminishing in frequency in the parietal, frontal, nasal and orbital regions. Very occasionally a nasopharyngeal encephalocele is mistakenly removed as

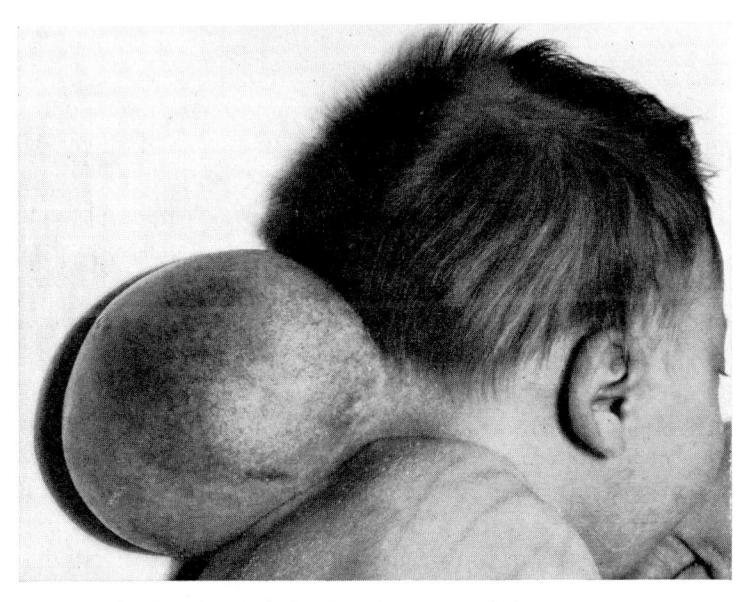

FIG. 2.9. Occipital encephalocele: a large encephalocele with a relatively narrow neck. The sac contained some disorganized cerebellar tissue and an extension of the fourth ventricle.

a polyp with dire consequences. The size varies greatly from small and inconspicuous to sacs larger than the head from which they arise. The covering of the sac may consist of full thickness integument, which may or may not show the usual anomalies, or of membrane (Fig. 2.9). The latter appears as a bluish semi-transparent structure variable in extent generally near the fundus. It is unusual for central nervous system tissue to be present on the surface as in the myelocele.

The contents may be fluid only, in which case it is a true cranial meningocele. Often, however, brain showing various abnormalities herniates through the skull defect to form an encephalocele. Part of the ventricular system may also enter the sac. The distinction between meningocele and encephalocele is not easy clinically. Solid tissue may be felt.

Transillumination may show solid contents. An x-ray of the skull will demonstrate the bony defect. It will also show craniolacunia and the small skull often associated with an encephalocele. A little air injected into the ventricle will demonstrate hydrocephalus, which generally accompanies an encephalocele. Occasionally air can be manipulated into the sac. It is often not possible to be sure what lesion is under consideration until operative exploration.

Prognosis and Treatment
The cranial meningocele carries a good prognosis as there is usually no associated hydrocephalus or malformation; they should all survive and have few sequelae. Removal of the sac preferably within a few weeks of birth with some form of repair of the defect is a simple matter unless it is a nasal, frontal or orbital lesion when extensive plastic surgery may be required.

The encephaloceles present a different problem. Many of the infants have a degree of microcephaly as well as hydrocephalus and other cerebral anomalies. Large sacs present a nursing difficulty as the skin and membranes easily become chafed and infected with the ensuing danger of meningitis. Occasionally a sac bursts. The bizarre and unsightly appearance, as well as the nursing problems, make it desirable to remove the sac soon after birth, although it is rare for the anomaly to be correctable in any way; any considerable bulk of cerebral tissue, even if morphologically normal in appearance, cannot be replaced within the cranium without running the risks of raising intracranial pressure to dangerous levels and distorting important structures such as brain stem, sinuses, or draining veins. The procedure generally adopted is to carry out a radical removal of the sac and cover the defect with fascia or dura and scalp. The incidence of post-operative deaths from various causes such as hydrocephalus and meningitis is high. Many of the survivors have varying degrees of mental defect.

Spinal Dermal Sinus and Dermoids

Sinuses may occur anywhere along the spinal axis in the midline but are found most frequently in the lumbosacral region (Fig. 2.10). They are due to faulty separation of the neuro-ectoderm from the endoderm and represent the posterior neuropore, this being one of the last places of separation between the two layers.

In one series of newborn infants 1·4 per cent were found to have lumbosacral sinuses, another 2·8 per cent had dimples while many more had shallow depressions.

The sinus is seen on the surface as a dimple, which becomes more obvious in the newborn by moving the skin. It is sometimes surrounded

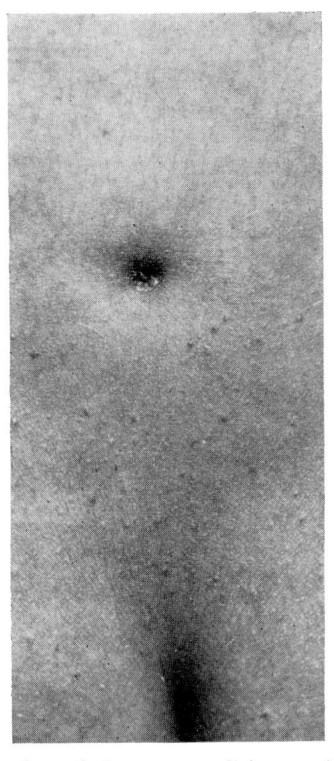

FIG. 2.10. Lumbar dermal sinus: a small inconspicuous sinus, which had been infected. Some dried-up discharge can be seen. On exploration this tract extended as far as the dura.

by hypertrichosis and port-wine stained skin. When it is examined closely, it is found to be lined by squamous epithelium and may end at any point down to the spinal cord. Most frequently, however, the sinus ends before reaching the vertebral column. When, especially after puberty, the epithelium of such a sinus grows hair, it is sometimes called a pilonidal sinus and may be mistakenly regarded as a separate entity. Some of the sinuses are associated with spina bifida occulta. Occasionally one is associated with dermoid, lipoma or even teratoma, any of which may produce cord pressure symptoms if situated within the spinal canal.

These sinuses sometimes become infected and discharge. A dermoid may become converted to an abscess, while communication with the dura or cord may lead to meningitis. For this reason a search for such sinuses should be made in cases of unexplained meningitis.

When infection has occurred the treatment should be radical excision of the tract, together with any tumour with which it may be associated. This must be considered a major operative procedure. Surgery should not be undertaken until infection has been completely controlled by antibiotics. There may be a case for the removal of some of the deeper sinuses as a prophylactic measure.

Occipital Dermal Sinus and Dermoid

The other comparatively common site for the sinus is in the midline of the occipital region representing the anterior neuropore. Most of these end blindly before reaching the occipital bone and are harmless. Some do pass through a small often obliquely placed defect in the occipital bone to end extradurally, in the subdural space or even within the cerebellum. They then constitute a real danger, if they become infected. Associated with the sinus may be the intradural or extradural dermoid. A well-positioned x-ray may demonstrate the small tract, while the presence of the dermoid may be suggested by some rarefaction of the occipital bone overlying the dermoid. Both sinus and dermoid should be removed. In about half the recorded cases of midline posterior fossa dermoids no associated sinus could be found.

HYDROCEPHALUS

Hydrocephalus not associated with spina bifida cystica is a relatively rare condition. The incidence at birth is given variously between 0·3 and 2 per thousand births. That in South Wales is about 0·5 per thousand births. However, as many cases and especially the acquired ones, do not manifest themselves until later, a higher incidence is recorded if estimated at 5 years of age. When all the cases of hydrocephalus are considered then those associated with spina bifida cystica outnumber the others greatly and the incidence will show a geographical distribution similar to that of spina bifida cystica.

ABNORMALITIES OF THE CENTRAL NERVOUS SYSTEM 51

When the hydrocephalus is associated with spina bifida cystica the empirical risks given in the appropriate section apply. Exclusive of these cases, the empirical risks of a child with a central nervous system malformation, after an index patient with hydrocephalus, are low. There is, however, a small proportion of cases in which the primary malformation is a stenosis of the aqueduct of Sylvius where the family history shows that a sex-linked recessive gene is determining the condition. The Dandy–Walker syndrome behaves in at least some families as a recessive condition. In these cases the family risks consequent on this form of inheritance apply.

PATHOLOGY

Theoretically hydrocephalus may result from over-production, or failure of absorption, of cerebrospinal fluid or from obstruction to its circulation (Table 2.1). Over-production occurs in cases of choroid

TABLE 2.1
Causes of hydrocephalus. Some of the more abstruse causes have been omitted for clarity's sake

Over-production of C.S.F.	Choroid plexus papilloma and villous hypertrophy
Obstruction to C.S.F. pathway	*Within ventricular system:* Foramina of Monro, Aqueduct, Exit foramina. *Subarachnoid space:* Arnold–Chiari malformation, Basal cistern block
Defective absorption of C.S.F.	? Venous sinus thrombus

plexus papilloma, a rare tumour which is functionally active and which is occasionally present at birth causing hydrocephalus then or soon after, but is generally seen in an older age group. Failure to absorb cerebrospinal fluid, thought to occur in dural venous sinus thrombosis, is not well authenticated. Obstruction to the cerebrospinal fluid pathway is pathologically and numerically the most important cause and all cases of hydrocephalus due to a malformation fall into this group. Blockages, which may be multiple (Table 2.2A, B), tend to occur at points of narrowing of the pathway, both within the ventricular system, in the aqueduct of Sylvius or at the exit foramina of the fourth ventricle and in the subarachnoid space around the tentorial opening or the basal cisterns. The cerebrospinal fluid pathway proximal to the obstruction then dilates, so that in cases of aqueduct block the lateral and third ventricles expand, while with basal cistern block the whole ventricular system as well as some of the basal cisterns become dilated.

TABLE 2.2A
Aetiology of hydrocephalus (100 post-mortem examinations)

Malformation:		46
Alone	14	
With infection	30	
With trauma	2	
Inflammation:		50
Infection alone	17	
Trauma alone	22	
Unknown (probably infection or trauma)	11	
Tumours		4

TABLE 2.2B
Site of block causing hydrocephalus
(100 post-mortem examinations)

Isolated sites:		50
Aqueduct	10	
IV ventricle foramina	7	
Basal cistern block	21	
Arnold-Chiari malformation	12	
Multiple sites:		48
Basal cistern block with block at foramina of Monro, aqueduct or IV ventricle	20	
Arnold–Chiari malformation with blocks at foramina of Monro, aqueduct, IV ventricle or basal cistern	28	
No block (over-secretion)		2

Aqueduct of Sylvius Malformations

The aqueduct of Sylvius may be the site of stenosis or forking. The former is uncommon and may be associated with other malformations of the brain. The shape of the aqueduct is usually preserved but the channel is reduced in diameter though often it has a crenated and irregular outline. The ependymal lining remains intact, with surrounding brain tissue free from gliosis. Forking, on the other hand, is a common anomaly, frequently associated with spina bifida cystica; the aqueduct is usually divided into a large dorsal and a number of smaller ventral channels. One of these generally communicates with the third and fourth ventricles while the rest end blindly. These channels have an intact ependymal lining and there is no gliosis between them.

Arnold–Chiari Malformation
Nearly all myeloceles except some of those situated low down in the cerebrospinal axis have an anomaly of the hind brain which takes the form of an Arnold–Chiari malformation (Fig. 2.11). This consists of a midline tongue of vermis of the cerebellum, extending for a variable distance down the spinal canal, and an elongated abnormal medulla descending beyond the foramen magnum. Lying between the cerebellum and the pons and medulla is a long and often narrow fourth ventricle which may have a pouch-like caudal prolongation with the choroid plexus generally forming a compact mass near the tip of the cerebellar tongue. In addition, the cerebellum may be small and poorly lobed. The medulla may be kinked backwards upon the cord and the upper spinal nerve roots take a cranial course. The whole malformation is covered by congested meninges, which in time become thickened and fibrosed. The malformation may be only very slight with a cerebellar tongue measuring no more than 2 mm long; occasionally there is only a lengthened medulla extending for a variable distance down the spinal cord with a normal cerebellum. The Arnold Chiari malformation must be differentiated from cerebellar herniation where the tonsils descend down the spinal canal laterally and where there is no medullary component unless medullary coning is present as well.

Association of the Arnold–Chiari malformation with other congenital anomalies of the central nervous system is common. Aqueduct forking is seen in about 25 per cent of cases; the thalamic bodies may be fused to a variable degree forming a large inter-thalamic bar; a hypoplastic falx and great longitudinal fissure together with interdigitation between the two cerebral hemispheres is common. Ectopic subependymal grey matter and microgyria is sometimes seen while in many cases there is an upward herniation of the cerebellum through the tentorial opening. The spinal cord often shows hydromyelia, diastematomyelia and cysts.

The aetiology of the hydrocephalus associated with spina bifida is two-fold. Aqueduct anomalies will in themselves lead to hydrocephalus; so will the Arnold–Chiari malformation by virtue of the overcrowding

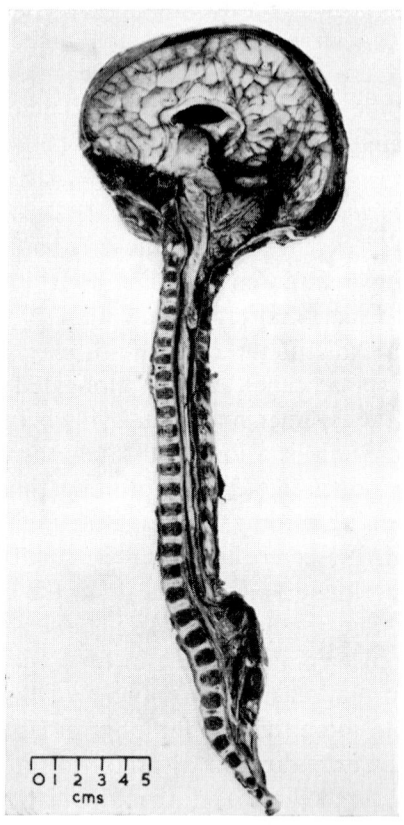

FIG. 2.11. A hemisected cerebrospinal axis showing moderate hydrocephalus, a typical Arnold–Chiari malformation and a lumbosacral myelocele. There is considerable vascular engorgement in the posterior fossa. The elongated medulla is kinked upon the cord which also shows hydromyelia.

(By courtesy of the Editor of the *Annals of the Royal College of Surgeons*.)

of structures in the often small malformed posterior fossa and the upper spinal canal, causing compression of the basal cisterns. The hyperaemia and eventual thickening and fibrosis of the meninges surrounding the malformation will further interfere with an already embarrassed cerebrospinal fluid circulation. Thus a large proportion of cases of spina bifida cystica already have an established hydrocephalus when born, although this may not be obvious as many have a normally sized or even small head. More important in these cases is ascending meningitis from the raw unepithelialized spina bifida sac causing post-inflammatory obstructions superimposed upon congenital narrowing.

Atresia of the Fourth Ventricle Exit Foramina
Occasionally a developmental atresia of the foramen of Magendie is

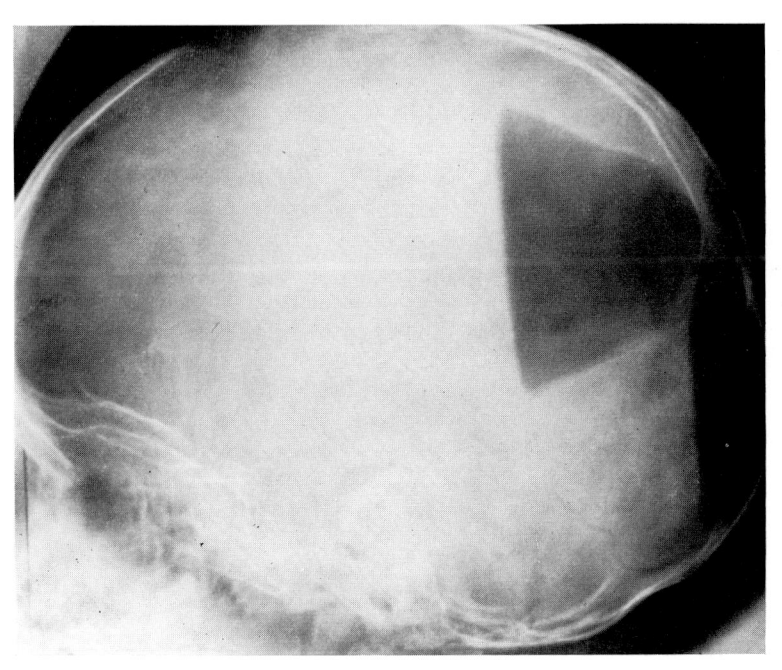

Fig. 2.12. Dandy–Walker syndrome. There is considerable bony enlargement of the occiput and the posterior fossa, the lateral sinus groove and torcula lie abnormally on the skull vault. The ventriculogram shows marked hydrocephalus with air in the posterior horns which occupies almost the whole space within the posterior fossa and in an enormously dilated fourth ventricle.

seen, leading to an enormous dilatation of the fourth ventricle and an abnormal development of the cerebellum. In this condition, which is also known as the Dandy–Walker syndrome, apart from severe hydrocephalus with marked bony enlargement of the occiput (Fig. 2.12) the patients always show considerable truncal ataxia in addition to the usual neurological features.

Inflammations

Post-inflammatory hydrocephalus with obstruction in the aqueduct, exit foramina or basal cisterns (Fig. 2.13), even in the absence of spina bifida cystica, is relatively common. Bleeding into the cerebrospinal

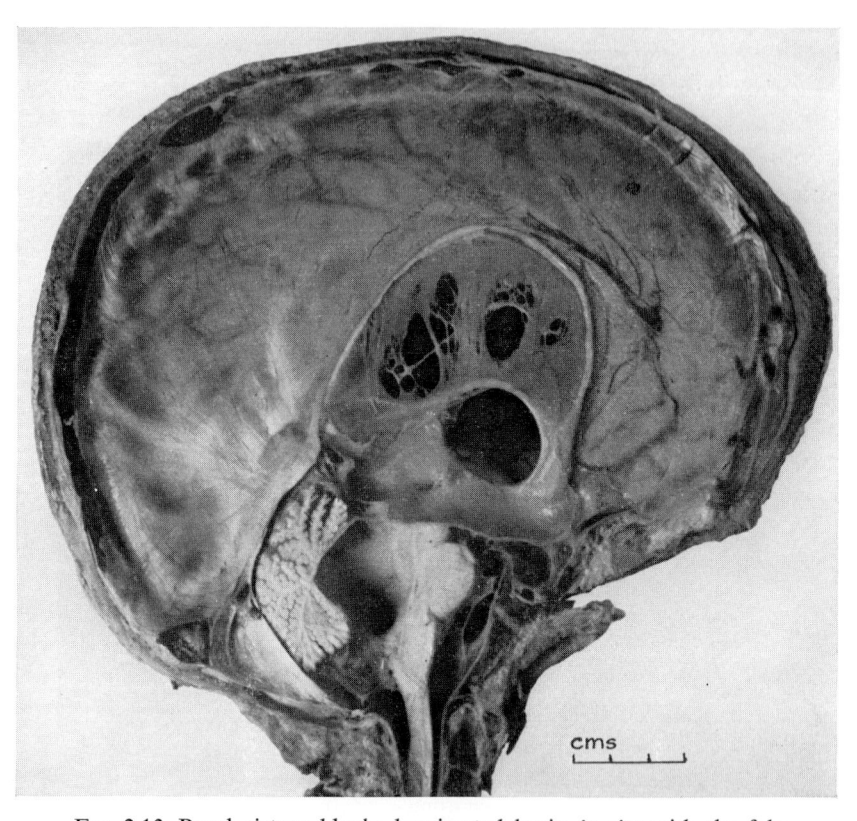

FIG. 2.13. Basal cistern block; hemisected brain *in situ* with the falx cerebri and tentorium left in position showing dilated basal cisterns (cisterna magna pontis and interpeduncularis), dilated exit foramina, fourth ventricle, aqueduct and third ventricle. The dilated lateral ventricle can be seen through the attenuated septum pellucidum and dilated foramen of Monroe.

pathway which may lead to inflammatory reaction and then to blockage most commonly results from birth trauma or anoxia especially in the premature; but it may also occur without any apparent perinatal difficulties. It may also follow head injuries. Meningitis, especially if not treated promptly, may also cause hydrocephalus. Both birth 'injury' sufficient to cause C.S.F. haemorrhage and meningitis may be accompanied by parenchymal brain damage. In an appreciable number of cases of basal cistern block, which must be of inflammatory origin, with progressive hydrocephalus becoming obvious in the first few weeks of life, there is however no history of either birth trauma or of meningitis.

Gliosis of the Aqueduct
This is a rare cause of aqueduct block due to overgrowth of the subependymal glia. It is seen in childhood rather than infancy. There is never any history of inflammation and the condition is probably hamartomatous.

Tumours
Any intracranial tumour, but especially those of the brain stem and cerebellum, may cause obstructive hydrocephalus. Occasionally medulloblastomas or choroid plexus papillomas, which must have been present at the time of birth, cause hydrocephalus early in life.

CLINICAL FEATURES
There is no difficulty in diagnosing an advanced case, but early hydrocephalus is not always recognized. The feature which most commonly brings patients to the doctor is undue head enlargement, sometimes accompanied by irritability or failure to progress. It is surprising, however, how frequently a mother will not be aware of quite marked head enlargement until it is pointed out to her. The normal infant's head should not grow more than 2·5 cm in each of the first 2 months and very much less subsequently (Table 2.3 and Fig. 2.14). Growth beyond this rate should arouse suspicion. However, the skull of a severely premature infant which may be only 25 cm in circumference at birth will enlarge very rapidly at first but maintain the normal shape and show no other features of hydrocephalus. On the other hand in some cases of spina bifida cystica quite marked hydrocephalus is often present although the head may be of normal size or even be microcephalic. The head of a hydrocephalic infant tends to be globular in shape, rather soft with prominent parietal bones and perhaps a slightly protuberant forehead. Other features such as large and bulging fontanelles, unduly wide sutures sometimes with Wormian bones, prominent scalp veins and the 'crack-pot' note on percussion occur in advanced cases. The fontanelle tension is usually high but may not be so if the skull is soft, if

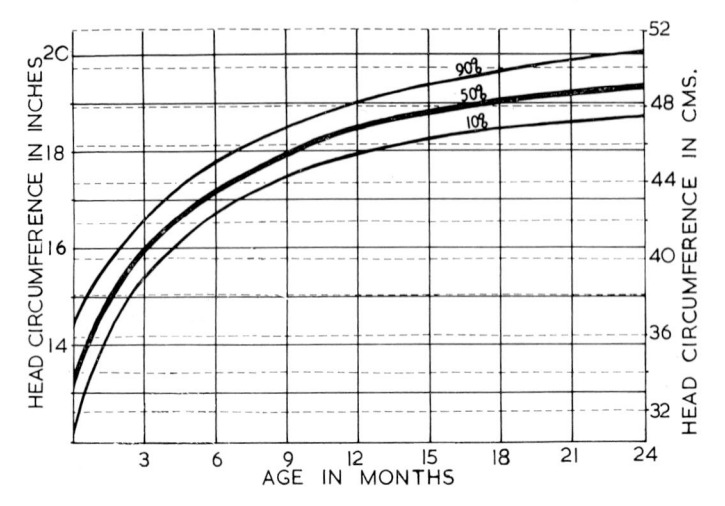

FIG. 2.14. Normal headgrowth: a graph showing the normal headgrowth from birth to 2 years. The 10th, 50th and 90th percentile lines are included, but these are computed from the mean of the values for boys and girls.

TABLE 2.3
The mean head circumference of boys and girls up to the age of 10 years, taken from various sources

Age months	Boys		Girls	
	in.	cm	in.	cm
0	13·6	34·5	13·2	33·5
1	14·7	37·2	14·4	36·7
2	15·4	39·2	15·2	38·6
3	16·0	40·9	15·7	40·0
4	16·3	41·8	16·0	40·7
6	17·3	43·9	16·8	42·8
9	18·1	46·0	17·6	44·6
12	18·7	47·6	18·9	45·0
15	18·8	48·0	18·3	46·5
18	19·2	48·7	18·5	47·1
Years				
2	19·6	49·7	18·9	48·1
2½	19·9	50·2	19·2	49·8
3	20·0	50·4	19·4	49·3
5	20·0	50·6	19·8	50·0
10	20·9	52·4	20·5	51·4

the cerebrospinal fluid has been leaking from an associated spina bifida sac, or if the infant is severely dehydrated. Slight increase in tension is difficult to assess, especially if the infant is restless or upset.

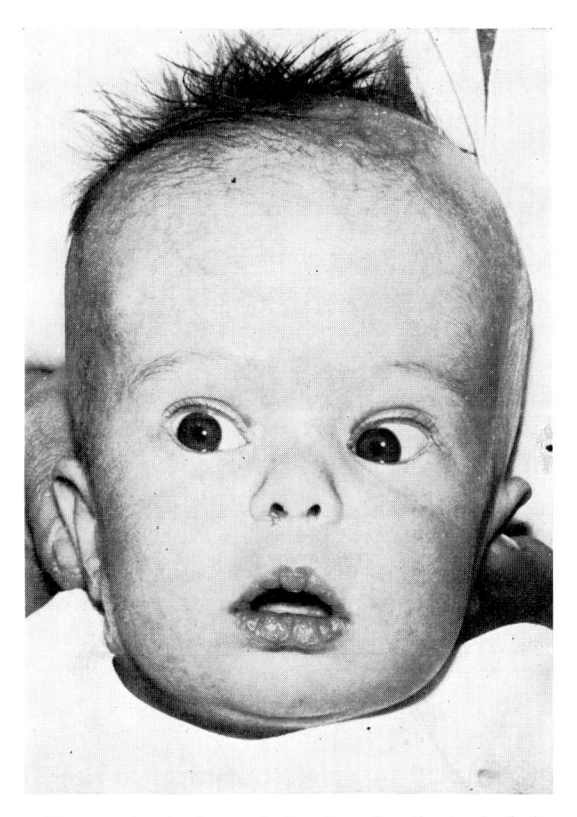

FIG. 2.15. Progressive hydrocephalus showing the typical shape of the head, the full fontanelles, the distended scalp veins and the setting sun appearance of the eyes.

As the disease advances the eyes tend to become displaced downwards and show the 'setting-sun' appearance when part of the iris is hidden by the lower lid and the sclera is visible above (Fig. 2.15). In addition there may be loss of interest in the surroundings though often mental and physical processes are preserved remarkably well in spite of very severe thinning of the cortex. Irritability, spasticity of the limbs, vomiting and convulsions are late signs.

The appearance of the fundus is deceptive. The optic discs are often pale suggesting optic atrophy, but blindness is comparatively uncommon in hydrocephalus. Papilloedema is rarely seen in infantile hydrocephalus and its presence should suggest an intracranial tumour as the underlying cause of the condition.

Other conditions to be remembered in the diagnosis of a child with a large head are rickets (now rare), cerebral abscess, porencephalic cysts under tension, subdural hygroma or haematoma (which would be needled during the subsequent investigation), achondroplasia, megalencephaly and of course the hereditary large but normal head.

INVESTIGATION

Clinical, X-ray and Spinal Fluid Examination
A full examination of the central nervous system should be carried out. This ought to include the usual cranial nerve examination and especially a careful assessment of vision and hearing and an inspection of the fundi, the testing of power, co-ordination and sensation, and the elicitation of the tendon and other reflexes. Some assessment of development, orientation and intelligence should also be attempted.

The further investigation of hydrocephalus should begin with carefully charted head measurements at regular intervals, to determine the rate of enlargement of the skull. This will indicate the urgency of further investigation and of treatment. A plain radiograph of the skull may yield valuable information. The vault is large compared with the facial bones, the sutures are generally separated and in the young the skull bones are thin while in the older children they may present an excessive copper-beaten appearance. In cases of spina bifida cystica, especially where the skull is small or relatively normal in size the bones may show cranio-lacunia (areas of very severe thinning) or even cranio-fenestra (complete deficiencies in the skull bones). A hollow posterior fossa in the absence of spina bifida cystica suggests an aqueduct lesion. Calcifications are rarely found but when present suggest toxoplasmosis; a rare but well-authenticated cause of hydrocephalus.

A full examination of the cerebrospinal fluid should next be made; also the lateral angles on the anterior fontanelle should be needled for subdural effusions and haematoma in infants. It is always wise to perform a ventricular puncture through the lateral angles of the anterior fontanelle (or burr holes) and slowly remove some cerebrospinal fluid in order to reduce the tension. At the same time an estimate of the thickness of the cortex may be made by observing the depth at which the needle enters the ventricle. A lumbar puncture may sometimes be most difficult especially in cases of block of the exit foramina where the cerebrospinal fluid may be at a low pressure in the thecal space, and in cases of myelocele where the cord extends at least as far as the sac. Old or fresh blood or xanthochromia in the cerebrospinal fluid indicate an antecedent haemorrhage. Increase in the number of cells and a raised protein content suggest an earlier infection, whereas a raised protein content alone could indicate a tumour.

It cannot be emphasized too strongly that any punctures involving the cerebrospinal fluid circulation, such as ventricular or lumbar puncture, and air encephalography, are potentially dangerous in hydrocephalic infants; they may react very violently to such procedures and a quiescent case may become rapidly progressive. Special care must be exercised in cases with an aqueduct block and a high ventricular pressure as a pressure cone may be precipitated by a lumbar puncture. Clumsy needling through the anterior fontanelle can produce subdural or intracerebral haemorrhage. For these reasons such patients should always be investigated with circumspection and in a place where prompt action can be taken in case of mishap or rapid deterioration.

Dye Studies
These have no place in modern neurosurgical practice.

Encephalography
Contrast encephalography is an essential part of the investigation of hydrocephalus, not only in order to locate accurately the position and extent of the obstruction, and to give a clear idea of the thickness of the cortex, but also to exclude tumour as the underlying cause of the condition. Porencephalic cysts and other evidence of parenchymal brain damage may be demonstrated and subdural collections of fluid visualized. Numerous techniques are available including lumbar air encephalography and air bubble, subtotal air replacement and myodil ventriculography. This is not the place to discuss the merits or special applications or for describing the techniques of each of these methods. Such investigations should always be carried out and interpreted by a neuroradiologist using special equipment, as incomplete or unsatisfactory radiographs are misleading, and dangerous.

Angiography
This is a difficult investigation and of only limited value in hydro-

cephalus, even though the vascular patterns are very characteristic. On occasion it may be an essential technique for demonstrating a tumour such as a choroid plexus papilloma.

Echoencephalography
This can be used to gauge the thickness of the pallium and to confirm the midline structures of the brain.

Electroencephalography
This is of limited assistance in hydrocephalus.

NATURAL HISTORY

Since hydrocephalus is a condition with a number of different causes, the disease is not uniform in character. When it is due entirely to a malformation such as an aqueduct stenosis or a severe Arnold–Chiari malformation, hydrocephalus is usually obvious at birth. Many such cases have difficult deliveries and in some cases the head has to be perforated for the infant to be born. In other instances, especially in those associated with spina bifida cystica, although the head may be of normal size (or even smaller than it should be), considerable hydrocephalus may be found on investigation. Many cases of spina bifida cystica develop ascending meningitis and this rarely appears later than 6 months of age, as by then the sac has generally become epithelialized, thus excluding infection. Should such a case have escaped hydrocephalus by that age, it is unlikely to develop it later. When hydrocephalus is due to birth haemorrhage, the condition is often not noticed for 4–6 weeks after delivery but generally cannot fail to be obvious by the age of 4–6 months. On the other hand, hydrocephalus following meningitis may develop at any age, but generally within a short time after the illness (Fig. 2.16).

Many cases progress rapidly with unremitting head enlargement. In the absence of treatment the patients lose interest in their surroundings, terminal spasticity, vomiting, pressure sores and occasionally blindness develop. Death occurs commonly from bronchopneumonia, cardio-respiratory failure and, in cases of spina bifida cystica, intracranial infection, often before the patient is a year old. Other cases may progress rapidly for a while and then stabilize, but not before the head has become too large to be supported or before much additional brain damage has occurred. These cases are often placed in an institution or the long-suffering families nurse them with their severe spasticity, inco-ordination and often mental defect and general helplessness. However, a recent investigation of 182 unoperated cases seen by one surgeon has shown that in a considerable number of cases (43 per cent) the hydrocephalus arrested spontaneously much earlier before severe brain damage has

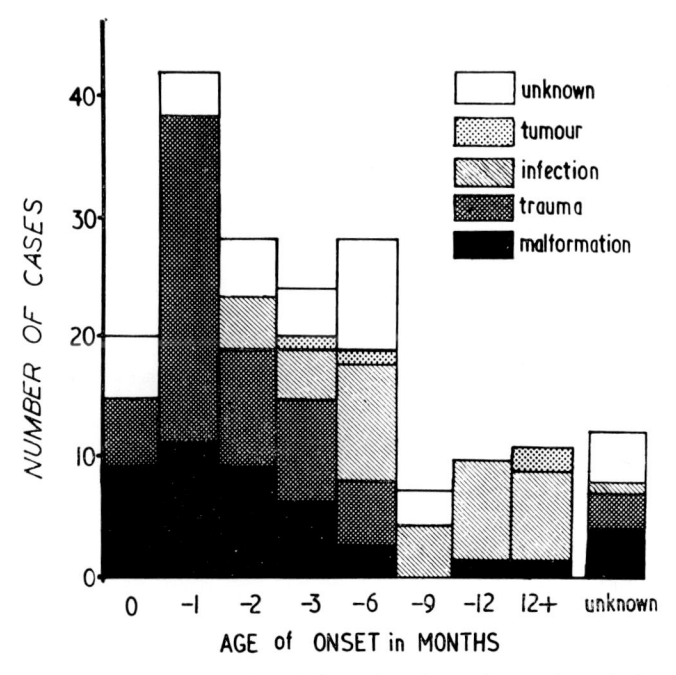

FIG. 2.16. Onset of hydrocephalus: the chart shows the relationship between onset and aetiology in 182 cases.
(By courtesy of the editor of the *Postgraduate Medical Journal*.)

been caused and in nearly all of them was still spontaneously arrested 7 years later. When a life table is computed from these data on actuarial principles it is found that over 20 per cent of the cases of hydrocephalus can be expected to survive at least into the third decade. A life chart makes this quite clear (Fig. 2.17). Most of the deaths occur during the first 2 years of life, though a few do die subsequently.

There may be some uncertainty about the exact time at which natural arrest takes place, as this tends to be a gradual process. Three or four consecutive head measurements, read at monthly intervals, remaining the same, are a good indication, especially if this should coincide with a noticeable improvement in the general condition of the child and a period of rapid physical and mental development. In most cases spontaneous arrest will occur by the age of 2 years. Careful head measurements should, however, be continued at regular intervals. In many children the head size remains stationary until the child has grown sufficiently for the head to be 'normal' in relation to the rest of the body, before growing again, but now at the normal rate. In some, the head will begin to grow again before the rest of the body 'has caught up' with

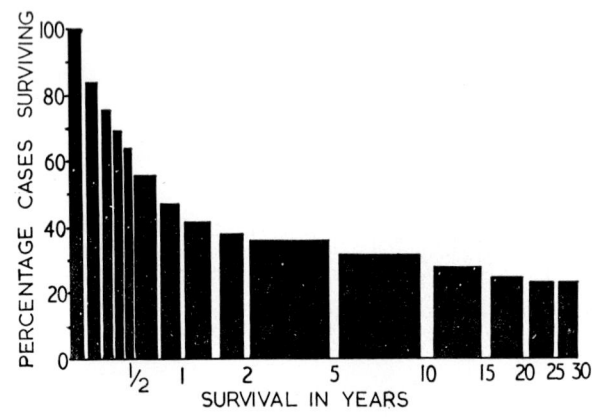

FIG. 2.17. Life chart for 182 cases of hydrocephalus: this, worked out on actuarial principles, shows the life expectancy of the series to be a survival to adult life of 25 per cent. With this chart it is possible also to compute the life expectancy of a child seen at later ages, e.g. one seen at 2 years has a 65 per cent chance of surviving into adult life.

the skull, but head growth runs parallel to the normal growth curve. In others, especially these in whom the skull has become very large, head growth never resumes. In all cases the large head becomes less conspicuous with time, though the characteristic shape can usually be recognized. Should the rate of growth of the skull exceed the normal rate at any time, or should the general condition deteriorate, or physical and mental development cease, the patient must be watched very carefully and recommended for investigation and surgery, if the trend continues for more than 2 or 3 months. Indeed hydrocephalus, whether arrested spontaneously or by surgical means, may become rapidly progressive again following head trauma, a general infection, or for no apparent reason. Occasionally this occurs so acutely that the patient who was perfectly well may develop status epilepticus and die within hours if nothing is done.

Neurological and Psychological Sequelae

Hydrocephalus associated with spina bifida forms a somewhat special subject as children with spina bifida tend to have considerable physical disability with relatively little intellectual impairment unless their hydrocephalus has become severe. The seventy cases of hydrocephalus

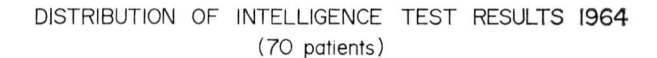

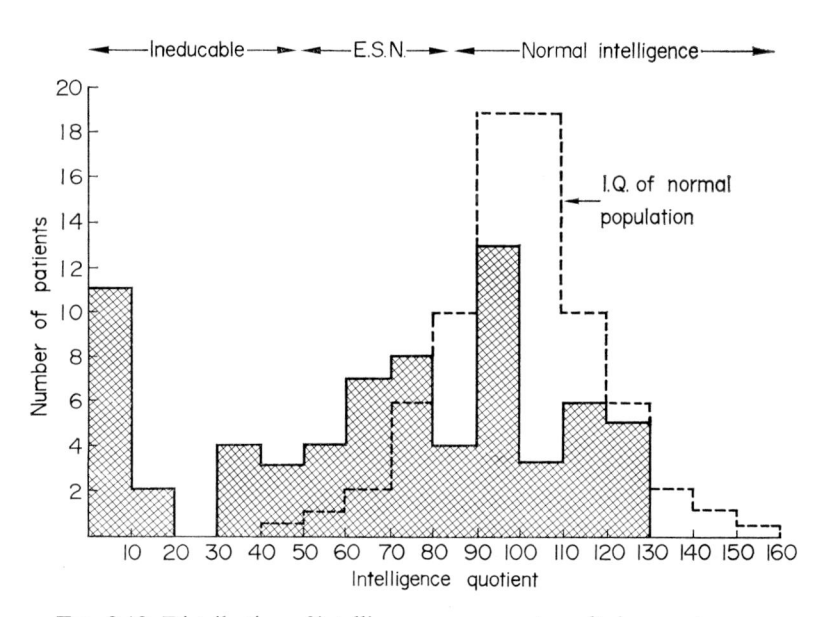

Fig. 2.18. Distribution of intelligence assessment results in seventy cases of hydrocephalus: the average I.Q. is 60. Although many have I.Q. results within the normal range, some are severely or grossly retarded.
(By courtesy of the Editor of *Archives of Neurology*.)

not associated with spina bifida from the investigation referred to earlier were investigated from the point of view of the sequelae. It was found that over 40 per cent were of normal intelligence, a further 30 per cent were educable with the remainder severely retarded; the whole series had a mean intelligence quotient of 68. Although there were fourteen children with intelligence quotients (I.Q.) above 100, thirteen had quotients which were below 20, (Fig. 2.18). Neurological features such as spasticity were almost always worse in the legs than the arms; ataxia and imbalance and clumsiness of fine finger movements and tremor of the hands always tended to be more severe in the more markedly hydrocephalic children. The spasticity and the imbalance and ataxia in the more severely affected patients amounted almost to a combination of cerebellar ataxia and spastic diplegia.

There was a close correlation between intellectual performance and physical disability caused mostly by the neurological sequelae but also by squints, etc.; those children who were mentally retarded were physically disabled as well. Relationship between the severity of the hydrocephalus and the intelligence was also quite close, with those who were more severely hydrocephalic being more retarded. There were, however, a number of striking exceptions including several children whose cerebral cortex was less than 1 cm in thickness and who had a normal intellect. Several with relatively mild ventricular dilatation were very retarded. These must have suffered severe brain damage as a result of the condition that led to the hydrocephalus, as must have been the case of most of those with very low intelligence. The older children, on the whole, tended to have a slightly higher intelligence quotient and be slightly less physically handicapped, suggesting that with age and training these children do compensate for some of the sequelae of hydrocephalus.

More subtle damage is caused by hydrocephalus apart from a reduction of the intelligence quotient. Scatter in the scores in the various subtests, recognized as a feature of brain damage, was more constantly present and usually more severe in the grosser hydrocephalics. Similarly the more severe hydrocephalics tended to show the shallow intellect sometimes called the 'cocktail party syndrome' where the patients had a good verbal performance, unmatched by other modalities of intelligence and were able to recite without much understanding of what they were saying. Other signs of mental difficulty, such as being easily upset, and failure to match performance with ability, though somewhat more common among the severer hydrocephalics, were less constant. Other evidence of damage, not usually detected by our intelligence tests, such as lack of confidence and self-reliance and inability to deal with complex problems of life needed to make a success of life and to keep a job, was also seen.

TREATMENT

Surgery should be undertaken with the above figures in mind, with the surgeon keeping definite aims before him, which should be primarily to prevent additional brain damage from the dilating ventricular system. Damage brought about by the condition leading to the hydrocephalus or that already produced by ventricular distension cannot be undone.

A plea is made that the spontaneous arrest figures should not be used as an argument against resolute early surgery. There ought to be little argument about the desirability of early surgical treatment in cases of progressive hydrocephalus. The slowly progressive case presents a more difficult problem, but this too should be operated upon without waiting for spontaneous arrest to occur as additional brain damage may result. In the cases where the condition does not seem to be progressive an expectant policy may be adopted as most of these are probably, in fact, arrested. If arrest has taken place then the patient should not be subjected either to surgical intervention or to investigation, as this in itself may precipitate progressive hydrocephalus once more.

In 1957 a satisfactory ventriculo-auricular shunt was introduced by Pudenz who used silicone rubber tubing and a slit core valve at the distal and lying within the right atrium. At about the same time Spitz reported the results of using a valve invented by Holter. This was a unidirectional valve depending on a fine slit in two silicone rubber tubes situated within a silicone tube 2·5 cm long (Fig. 2.19). Several types, draining fluid at differing pressures, are now available but that draining cerebrospinal fluid at a pressure of 25 mm of water seems to be most used. The procedure is very simple and is applicable for all types of hydrocephalus, irrespective of the site of the block. Through the right parietal burr hole a ventricular catheter leads to the valve, which is stitched in place to lie under periosteum behind the ear. A soft whip-like venous catheter leads from the distal end of the valve subcutaneously to the divided and tied jugular vein. The length of this tube is carefully determined from previously taken standard radiographs, so that the distal end lies just within the right atrium. Alternatively the position of the catheter in the right atrium can be confirmed by a method which employs the electrocardiogram (E.C.G.) The catheter is slowly moved down the superior vena cava when filled with hypertonic saline solution, and the other end of the tubing is connected to the E.C.G. machine. When the tip of the catheter passes the sino-auricular node the 'P' wave in the E.C.G. becomes bifid. The end-point obtained by this method is very accurate and the method itself quick and convenient.

Drainage is gradual with no danger of sudden fall on the intracranial pressure. Operative mortality is very low and the procedure is well tolerated, even by the very young. Results so far published suggest that the operation is successful in about three-quarters of cases, a very considerable advance on any other method. The value does not function well when the C.S.F. has a high protein content, and of course if there

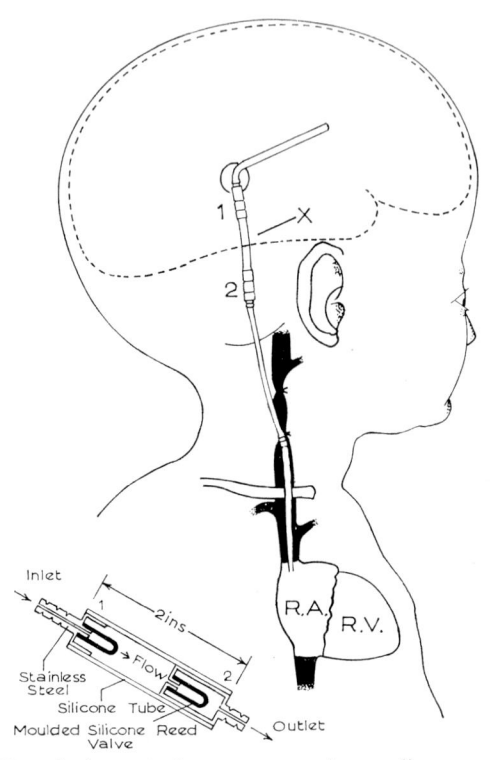

Fig. 2.19. Ventriculo-auricular anastomosis: a diagrammatic representation of the operation. The inset shows the details of the Holter valve.

(The main diagram is published by permission of Mr G. H. MacNab and the inset by permission of the publishers and editor of *Recent Advances in Paediatrics*.)

are many cells and there is debris. Difficulties sometimes arise from thrombosis in the jugular vein or superior vena cava, when the distal tube is too short. Occasionally thrombosis occurs within the right atrium. Rarely a patient develops multiple pyaemic abscess. More troublesome is the development of a persistent low-grade staphylococcus albus septicaemia from the valve. This cannot be controlled, except by removal and eventual replacement of the valve.

GENERAL MANAGEMENT

Hydrocephalics should be treated like 'normal' children as far as possible at least when the intellect is not too impaired, and complications dealt with as they arise and not anticipated. Most of the general principles applicable to children with spina bifida cystica apply to those with hydrocephalus only as well.

MALFORMATIONS CAUSING MENTAL DEFICIENCY

A number of congenital malformations are associated with mental deficiency. Those primarily of the central nervous system, and which make their appearance early in life, will be dealt with here. Down's syndrome (mongolism) and those having a known metabolic disorder as a basis are discussed elsewhere.

MICROCEPHALY

Features and Diagnosis

Microcephaly is an uncommon condition occurring in less than 1 per thousand births. The infant is born with either a normal or slightly small head, which subsequently fails to grow. A skull of a full-term infant which is 31·25 cm in circumference at birth, instead of 33 cm, will measure only 35 cm at 6 months, instead of 43·75 cm, and perhaps 36·25 cm at a year, instead of 46·25 cm, and will rarely grow beyond 42·5 cm. At the same time the face develops normally, giving the infant the typical appearance of a small head, with a large face, a receding forehead, and a loose, often wrinkled, scalp (Fig. 2.20). The fontanelles, which are usually small at birth, close within a few weeks and the sutures unite by 12 months. Though physical development is fairly normal, microcephalics are generally grossly retarded mentally and many never learn to walk properly or to speak. About 30 per cent suffer from convulsions; many are irritable, restless and destructive. On the other hand, some may learn to perform simple jobs. As with all mentally deficient subjects, they are prone to intercurrent infection from which they may die.

True microcephaly has, however, to be distinguished from the relative microcephaly resulting from severe intracranial lesions occurring at or soon after birth, as a result of birth trauma, anoxia or meningitis and also from that seen in association with spina bifida cystica. In true microcephaly, the history will help and also the dentition is usually delayed, which is not a feature of the relative microcephaly seen in the

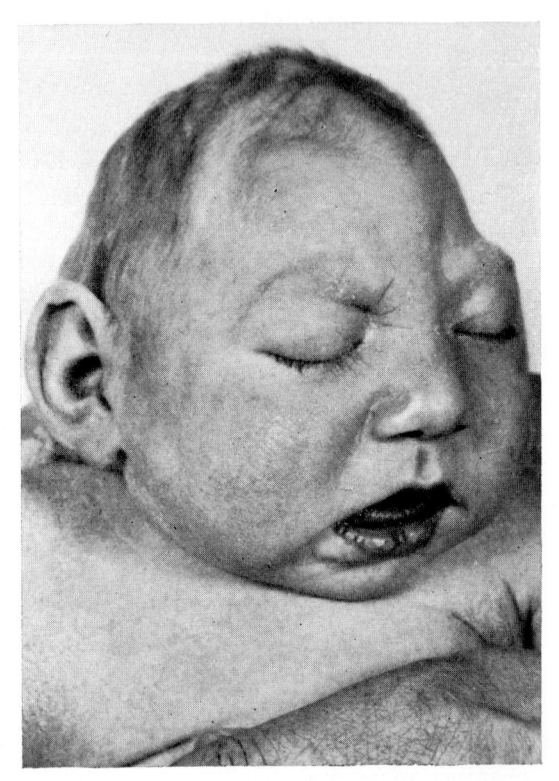

FIG. 2.20. Microcephaly: typical example with a normal-sized face and small vault covered with loose-wrinkled scalp.

other conditions. An x-ray of the skull, showing lacunation and fenestration, will help in those where there is spina bifida. Differentiation from craniosynostosis has also to be made.

Genetics and Aetiology
A substantial proportion, perhaps about a half, of cases of severe microcephaly, having skulls which are short, low and narrow, are homozygotes for an autosomal recessive gene. The risk of a second microcephalic

child is, therefore, of the order of 1 in 8; this becomes 1 in 4 if there is other genetic evidence, such as parental consanguinity or an older microcephalic sib, that an autosomal recessive gene is responsible. The aetiology of the others is obscure. Roentgen therapy during early pregnancy can definitely cause the anomaly and it has been reported after maternal rubella during the first 3 months.

Pathology
The brain is much smaller than normal and usually weighs between 500 and 600 g (normal 1200–1400 g) with small but normally shaped cerebral hemispheres that do not cover the relatively normal cerebellum. The simple convolutional pattern is reminiscent of that of the anthropoid ape or of a 5 months foetus. Microscopically the cortical cells are relatively normal, but tend to be arranged in cords. Some cases show considerable arteritis with ulegyria. Rarely heavy calcium carbonate deposits are found in the cortex and nuclei, together with myelin breakdown material, reminiscent of a destructive process.

MEGALENCEPHALY

Features and Diagnosis
Individuals are found with very large brains weighing between 1600 and 2800 g in the adult (normal 1400 g). Although this weight is very occasionally associated with exceptional intelligence, nearly all these patients are mental defectives.

At birth the head of the megalencephalic, who is usually a male, may be large, though as a rule not large enough to attract notice. The fontanelles are large and the sutures wide, and soon the skull begins to enlarge rapidly and assume a typical hydrocephalic shape, with the fontanelles and sutures remaining open. The patients, however, do not show the eye signs of hydrocephalus. Mental and physical development is severely retarded and most cases suffer from convulsions. The retardation is not progressive except in a few cases but, like most severe defectives, they die early from intercurrent infection or in a convulsion.

The diagnosis can only be established with certainty by ventriculography, when a normal or even small ventricular system is demonstrated, though the condition may be suspected when a thick cortex and cerebrospinal fluid under normal pressure is found in a severely retarded case of 'hydrocephalus'.

Pathology
The brain is large, heavy and firm with convolutions more complex and larger than normal. Microscopically there is no evidence of degeneration but in most cases the cortex shows numerous lamellae of well-formed neurones and broad zones of nerve fibrils. There is generally a great excess of glia especially in the sub-cortical white matter. The brain stem and cerebellum do not show obvious changes. Occasionally one cerebral hemisphere only is affected.

Megalencephaly seems to be due to a heterogeneous group of entities. In many instances it is possible to obtain a family history of mental retardation and sometimes there are several cases in one family. Some regard the condition as neoplastic.

Agenesis of Corpus Callosum

This condition has been known to pathologists since the beginning of the century, but it was not until 1934 ,when Davidoff and Dyke described characteristic findings on pneumoencephalography, that it came to be recognized clinically.

Features and Diagnosis
From the clinical standpoint this is an ill-defined condition generally presenting with Jacksonian convulsions, which do not respond to anticonvulsant therapy. The majority of cases show severe, but non-progressive mental retardation, both mental and physical, with particularly marked disturbance of speech. About half the cases suffer from hydrocephalus.

The diagnosis rests almost entirely on pneumoencephalography. In nearly all cases the air pictures show a large dorsally displaced third ventricle, separating the lateral ventricles. Most show, in addition, sharply angular 'bat wings' lateral ventricles with concave medial walls and the posterior horns are often moderately dilated. Elongated intraventricular foramina, and an abnormal radial arrangement of the sulci on the medial surface of the hemispheres, may also be demonstrated. An internal hydrocephalus is seen in a large proportion of cases (Fig. 2.21) and some have external hydrocephalus as well.

Pathology
The brain, often lighter than normal, may show complete agenesis of

the corpus callosum or only partial agenesis with the very anterior portion intact but thin. The gyri on the medial surface of the cerebral hemispheres have a radial arrangement with the cingulate gyrus buried below the surface. The septum pellucidum is absent and the fornix is abnormal with a very large bundle of fibres, which probably represent those that normally cross over in the corpus callosum. The space between

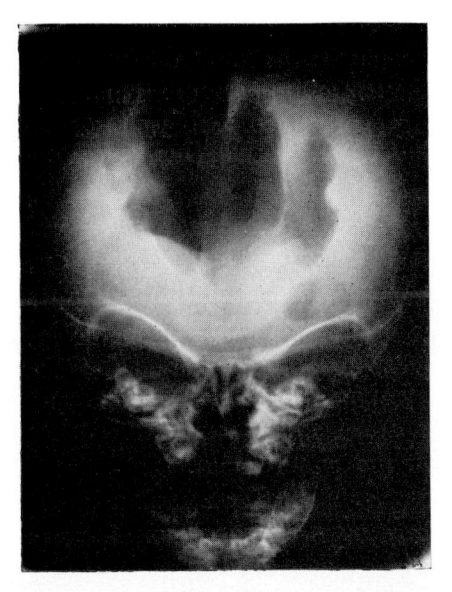

Fig. 2.21. Agenesis of the corpus callosum with hydrocephalus: the lateral ventricles are severely dilated, the latter particularly. The skull has the typical hydrocephalic shape.

the cerebral hemispheres is generally occupied by the large third ventriole, but occasionally a lipoma, cyst or meningioma takes its place. Microscopically the only abnormal findings are a thick, highly cellular granular layer of the cortex and absence of the usual laminations in the calcarine fissure.

Aetiology
The corpus callosum does not develop until the twelfth week, when the first fibres appear anteriorly near the lamina terminalis. Fibres then cross further back and the structure is fairly complete by 22 weeks. An interference with this process could readily account for all the features. The cause of this disturbance is not known except that in man, at any

rate, it does not appear to be inherited. Some cases of agenesis when associated with cleft palate and some form of arhinencephaly may have a trisomy of the 13/15 (D) chromsomes.

DESTRUCTIVE LESIONS OF THE BRAIN

Damage to the foetal central nervous system may lead to complete resorption of the damaged portion, as in hydranencephaly. In porencephaly it is, however, very difficult to know where to draw the dividing line between a 'congenital' lesion and one that is acquired, as there is a complete gradation between one and the other.

HYDRANENCEPHALY

Pathology and Aetiology
In this condition the greater part of the cerebral hemispheres is completely

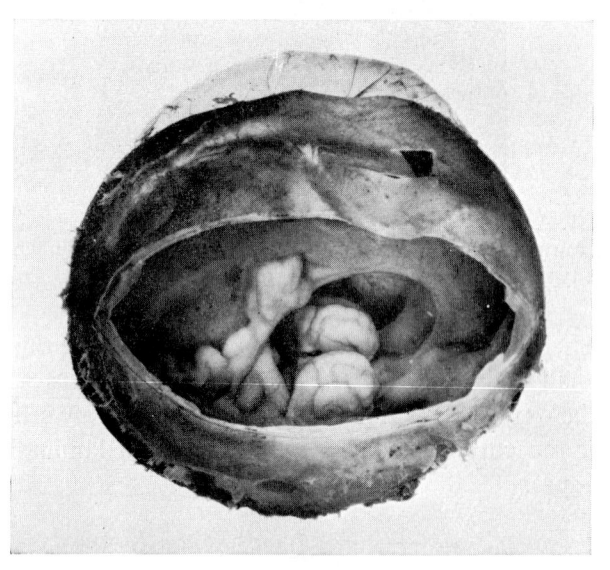

FIG. 2.22. Hydranencephaly: a post-mortem specimen with part of the skull and membranes cut away on the right side revealing the ventricular cavity where it is possible to identify the basal ganglia masses, part of the occipital lobes, and the choroid plexus. Bone only was removed on the left, allowing the thin glial membrane with thin blood vessels coursing over it to bulge.

destroyed, and is represented by only a thin membrane of condensed glial fibrils on the ventricular surface and arachnoid externally. This membrane encloses large ventricles, at the base of which can usually be seen normal choroid plexus and relatively normal basal portions of the temporal and occipital lobes. The hippocampi and amygdaloid nuclei, the brain stem and the cerebellum are usually preserved (Fig. 2.22). The cerebrospinal fluid pathways are generally intact, though sometimes

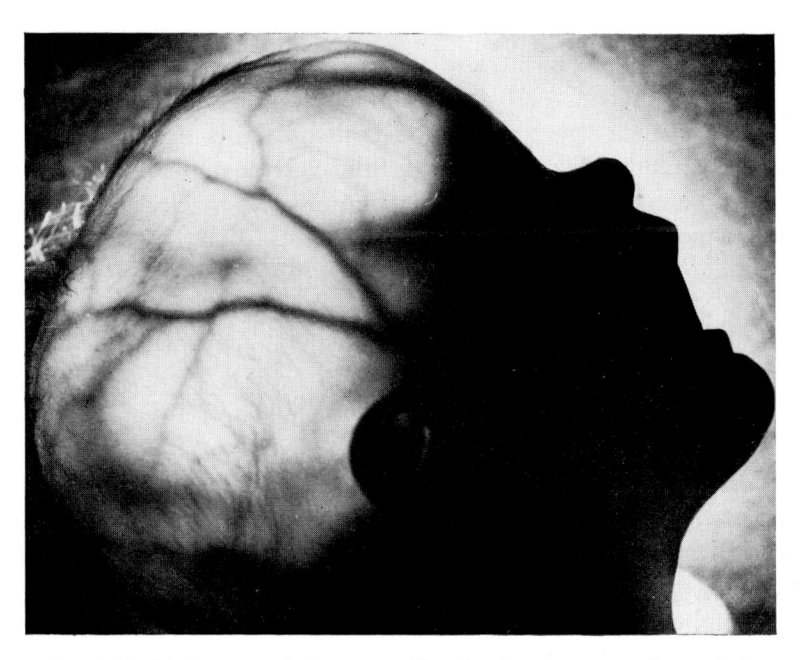

Fig. 2.23. Hydranencephaly: transillumination causes the whole skull to light up 'like a lamp' showing up the blood vessels in sharp relief. The vault of the skull is not unduly enlarged compared with the face.

aqueduct stenosis is present. The cerebrospinal fluid is either normal or xanthochromic.

The aetiology is obscure but there is some evidence that it is caused by obstruction to the blood flow in the areas supplied by the internal carotid arteries which may be occluded. This would have to occur early enough in foetal life for the affected brain tissue to be completely absorbed. There seems to be no connection between anencephaly and hydranencephaly.

Features and Diagnosis
These infants generally appear normal at birth; they feed normally and have been known to smile. Anxiety is usually not felt for 4–8 weeks, when the head may enlarge and become globular, the infant is noted to be backward and tends to become irritable and to have convulsions. They usually die of intercurrent infection at the age of 3–4 months, though cases have survived for 3 years. The developmental age always remains at the newborn level.

The diagnosis is made by transillumination of the head when, in a suitably darkened room, the entire cranium lights up like a lantern (Fig. 2.23) and the glow is transmitted through the pupils. Confirmation may be obtained by pneumoencephalography and by electroencephalographs which show complete absence of electrical activity in all leads.

PORENCEPHALY

This includes both obviously destructive lesions and distortions of growth.

Pathology
A lesion which is probably developmental in nature is the bilaterally symmetrical schizencephaly of Yakovlev, where a deficiency of the cerebral hemisphere occurs, involving the whole depth of the cortex, especially in the region of the primary fissures, the frontal and the parietal lobes. The cysts are often lined by heterotrophic grey matter and there is never any evidence of destruction of brain tissue. It is probably due to localized agenesis before the end of the second month of foetal life.

A different picture is presented by the more common localized and asymmetrical destructive lesion resulting from vascular occlusion or some encephalitic process occurring antenatally, or from birth injury. The position and extent of the lesion is very variable. It often does not communicate with the ventricular system and is separated from it by the ependyma and the subependymal glia. The overlying meninges are generally densely adherent. The cyst is often lined by a glial membrane and when 'non-communicating' it contains yellow serous fluid. Altered blood may be found in it and haemosiderin in the wall.

ABNORMALITIES OF THE CENTRAL NERVOUS SYSTEM

Features and Diagnosis

The Yakovlev type appears to be associated with double hemiplegia and dementia.

In localized porencephaly the clinical features are very variable. Frequently no symptoms are apparent for several months after birth, when it may be noticed that there is mental retardation, variable flaccid paralyses and physical underdevelopment. Convulsions referable to the affected side may occur.

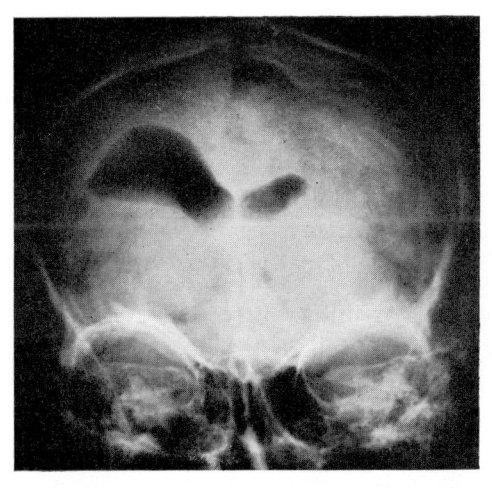

Fig. 2.24. Porencephaly: a ventriculogram showing a cyst communicating with the lateral ventricle.

The diagnosis rests on the ventriculographic findings in cases where the cyst communicates with the ventricular system (Fig. 2.24).

MISCELLANEOUS MALFORMATIONS

Miscellaneous malformations are occasionally met, for which there is only symptomatic treatment.

MICROPOLYGYRIA

This is a common malformation of the cerebral cortex, characterized by broad irregular granular gyri, with the grey matter extending in a festoon-like manner deep into the brain substance from the apex of the gyrus. The anomaly may be localized or involve the whole of one or both cerebral hemispheres. This has to be differentiated from what is sometimes called polygyria, where an excessive formation of secondary gyri may complicate an otherwise normal convolutional pattern. Microscopically two main varieties of micropolygyria are recognized. In the first there is non-separation of the molecular layer between the folds and a failure of the molecular layer to be arranged in a laminar pattern. In the second variety the molecular layer is divided into four thick bands of nerve cells.

These patients show varying degrees of mental deficiency and may suffer from epilepsy. If the lesion involves the motor cortex, cerebral diplegia and hemiplegia may be present, as then the pyramidal tracts tend to be deficient.

Pachygyria, Lissencephaly and Agyria

In these inter-related conditions there is a severe reduction or absence of the secondary convolutions, over part of the whole of the cerebral hemispheres, together with an increase in the depth of the cortical grey matter. In an extreme case the only sulcus present may be the Sylvian fissure, with the operculum poorly developed. Microscopically, severe abnormalities of the layers and immaturity of the neurones is found. This malformation is explicable on the basis of a retardation of development at the third or fourth month. Clinically, these malformations are associated with spastic diplegia.

Cerebellar Malformations

Complete absence of the cerebellum probably does not occur. Careful examination will generally reveal a small vestige of cerebellar tissue. Hypoplasia, however, is quite common. Other cerebellar malformations such as cerebellar rachischisis, due to partial or complete aplasia of the vermis, and cerebellar microgyria, are sometimes encountered. These anomalies are normally seen associated with other severe malformations.

There may be a variable degree of inco-ordination and tremor, but cerebellar hypoplasia may also be found at autopsy as an incidental finding.

SKELETAL TISSUE DISORDERS

Only two conditions affecting the central nervous system, craniosynostosis, and skull and scalp defects, will be included.

CRANIOSYNOSTOSIS

Aetiology

Sutures are normally un-united at birth and a fibrous union occurs by the fifth or sixth month, but bony union is not completed until the sixth or seventh decade. In craniosynostosis, premature fusion of two or more cranial bones occurs. The cause of this uncommon condition is unknown but it is probable that genetic factors play a major part. It is commoner in males (85 per cent of all cases) and is frequently associated with other anomalies, particularly syndactyly. Nonetheless, other causes such as prenatal trauma or endocrine disturbance have been suggested. Histologically no abnormality of the bone has ever been found.

In some families, uncomplicated craniosynostosis is inherited as if due to a dominant mutant gene. However, if no relative is affected, the empirical risks of later sibs being affected is low.

Features

Deformity of the skull, the most important and the earliest feature, is often noticed soon after birth when it may at first be mistaken for excessive moulding. The suture line may be felt as a bony ridge and movement of the skull bones is not possible. Confirmation is by radiography which will show the prematurely united sutures, tangential views along the line of the suspected sutural fusion being particularly useful. The skull frequently shows associated digital marking. As the child grows the skull deformity becomes more obvious. Occasionally the skull becomes progressively thinned so that eventually the brain and meninges herniate through as false 'meningoceles'.

Many infants with suspected cranial deformities eventually prove to have minor asymmetries of no importance. Such asymmetries may be graced by the name of plagiocephaly and asymmetrical premature fusion of cranial sutures may result in this condition. Other conditions to be considered in the differential diagnosis of the asymmetrical head are hemiatrophy secondary to cerebral damage or agenesis, postural asymmetry and infantile subdural haematoma. Premature synostosis has also to be differentiated from microcephaly, where the sutures unite at the age of about 1 year and no pressure symptoms develop.

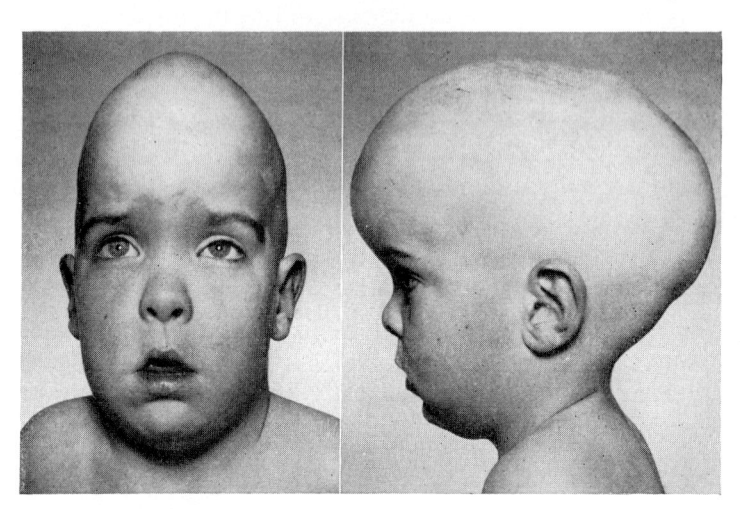

FIG. 2.25. Craniosynostosis: showing marked scaphocephaly due to fusion of the sagittal suture.

The clinical management of cases of premature sutural fusion has been complicated by synonyms and in describing these conditions it is wise to name the sutures prematurely fused as well as the resultant deformity. The type of deformity is dependent upon the sutures involved as the skull tends to expand in a direction parallel to the line of the closed suture. If the sagittal suture becomes closed (50 per cent of cases) the skull becomes scaphocephalic (syn. dolichocephalic) (Fig. 2.25) and when the coronal suture is prematurely fused (30 per cent of cases), the skull becomes brachycephalic (syn. oxycephalic). If in this latter condition the sagittal suture continues to remain widely open, the enlargement of the skull will be in an upwards direction to an unusual height (turricephaly). If the sutures in the immediate vicinity of the anterior fontanelle remain open when the more peripheral parts of the coronal and posterior part of the sagittal suture close, the upward growth of the skull occurs anteriorly and almost forms a point (acrocephaly). In mild cases where only one suture is involved the skull deformity may become less obvious with age probably due to the relative reduction of head compared to body size, to the growth of hair, etc.

Exophthalmos may occur in cases where early fusion of the coronal suture has occurred together with part of the sagittal suture and is probably due to compensatory over-expansion of the middle cranial fossa and consequent reduction in orbital volume. Generally it is only when more than one suture is fused at a very early age that papilloedema and other symptoms of raised intracranial pressure develop. Then the x-ray will show excessive convolutional markings and the child may have headache, blindness and mental retardation.

Treatment
When these symptoms and signs of raised intracranial pressure are present surgical relief is essential. The techniques employed vary; all involve an attempt to recreate permanent new 'suture lines' by removing a strip of bone at or alongside the prematurely closed suture and attempting to prevent reossification by an artificial barrier of polythene film, tantalum, wax or other material. All techniques work in the short term but in most cases reossification takes place after a year or two and further operations may have to be undertaken. This is why most neurosurgeons are becoming disinclined to operate on cases of craniostenosis without raised intracranial pressure where the only indications are cosmetic; although initially there was considerable enthusiasm expressed about such operations and their success.

Craniostenosis may be associated with other congenital anomalies:

Crouzon's disease, in this there is an associated beaked nose, hypoplasia of the maxilla and occasional abnormality of the digits. The skull and facial deformity is considerable and leads to a central prominence in the frontal region, marked exophthalmos with external squint while the maxillary hypoplasia causes the lower teeth to overlap the upper, leading to an apparent prognathism. The condition is an autosomal dominant.

Apert's Syndrome. Apert in 1907 described the association of syndactyly with acrocephaly and this was confirmed by Park and Powers in 1920. The syndactyly may be partial or complete involving all four extremities. Other abnormalities include synostosis of radius and ulna, absent radius, ankylosis or limitation of large joints, especially the elbow. Apert's syndrome has been reported in mother and child and in these cases was probably determined by an autosomal dominant gene, but the majority of cases occur sporadically as a result of a fresh mutation.

Hypertelorism and Waardenburg's Syndrome

Hypertelorism

The classical description of this abnormality has been given by Greig (1924). Basically there is distortion and deformity of that part of the sphenoid laid down in cartilage with consequent overgrowth of the lesser wings of the sphenoid. From birth the child is noted to have a broad forehead, an abnormally wide interocular distance, a broad root to the nose and an external squint. Other abnormalities described in Greig's series included: cleft lip and palate, mandibular asymmetry, deafness and microphthalmos. Mental defect is frequently present. The abnormality may be present in families but it is more frequent for cases to occur sporadically without obvious genetic basis.

Waardenburg's Syndrome

Waardenburg has described an autosomal dominant syndrome in which he found hypertelorism and congenital deafness associated with a white forelock and different-coloured eyes.

Fisch has collected eighty-one cases of this syndrome, selecting thirty-five for careful analysis. He has shown that hypertelorism is not in fact a feature, but that the pupils of the two eyes are separated by the normal distance. An abnormality of the inner canthus is constantly present giving a resemblance to hypertelorism because folds of skin on either side of the nose widen the bridge while reducing the amount of sclerotic visible medially to the pupils. This fold is normally present in the Mongolian race (and in some normal white children). It should not be confused with the epicanthic fold seen in Down's syndrome. The hearing defect may amount to total deafness or may be limited to the lower and middle ranges with normal high-tone hearing. Unilateral deafness is usually moderate, while in bilateral cases only one ear may be totally deaf. The degree of deafness varies among the relatives. In one child who died, ear and brain studies which were carried out showed an absence of the organ of Corti in the cochlear canal with atrophy of the spiral ganglion and nerve. The auditory pathway was intact. The white forelock in the middle of or just to one side of the centre of the forehead may form a thick, well-outlined lock or may occur as a few white strands. The heterochromia of the iris consists of one brown with one persistent blue eye, or of partial brown pigmentation in both blue eyes. Fisch has noticed a similarity of profile in his cases with a depressed nasal bridge, sometimes a metopic suture, and a massive lower jaw. Nasal infections are frequent.

In some families there is dappled, part brown, part pigmented skin. One girl had congenital atresia of the lower part of the oesophagus which Fisch suggests as a possible cause of the wasting and early infant deaths recorded in a few of the affected families.

Cleidocranial Dysostosis

This is a relatively rare condition where there is increased width of the forehead associated with absence of the middle portions of the clavicles. This defect results in abnormal mobility of the shoulder girdles which should be immediately evident on clinical examination. The ossification defect responsible for this gap in the clavicles may also be present in the pubic symphysis although to a less obvious extent. The wide forehead always shows a vertical groove. Even in the neonatal skull it may admit two or three fingers. It is due to an abnormally wide gap between the two frontal bones; in addition the sagittal and metopic sutures may persist for an abnormal length of time. A wide gap between bones in the vault may of course be present in other conditions such as hydrocephalus, hypothyroidism and congenital syphilis but it is relatively easy to distinguish between these conditions and cleidocranial dysostosis. Both sexes are equally affected in this condition, which is compatible with normal intelligence and life span although some cases have been described with associated spastic tetraparesis and mental defect.

When a case is diagnosed search should be made for other associated anomalies, which may include coxa vara, spinal hemivertebrae and partial fusion of vertebrae. Absence of the lower part of the sacrum and coccyx has been described. The most striking x-ray change in the hands and feet is the presence of epiphyses at both ends of metacarpal and metatarsal bones.

Muscle abnormalities include absence of the clavicular portions of the trapezius, the sternomastoid and the pectoralis major. The condition is normally symptomless but pain and numbness in the ulnar area from pressure of the outer fragment of the clavicle on the brachial plexus has been reported.

Ossification continues late in life and the skull usually closes completely in the end. The mothers of the author's patients were diagnosed as having rickets in childhood (probably from what was thought to be delayed closure of the anterior fontanelle). A triangular depression with its apex emerging from beneath the hair margin in the middle of the forehead can sometimes be felt or seen when the mother herself lacks clavicles. An autosomal dominant gene is responsible.

Congenital Skull and Scalp Defects

Defects of the scalp are generally small, but occasionally may be so large as to pose a difficult problem for the plastic surgeon. They may be associated with an underlying defect of bone. The commonest position is at the vertex, in the region of the hair crown. The aetiology is unknown.

All but the smallest defect should be dealt with early and radically before the wound has become converted into an infected granulating sore with the danger of precipitating a severe haemorrhage from emissary sinuses or of causing meningitis. The lesion should be excised and closed when possible. Large defects should be kept clean and moist until a plastic repair can be effected.

Defects in the skull are rare. These should be left, perhaps with some protection such as a soft bandage or a protective cap, without surgical treatment. At about 6 years, when the time of maximum skull growth has passed, the defects may then be repaired by plating with tantalum.

SELECTED REFERENCES

APERT E. (1907) *Traité de maladies familiales et maladies congènitales.* Paris: Bailliére.

CARPENTER M.B. (1954) Agenesis of the corpus callosum–Study of 18 cases diagnosed during life. *Neurology* **4,** 200–10

CARTER C.O., DAVID P.A. & LAURENCE K.M. (1968) A family study of central nervous system malformations in South Wales. *J. Med. Genet.* **5,** 81–106

CROUZON O. (1912) Dysostose cranio-faciale hereditaire. *Bull. Soc. Med. Hop. Paris* **33,** 545

DAVIDOFF L.M. & DYKE C.G. (1934) Agenesis of the corpus callosum; its diagnosis by encephalography. *Amer. J. Roentgenol.* **34,** 1

DEKABAN A. (1959) *Neurology of Infancy.* Baltimore: Williams & Wilkins

FISCH L. (1959) Deafness as part of an hereditary syndrome. *J. Laryng.* **73,** 355

FORD F.R. (1960) *Diseases of the Nervous System in Infancy, Childhood and Adolescence,* 4th edn. Springfield, Illinois: Charles C.Thomas

GIROUD A. (1960) 'Causes and morphogenesis of anencephaly'. Ciba Foundation Symposium on *Congenital Malformations,* pp. 199–212. Wolstenholme G.E.W. & O'Connor C.M. (eds.). London: Churchill

GREENFIELD J.G., BLACKWOOD W., MCMENEMEY W.H., MEYER A. & NORMAN R.M. (1963) *Neuropathology*, 2nd edn. London: Edward Arnold
GREIG D.M. (1924) Hypertelorism. *Edin. Med. J.* **31**, 560
GUTHKELCH A.N. & RILEY N.A. (1969) Influence of aetiology on prognosis in surgically treated infantile hydrocephalus. *Arch. Dis. Childh.* **44**, 29
HAMBY W.B., KRAUSS R.F. & BESWICK W.F. (1950) Hydranencephaly, clinical diagnosis; presentation of 7 cases. *Pediatrics* **6**, 371–83
HAWORTH J.C. & ZACHARY R.B. (1955) Congenital dermal sinuses in children: their relation to pilonidal sinus. *Lancet* **2**, 10–14
HOPE J.W., SPITZ E.W. & SLADE H.W. (1955) Early recognition of premature cranial synostosis. *Radiology* **65**, 183–93
INGRAHAM F. & MAISON D.D. (1954) *Neurosurgery of Infancy and Childhood*. Springfield, Illinois: Charles C.Thomas
JACKSON I.J. & THOMPSON R.K. (1959) *Paediatric Neurosurgery*. Oxford: Blackwell
LAURENCE K.M. (1958) The pathology of hydrocephalus. *Ann. Roy. Coll. Surg. Engl.* **24**, 388–401
LAURENCE K.M. (1964) The natural history of spina bifida cystica: detailed analysis of 407 cases. *Arch. Dis. Childh.* **39**, 41–57
LAURENCE K.M. (1969) Neurological and intellectual sequelae of hydrocephalus. *Arch. Neurol.* **20**, 73–81
LAURENCE K.M. & COATES S. (1962) The natural history of hydrocephalus: detailed analysis of 182 unoperated cases. *Arch. Dis. Childh.* **37**, 345–62
LAURENCE K.M. (1966) Survival of untreated spina bifida cystica. *Develop. Med. Child Neurol.* Suppl. **11**, 10–19
LAURENCE K.M., CARTER C.O. & DAVID P.A. (1968) The major central nervous system malformations in South Wales. I. Incidence, local variations and geographical factors. *Brit. J. Prev. Soc. Med.* **22**, 146–60
LAURENCE K.M., CARTER C.O. & DAVID P.A. (1968) The major central nervous system malformations in South Wales. II. Pregnancy factors, seasonal variations and social class effects. *Brit. J. Prev. Soc. Med.* **22**, 212–22
LAURENCE K.M. & TEW B. (1967) Follow-up of 65 survivors from 425 cases of spina bifida born in South Wales between 1956 and 1962. *Develop. Med. Child Neurol.* **9**, Suppl. **13**, 1–3
LORBER J. (1961) Systematic ventriculographic studies in infants born with myelocoele and encephalocoele. *Arch. Dis. Childh.* **36**, 381–9
MACCARTHY D., LINDSAY M., MACNAB G.H., NASH D.F.E., GUTTMAN I., LAURENCE K.M., GUTHKELCH N. & JOLLY H. (1957) Discussion on the problems of spina bifida cystica. *Proc. Roy. Soc. Med.* **50**, 737–46
MACNAB G.H. (1958) 'Spina bifida', In Gairdner D. (ed.) *Recent Advances in Paediatrics*, pp. 201–13. London: Churchill
MACNAB G.H. (1958) 'Hydrocephalus', In Gairdner D. (ed.) *Recent Advances in Paediatrics*, pp. 214–26. London: Churchill
PARK E.A. & POWERS G.F. (1920) Acrocephaly and scaphocephaly with symmetrically distributed malformations of the extremities: a study of the so-called 'acrocephalosyndactylism'. *Amer. J. Dis. Child.* **20**, 235
PENROSE L.S. (1957) Genetics of anencephaly. *J. ment. defic. Res.* **1**, 4–15
POTTER E.L. (1961) *Pathology of the Foetus and the Newborn*, 2nd edn. Chicago: Year Book Publishers
RECORD R.G. & MCKEOWN T. (1949) Congenital malformations of the central nervous system: I. A. survey of 930 cases. *Brit. J. soc. Med.* **3**, 183–219
RECORD R.G. & MCKEOWN T. (1960), In Wolstenholme G.E.W. & O'Connor C.M.

(eds.) Ciba Foundation Symposium on *Congenital Malformations*, pp. 2–21. London: Churchill
RUSSEL D.S. (1949) Observations on the pathology of hydrocephalus. *Medical Research Council Special Report, No. 265.* London: H.M.S.O.
SPITZ E.B. (1959) Neurosurgery in the prevention of exogenous mental retardation. *Pediatric Clinics of North America* **6,** 1215–35
STOWENS D. (1966) *Paediatric Pathology*, 2nd edn. Baltimore: Williams & Wilkins

3

Abnormalities of the Cardiothoracic System

R.J.K.BROWN

This chapter is divided into two sections, the first dealing with congenital abnormalities of the respiratory tract and the second with cardiovascular anomalies. Only those anomalies which present problems in the newborn period will be considered. Intrathoracic anomalies of the alimentary tract, such as oesophageal atresia and diaphragmatic hernia, and anomalies of the larynx and neighbouring structures, are not included since they are considered elsewhere.

ANOMALIES OF THE RESPIRATORY TRACT

Clinically significant anomalies of the respiratory tract are rare. Yet although they are rare they are important since they may be clinically indistinguishable from the respiratory distress syndrome of the newborn due to hyaline membrane disease or meconium aspiration pneumonia. The symptoms produced by less severe lesions are varied and, though slight or absent most of the time, they are likely to be aggravated by the exertion of feeding or crying.

Respiratory tract anomalies are also important because of their frequent association with anomalies elsewhere. Thus hypoplasia of the lung is sometimes found together with lesions in the renal tract. An important example of this association is Potter's syndrome of renal agenesis, hypoplasia of the lung, a characteristic facies and skeletal abnormalities. Indeed, the combination of hypoplastic lung with a renal abnormality is so common that the presence of one of these lesions should always prompt a search for the other. The same is true of the association between gastro-intestinal duplications and abnormalities of the vertebral column. As one might expect, cardiac lesions are also found together with respiratory tract anomalies quite frequently. For example, somewhere between 10 and 20 per cent of cases of tracheo-oesophageal fistula are complicated by cardiac lesions.

Anomalies of the Trachea

True atresia of the trachea is happily very rare for it is incompatible with life.

Anomalies in and around the trachea which result in narrowing of its lumen will cause respiratory difficulty and stridulous breathing. Careful examination of the back of the throat followed by direct laryngoscopy and radiography will reveal the cause of laryngeal stridor in most cases, but if no cause is found at the level of the larynx, or above, then it must be presumed that the lesion is below the larynx. Under these circumstances, and if symptoms are severe, it may be necessary to proceed to bronchoscopy to determine the cause.

Lesions which are high up in the trachea produce a clinical picture which may be indistinguishable from laryngeal obstruction, but when the narrowing is low down it causes a low-pitched wheeze rather than stridor.

Tracheal stenosis may exist as a local narrowing or it may be caused by a web, a fibrous stricture, a malformed cartilage or cartilage bar, and all these lesions can be diagnosed by bronchoscopy.

Tracheal compression may result from cysts or tumours in the mediastinum or vascular rings. These may be detected on screening or radiography.

Tracheomalacia is a cause of narrowing along the whole length of the trachea. It is not a common condition but should be suspected in an infant with severe inspiratory stridor and sternal insuction who habitually lies with his head fully retracted (in order to widen the lumen of the trachea). X-rays, if taken on inspiration, show an obvious narrowing of the trachea throughout its length, but the inspiratory narrowing may be demonstrated best of all by cineradiography. Infants with this anomaly improve as they grow and the trachea enlarges and becomes firmer, but their condition may give rise to considerable anxiety in early infancy, and the severe obstruction may result in a permanent funnel-chest deformity. Oxygen therapy may be required for several weeks, and it is important to posture the baby so that the best possible airway is obtained. Prolonged airways obstruction may result in cardiac enlargement and possible right heart failure from pulmonary hypertension.

Treatment of other types of tracheal narrowing will depend upon the cause. Experience has shown that ligation or division of an anomalous artery to relieve tracheal compression has not always proved successful. This is because of an associated cartilage deficiency at the point of compression which may require resection or dilatation in order to produce a complete cure. (See p. 122 for further reference to vascular rings and tracheal compression.)

Anomalies of the Bronchi

Narrowing of a bronchus by a web, stenosis or compression may produce an audible wheeze but the physical signs will be localized to one lung or lobe of a lung. Treatment will depend very much upon the site and degree of the obstruction.

Anomalous branching of the trachea or bronchi is rarely of any clinical importance but may create confusion on bronchoscopy or bronchography.

Anomalies of the Lungs and Intrapulmonary Bronchi

Anomalous lobation of the lungs is of no clinical importance in the absence of other abnormalities. Some examples, such as the azygos lobe, are so common that they may be regarded as normal variants albeit genetically determined. Anomalous lobation is associated with other lesions in certain syndromes. In one such syndrome there is tri-lobation, situs inversus with laevocardia, congenital heart disease and agenesis of the spleen. (The *asplenia syndrome*: see p. 123.) Whether it occurs singly or as part of a syndrome, anomalous lobation never produces any symptoms.

Agenesis of the lungs is, of course, incompatible with life if it is bilateral, a state of affairs which is fortunately only found in anencephaly. Unilateral agenesis of the lungs produces no symptoms as a rule, but is usually discovered because of the many and varied associated anomalies which are commonly present. Sometimes these are so severe that they prove fatal, but the finding of pulmonary agenesis may give a lead to the discovery of associated lesions which are treatable. Unilateral pulmonary agenesis is more often on the left side and is commoner in the male.

Hypoplasia of the lungs may be unilateral or bilateral and may affect an entire lung or only one lobe, may cause confusion on bronchoscopy or bronchography but is otherwise of no importance. Lesions associated with pulmonary hypoplasia may be as numerous as with pulmonary agenesis, but the one factor common to them all is that they reduce the available space in the thorax and thereby interfere with the development of the lung on that side. For this reason hypoplasia of the lungs is found with diaphragmatic hernia, intrathoracic cysts and tumours, and cardiomegaly. Likewise, abdominal masses such as polycystic kidneys may produce a similar effect by elevation of the diaphragm. Reduction of the intrathoracic space by deformity of the spine may be the cause of pulmonary hypoplasia in some cases of anencephaly and in many achondroplastic dwarfs. It has been suggested that pulmonary insufficiency from this cause may be responsible for the high neonatal mortality in achondroplasia.

The close association between pulmonary hypoplasia and renal abnormalities has already been emphasized.

Cystic Anomalies of the Mediastinum

Almost all cysts in the mediastinum are due to congenital malformations but a great many do not present with symptoms until adult life. This applies to most examples of bronchogenic, pericardial, oesophageal and thymic cysts. In infancy gastro-intestinal duplications, cystic hygromata and teratomata are those most commonly encountered.

Gastro-intestinal duplications are the most common cystic malformations in the mediastinum in infancy. They nearly always cause symptoms in early life. Most of them arise from the oesophagus and a few may penetrate the diaphragm to enter the small intestine. When duplications communicate with the gastro-intestinal tract they may contain gas and so be mistaken for diaphragmatic herniae. One form of gastro-intestinal duplication is referred to by some authors as the neurenteric canal cyst. Although comparatively rare it is of particular interest because it is invariably associated with vertebral abnormalities such as spina bifida, hemivertebrae or fusion of vertebral bodies. In fact, the presence of such vertebral anomalies in a patient with a mediastinal cyst is diagnostic. The affected infants are usually male and often have abdominal intestinal

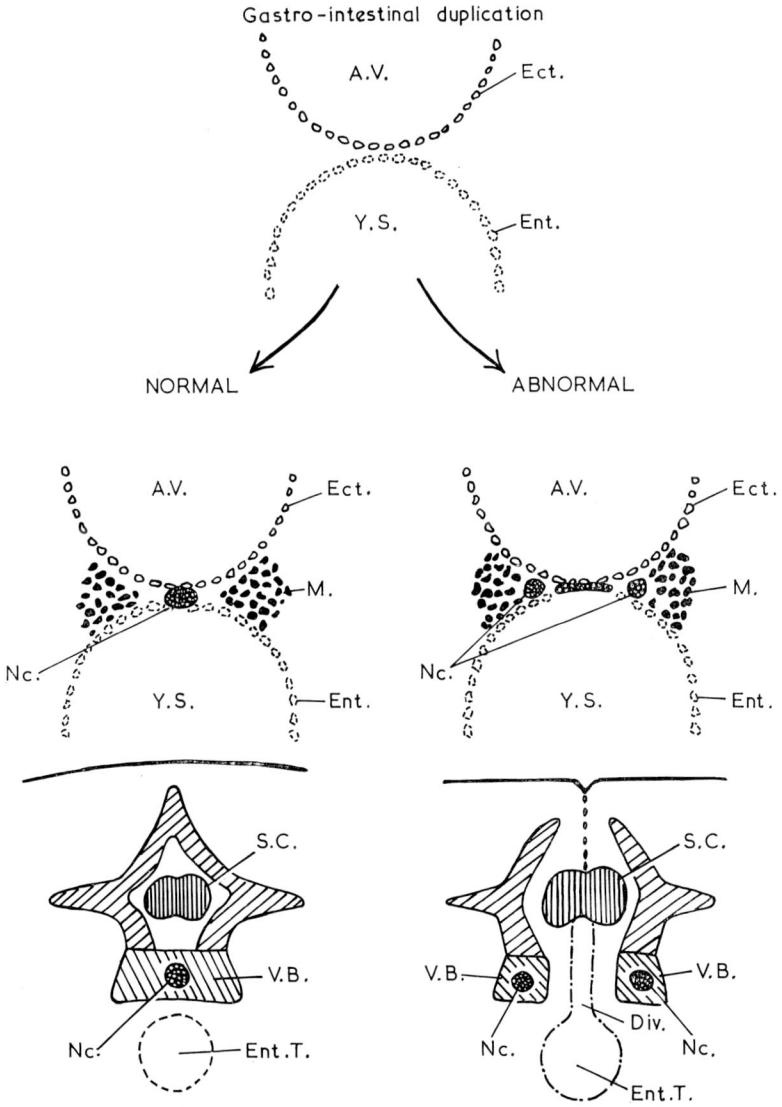

FIG. 3.1. Development of diverticulum from primitive entodermal tube, resulting from persistent adherence of ectoderm to entoderm. This also leads to division of notochord and vertebral body (after Forshall).

A.V.	amniotic vesicle	M.	mesoderm
Div.	diverticulum	Nc.	notochord
Ect.	ectoderm	S.C.	spinal chord
Ent.	entoderm	V.B.	vertebral body
Ent.T.	entodermal tube	Y.S.	yolk sac

duplication as well. The mediastinal cyst is lined by gastric or intestinal epithelium and is connected to a hemivertebra (almost always the second dorsal) by a cord or canal. Forshall has produced convincing evidence not only that the so-called neurenteric canal cyst is really a form of gastro-intestinal duplication but also that the associated abdominal intestinal duplication is really a direct continuation of the same process. Sometimes this is made obvious by the fact that the intrathoracic and

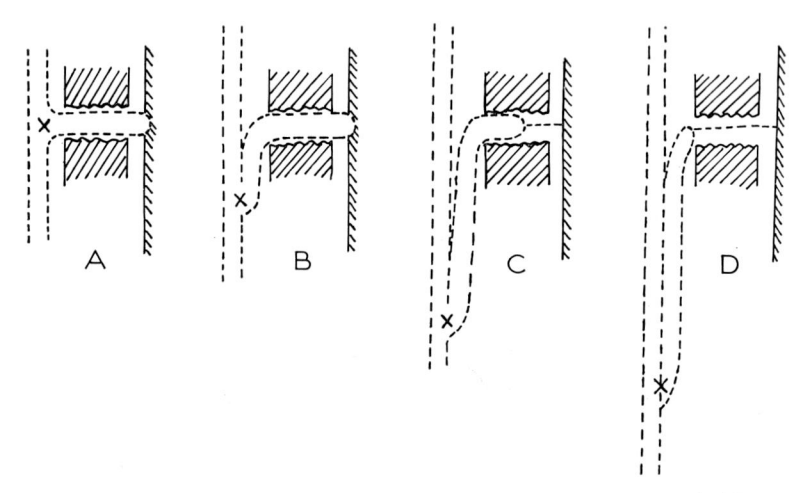

Fig. 3.2. Sagittal section of hypothetical diverticulum from primitive entodermal tube passing dorsally between hemivertebrae.

A, the diverticulum; B and C, progressive caudal growth of parent channel and diverticulum; D, release of diverticulum from vertebral body and closure of communication between parent channel and diverticulum, X (after Forshall).

intra-abdominal portions form a continuous tube. The diagrams (Figs. 3.1 to 3.4) should be studied in sequence to clarify this point.

Cystic hygroma is a relatively common mediastinal cystic malformation in children. It is multilocular and arises high up in the mediastinum. Diagnosis is made easy when it is associated with the cystic hygroma of the neck. These cysts exhibit a tendency to spontaneous regression, especially after surgery is attempted. This is fortunate since complete removal is rarely possible.

Teratomata and dermoid cysts are also relatively common forms of mediastinal cysts in infancy. They may be suspected because of their anterior position and the fact that they are the only cysts which commonly calcify.

Bronchogenic cysts are derived from ectopic bronchial buds but are nevertheless rarely found in children. However, they have been known to cause respiratory obstruction in infancy.

Anterior meningocele is a rare form of mediastinal cyst which is hardly ever found except as a manifestation of Von Recklinghausen's neurofibromatosis.

Treatment

The treatment for all mediastinal cysts is the same, namely, surgical removal whenever symptoms appear. In the case of gastro-intestinal duplication it is important to remember the possibility of association with intra-abdominal duplications and that these may be in direct communication.

Congenital Cystic Malformations of the Lungs

There may be solitary cysts or multicystic disease involving one or both lungs, multicystic disease being much more common. Most of the cysts are air-filled but a few are filled with fluid. The lining membrane of the cysts is usually bronchial epithelium which may simulate the lining membrane of the alveoli, making it difficult to distinguish the cysts from aquired lesions such as pneumatoceles in staphylococcal pneumonia.

A congenital cyst is most likely to produce symptoms if it possesses a valvular communication with the respiratory tract which causes it to increase in size and become a 'balloon cyst' which behaves much like a tension pneumothorax. This is exactly the way many acquired lesions behave also, and there is certain to be great difficulty in distinguishing congenital malformations from acquired lesions in most instances. Finding the disease very early in life favours a congenital aetiology—though staphylococcal pneumonia with cystic changes has been observed within a few days of birth—and the absence of regression following intensive medical therapy is also against acquired aetiology. Cysts of congenital origin are apt to enlarge rapidly to produce symptoms.

Solitary bronchogenic cysts occur in the lung and do not differ in any way from those found in the mediastinum. Fluid-filled at first they later become air-filled. It is necessary to follow the progress of affected infants into later life since subsequent development of polycystic disease of the lungs has been reported where only a single cyst was originally thought to be present.

It may be extremely difficult to differentiate a solitary congenital cyst from a lung abscess, a post-infectious cyst or pneumatocele, an emphy-

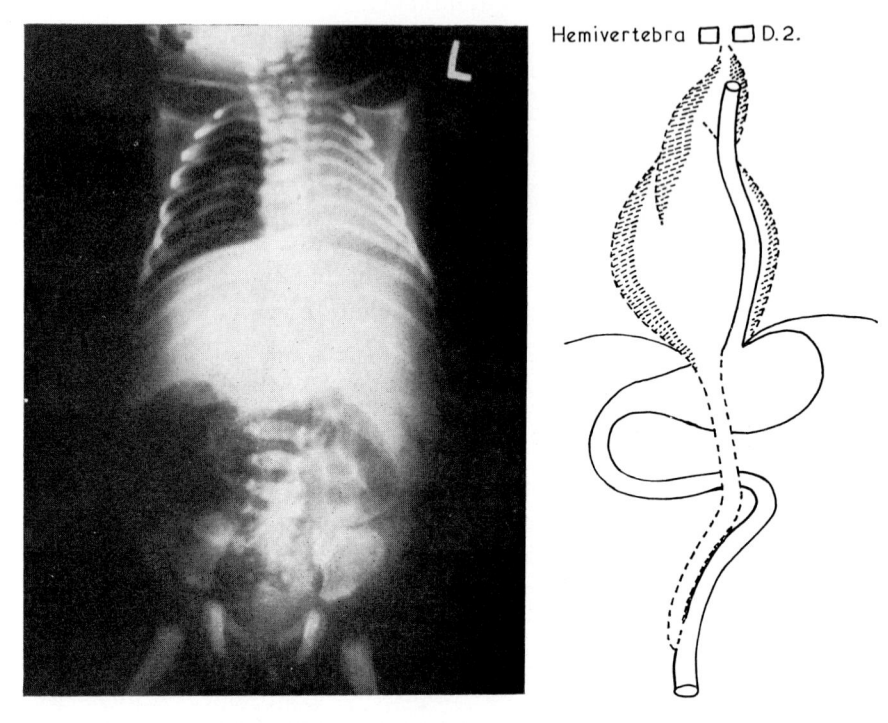

FIG. 3.3

FIG. 3.4

FIG. 3.3. X-ray showing translucent right hemithorax and displacement of the mediastinum to the left by a large intrathoracic cyst. Lower cervical and upper dorsal hemivertebrae are also shown (Miss Forshall's case).

FIG. 3.4. Diagrammatic representation of findings in Miss Forshall's prototype case (see accompanying x-ray). The thoracic element was still continuous with the abdominal element of the duplication. The diverticulum apparently originated from the 2nd dorsal vertebra which was a hemivertebra.

sematous bulla, a pneumothorax, an area of lobar emphysema, a diaphragmatic hernia, or intralobar sequestration.

Multiple cystic disease of the lungs is a term used to describe a diffuse cystic disease which sometimes occurs in infancy, in which the cysts are all quite small. This type has been described by Potter in association with anencephaly and tracheal atresia. It has also been found as a rare concomitant of arachnodactyly and of epiloia.

Congenital pulmonary lymphangiectasis, sometimes referred to as congenital pulmonary cystic lymphangiectasis, is a diffuse cystic condition of the lungs produced by a dilatation of the lymphatic channels. It has been well described by Laurence, who believes that it is due to a developmental defect of the intrapulmonary lymphatics, but the frequent

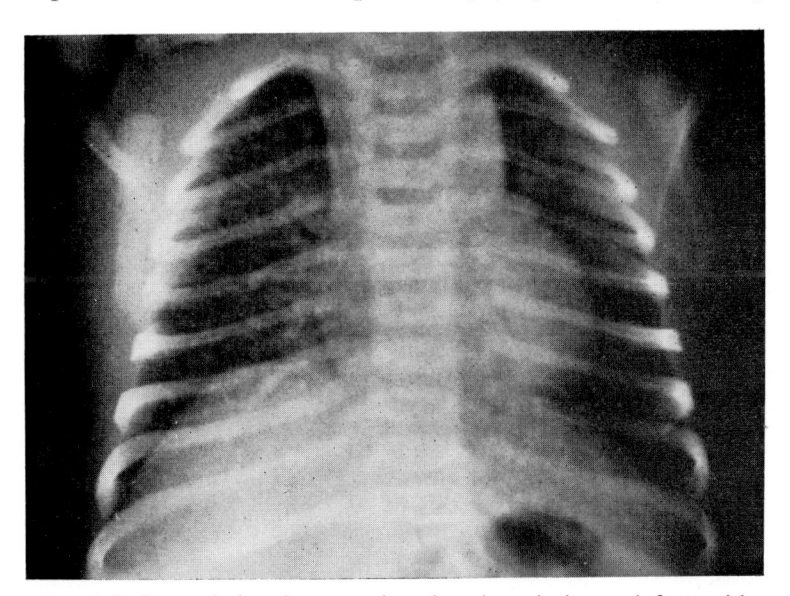

FIG. 3.5. Congenital pulmonary lymphangiectasis in an infant with total anomalous drainage of pulmonary veins which entered the superior vena cava via a small constricted common trunk. The x-ray shows an unusual coarse mottling throughout the lungs but does not clearly demarcate the cystic areas found at autopsy.

association of obstructive lesions of the left heart or total anomalous pulmonary venous drainage suggests that obstruction to venous return from the lungs may play an important part in the aetiology. Infants with this rare anomaly are very ill from birth and do not survive long. No treatment ever appears to influence the progress of the disease. The x-ray picture may sometimes closely simulate the picture of 'honeycomb lung'.

Congenital cystic adenomatoid malformation of the lung (or adenomatous dysplasia of the lung) is a rare and unusual malformation in which local obstructive emphysema is the principal cause of symptoms.

The disease usually involves one lobe, but it may involve several lobes or even the whole of both lungs. Diseased areas are large and contain many cysts which on microscopy are found to consist of thin-walled, irregular spaces lined by the same type of epithelium as that lining the bronchioles. Some severely affected infants have generalized oedema for no very obvious reason, though some people have attempted to explain it on the basis of obstruction to the great veins. A few of these infants are stillborn. Liveborn infants may become dangerously ill very soon after birth from rapid distension of the thin-walled cysts from obstructive 'emphysema'. The x-ray picture may be indistinguishable from congenital lobar obstructive emphysema (see below) when only one lobe is involved, but usually multicystic areas can also be made out which provide the clue to the correct diagnosis. Typically, however, the x-ray shows an enlarged lung on the affected side containing a soft tissue mass in which are numerous air-containing structures.

Intralobar sequestration of the lung is an unusual form of cystic anomaly. The name implies that there is no communication with the remainder of the respiratory tract, but there is often an indirect communication for many of the cysts contain air or air together with fluid. The lesion consists of an area of cystic malformation, typically in the lower lobe and more commonly on the right. The arterial supply is systemic, usually by a single large vessel from the aorta or one of its main branches.

Although this anomaly is present from birth its existence remains unsuspected until there is superadded infection which commonly occurs much later in childhood. If, however, the lesion is suspected, perhaps because of an unusual radiographic picture, then angiocardiography will provide the best diagnostic confirmation (preferably a retrograde aortogram via a catheter in a femoral artery). In the differential diagnosis probably the most important lesion is herniation of the stomach through the diaphragm on the right side which may produce a strikingly similar x-ray picture. Intralobar sequestration is likely to lead to repeated episodes of lung infection and it may be complicated by serious haemoptyses. Therefore, once the diagnosis is made the affected portion of lung is best removed surgically, bearing in mind the presence of the large systemic artery which could lead to serious haemorrhage if accidentally severed.

Extralobar sequestration of lung is really an anomaly of tracheobronchial branching but the sequestrated lobe is not connected to the respiratory tract. If there is a connection the lesion is really an accessory lung. Almost all examples of extralobar sequestration have been left-sided in contrast to intralobar sequestration which is typically right-sided. The sequestrated lung is usually cystic and supplied by systemic arteries, but infection is rare. As a rule the x-ray shows a dense mass in the region of the left lower lobe. There is a frequent association with diaphragmatic hernia.

Treatment of cystic malformation of the lung. It is usual to wait until important symptoms develop. Where the lesions are complicated by infection this must be treated with antibiotics whether or not surgery is contemplated. Surgical removal of cystic lesions will only be possible when the disease is sufficiently localized.

Lobar Obstructive Emphysema

This condition may simulate lobar cystic disease. The diagnosis may be suspected when severe respiratory distress occurs shortly after birth with wheezing, insuction and cyanosis, and physical examination reveals an area of hyperresonance with diminished breath sounds. Radiography shows striking expansion and translucency of the involved lobe pushing the mediastinum over to the opposite side and sometimes herniating through the anterior mediastinum. Other conditions to be considered in the differential diagnosis are pneumothorax, pneumomediastinum, and atelectasis with compensatory emphysema. The lesion results from a check valve obstruction and is not due to a localized hypertrophic emphysema. In about half the cases this obstruction is quite obvious and consists of such things as a mucosal fold, a web, a cartilaginous defect, or pressure from anomalous vessels. In the remainder no definite bronchial obstruction is revealed but it is thought that there must be a localized chondromalacia which permits the bronchial walls in the area to collapse together on expiration. It is the left upper lobe which is most often affected. Treatment is expectant until the severity of symptoms makes surgical removal of the affected lobe essential. If acute symptoms do not develop, the condition tends to improve spontaneously as the infant grows.

Hamartoma of the Lung

The term hamartoma of the lung has been used to describe masses of mesenchymal tissue in the lung which may or may not contain air passages. The tissue includes fat, muscle, connective tissue, cartilage and blood vessels. The lesion is present at birth and tends to grow in proportion to the growth of the body, in contrast to the uncontrolled growth of a true neoplasm. It is thus almost certainly a congenital malformation. Symptoms vary according to the size of the mass which is sometimes large enough to cause death in the newborn period.

ANOMALIES OF THE CARDIOVASCULAR SYSTEM

It is difficult to assess the frequency of congenital malformations of the heart and great vessels, but it is generally agreed that between 0·5 and 1 per cent of all newborn infants have a significant anomaly of these structures. Not all these malformations will declare their presence in the newborn period, many of them remaining asymptomatic until the child is much older. However, a better understanding of the suspicious signs and symptoms should enable more lesions to be diagnosed during the newborn period. Until quite recently it was estimated that 75 per cent of all infants with significant congenital heart disease died before their first birthday. Obviously it is in this age group that we need to concentrate our efforts in the future to perfect methods of early diagnosis and the means for carrying out surgical treatment on the small infant with a severe malformation.

It is the purpose of this section to detail the more important malformations causing symptoms in the newborn period and to indicate their main diagnostic features. For more detailed information the reader is referred to the many excellent books devoted to congenital heart disease.

Signs and Symptoms of Congenital Heart Disease

The presence of a congenital cardiac anomaly may be suspected in the newborn infant because of cyanosis, respiratory distress, some abnormality of the pulses, cardiac enlargement, a cardiac murmur, or the occurrence of heart failure. Its presence may also be suspected when there are other anomalies or syndromes whose association with cardiac disease is well recognized. Typical examples are mongolism, arachnodactyly, the syndromes of webbing (e.g. Turner's syndrome), congenital cataracts, cleft palate, hypertelorism, polydactyly or syndactyly. Recognition of these associated conditions is not only helpful in arousing suspicion of heart disease, but in suggesting a probable diagnosis in some cases. Possibly 30 per cent of all mongols have congenital heart disease and, although almost all types of lesion have been described, the commonest lesions are ventricular septal defect and the atrioventricular canal defects. There is a high incidence of atrial septal defects with arachnodactyly. In Turner's syndrome, with a sex chromosome anomaly, coarctation of the aorta or hypoplastic aortic malformations are relatively common, but in those cases in which the phenotype matches the appropriate sex karyotype pulmonary stenosis is most commonly found. Polydactyly or syndactyly are most likely to be associated with a ventricular septal defect.

Aetiology

The relative frequency of genetic and environmental influences in the aetiology of cardiac anomalies is difficult to determine but genetic factors are not, in general, of great importance in the aetiology of congenital heart disease. The monozygous co-twins of index cases are usually not affected. Nevertheless, relatives of index patients are more often affected than would be expected to occur by chance, and the malformation is usually of the same type in the relative as in the index patient. The empirical risk for a later sib of an index patient with congenital malformation of the heart is of the order of 1 in 50. Risks cannot yet be quoted for individual types, but they appear to be somewhat higher than 1 in 50 for pulmonary valve stenosis and somewhat lower for intraventricular septal defect.

There are, however, individual families in which the risk is considerably higher. In addition, where the congenital heart disease is part of a syndrome (as in Marfan's syndrome or Ellis–van Creveld syndrome), the family risks are those of the main syndrome. Table 3.1 shows that teratogenic agents are likely to produce serious malformations only if they operate during the first 10 weeks.

Cyanosis

Cardiac malformations comprise only a few of the many different causes of cyanosis in the newborn infant and before considering them in detail

TABLE 3.1
Table of cardiac development in terms of somites, length in millimetres and calendar age of foetus (after Schnitker)

No. of pairs of somites	Crown rump length in millimetres	Age in weeks	Stage of development of cardiovascular system
3	1·38–1·50	3·0	Cardiogenic plate reversing vitelline veins, and two primitive aortae formed
7	2·0		Six pairs of aortic arches begin development
8	2·30–2·50	3·5	Embryonic blood vessels a paired symmetrical system; heart tubes fuse and bend S-shaped; beat begins
10	2·67		
17	2·65–2·75		
20	3·00–3·20		
24	3·50		
30	4·00–4·25		
38–40 (completed)	5·00	4·0	Pericardial cavity open to pleuro-peritoneal cavity; parts of heart bulbus, ventricle, atrium, and sinus venosus distinct; paired aortae fuse; aortic arches and cardinal veins completed
	8·0	5·0	Myocardium condensing; cardiac septa appearing: bulbus cordis merging into right ventricle. Fusion of endocardial cushions to form A-V ostia
	12·0	6·0	Septum primum fused with endocardial cushions; foramen ovale present; endocardial cushions fuse to separate R. & L. A-V canals; atrial septum secundum begins; atria balloon over bulbus; bulbus absorbed into R. ventricle; aortic septum divides bulbus arteriosus into aorta and pulmonary artery; 2nd aortic arch degenerates, 5th and 6th appear, and then 6th degenerates; pulmonary arteries and veins are present
	11·0–16·0	7·0	Aortic septum reaches heart; atrium and ventricle partitioned; cardiac valves present; sinus venosus taken up into R. atrium; orifices of superior and inferior venae cavae distinct; atrial septum secundum larger
	16·0–22·0	8·0	Formation of pars membranaceum; A-V valves nearly complete; coronary artery branches may be identified; A-V bundle is represented
	23·0–26·0	9·0	A-V valves complete, and semilunar valves nearly complete; A-V bundle of His now distinct
	27·0–birth	10·0–birth	Heart in its miniature size complete with interatrial communication and ductus arteriosus present and normal. Heart continues to grow and descend as neck elongates

ABNORMALITIES OF THE CARDIOTHORACIC SYSTEM 101

it may be helpful to discuss the differential diagnosis of cyanosis:

I. *Cyanosis due to Abnormal Forms of Haemoglobin*
   (a) *Methaemoglobinaemia.* This produces a rather characteristic slate-blue cyanosis which can be recognized with experience. Although a high content of methaemoglobin in the red cells may produce some respiratory embarrassment by interfering with oxygen exchange, the degree of cyanosis is out of all proportion to these symptoms, and, unlike the cyanosis of congenital heart disease, it never results in clubbing of the fingers. The diagnosis is made by spectrophotometry or by diagnostic tests with methylene blue or ascorbic acid (see below).

Congenital methaemoglobinaemia is inherited. Two types have been fully investigated. In one type, due to a recessive mutant gene, there is a deficiency of a coenzyme factor. There is normally a tendency for haemoglobin to be oxidized to methaemoglobin in the body, but the coenzyme factor accelerates the reduction of the methaemoglobin back to haemoglobin by Coenzyme 1. When the coenzyme factor is absent nearly 40 per cent of the red cells may contain methaemoglobin and be incapable of carrying oxygen, in spite of the action of other reducing substances in the blood such as ascorbic acid or glutathione. In the second type there is a genetically determined variant of haemoglobin present (haemoglobin M), the inheritance being dominant (this type does not respond to injections of methylene blue).

Acquired methaemoglobinaemia may be caused by a variety of chemicals. In newborn infants it has occurred when well-water containing nitrites has been used for making up feeds. It has also resulted from the absorption through the skin in the napkin area of aniline dyes contained in the marking ink used for laundry marks. Some outbreaks of cyanosis among newborn infants in maternity hospitals have been traced to this cause. In one outbreak known to the author the full name of the hospital contained no less than forty-four letters, and when these were written in large capitals on the napkins the amount of ink used was considerable!

Treatment. Ascorbic acid and methylene blue reduce methaemoglobin to haemoglobin and they may be used for diagnosis and for treatment. An intravenous injection of methylene blue in a dose of 1–2 mg per kg body weight will cause rapid disappearance of cyanosis and is a very useful quick diagnostic test; 3–5 mg per kg daily in divided doses given by mouth will keep a patient free from cyanosis. Similarly, large doses of ascorbic acid, 200–500 mg daily in divided doses, will reduce the

H

methaemoglobin content from 40 per cent to 10 per cent and so abolish the cyanosis.

(b) *Sulphaemoglobinaemia.* As a hereditary disease this is extremely rare. In an acquired form it is slightly more common and results from the ingestion of large amounts of sulphur and the production of hydrogen sulphide in the bowel by bacterial action. The colouring is similar to that produced by methaemoglobin but the pigment can be distinguished by spectrophotometry.

II. *Cyanosis due to an Abnormal amount of Reduced Haemoglobin*
A minimum of 6·5 c.c per cent oxygen unsaturation in the capillaries is necessary before cyanosis becomes evident and this represents approximately 5 per cent reduced haemoglobin (1 g per cent reduced haemoglobin $\equiv$ 1·34 c.c per cent oxygen unsaturation). When the haemoglobin level is 15 g per cent the oxygen capacity of the blood is 20 c.c per cent ($15 \times 1\cdot34$). Arterial blood is normally about 95 per cent saturated and, therefore, has an oxygen content of 19 c.c per cent or an unsaturation of 1 c.c per cent. Mixed venous blood is normally 70 per cent saturated representing an oxygen content of 14 c.c per cent or an unsaturation of 6 c.c per cent. The average unsaturation of capillary blood is taken as the mean unsaturation of the arterial and mixed venous bloods, i.e.

$$\frac{A+V}{2} = \frac{1+6}{2} = 3\cdot5 \text{ c.c per cent unsaturation.}$$

If the arterial blood is only 75 per cent saturated cyanosis will appear, for the arterial oxygen content then becomes 15 c.c per cent representing an unsaturation of 5 c.c per cent and the oxygen content of mixed venous blood 10 c.c per cent or 10 c.c per cent unsaturation (the average oxygen utilization by the tissues being 5 c.c per cent), so that the calculation becomes:

$$\frac{A+V}{2} = \frac{5+10}{2} = 7\cdot5 \text{ c.c per cent unsaturation.}$$

This level of oxygen unsaturation in the capillaries is well above the critical level for cyanosis.

If the subject is anaemic it requires a greater degree of oxygen unsaturation of the arterial blood to produce cyanosis. Suppose the haemoglobin level is only 10 g per cent. The oxygen capacity will then be only 13·4 c.c per cent ($10 \times 1\cdot34$) and similar calculations to those above will show that the arterial oxygen saturation would need to be as low as 70 per cent to produce cyanosis, and if the anaemia is very severe it may never be possible to have the minimum of 5 g per cent reduced haemoglobin in the capillaries. On the contrary if the subject is polycythaemic cyanosis appears even when the arterial oxygen saturation is relatively high. For instance a haemoglobin level of 20 g per cent provides an oxygen capacity of 26·8 c.c per cent ($20 \times 1·34$), at which level cyanosis will appear when the arterial oxygen saturation is only a little below 90 per cent.

There are three main reasons why an abnormal amount of reduced haemoglobin may be present in the capillaries:

(i) All the blood passes through aerated lung tissue but oxygenation in the lungs is incomplete, i.e. there is decreased alveolar ventilation.

This may be due to (a) obstruction of the respiratory tract, e.g. from mucus or as a result of laryngeal or tracheal stenosis, or (b) structural changes in the lungs such as emphysema or fibrosis or (c) a reduction in the number of normally functioning alveoli, e.g. pulmonary hyaline membrane, atelectasis, cystic disease of the lungs. Cerebral causes in the newborn will also usually operate by interfering with normal pulmonary expansion.

(ii) There exist unaerated veno-arterial shunts allowing appreciable amounts of reduced haemoglobin to pass from the right heart to the arterial blood.

This will occur (a) when blood flows through an extensive area of collapsed or consolidated lung (at least one-third of the cardiac output must be so shunted to cause cyanosis), (b) when there is a pulmonary arteriovenous fistula or (c) in congenital heart disease.

(iii) There is increased reduction of oxyhaemoglobin in the tissues.

This is usually due to capillary stasis. Localized cyanosis of this type is exemplified by the cyanosis seen in the face and distal portions of the extremities in the first few hours after birth. Generalized cyanosis of this type occurs in heart failure where increased venous pressure slows down the local rate of blood flow, and in the capillary stasis of polycythaemia or peripheral circulatory failure. A generalized mottled, cyanotic appearance of the skin is seen in many cases of severe infection such as septicaemia. Vasomotor instability is another cause of cyanosis of this type.

The so-called harlequin colour change in newborn infants is presumably a form of vasomotor instability, but instead of cyanosis one usually sees a unilateral flushing of the skin which ceases abruptly in the midline, and affects the dependent half of the body when the baby is lying on its side (suggesting that gravitational effects are involved). It does not appear to have any clinical significance although in some cases it has been thought to have been associated with a mild transient cerebral disturbance.

Undoubtedly cyanosis in the newborn is most commonly associated with some form of respiratory difficulty. Whereas the cyanosis in such cases may be due in some measure to reversal of shunts through foetal channels (ductus arteriosus and foramen ovale) such cases are not to be considered as examples of congenital heart disease and must be differentiated from them. Lessening of cyanosis with adequate oxygen inhalation, and radiological evidence of unaerated lung will help to settle the issue in most cases. However, sometimes within a few hours of birth the baby develops signs and symptoms of respiratory distress associated with cyanosis, cardiac enlargement and evidence of congestive cardiac failure. This appears to be due to a failure of adaptation to the circulatory adjustments consequent upon birth, and may be precipitated by delayed onset of respiration, asphyxia, atelectasis or, perhaps, aspiration of liquor amnii at birth. Usually oxygen and digitalis therapy will alleviate the symptoms promptly, but the clinical picture can be indistinguishable from transposition of the great arteries for which urgent treatment would be required (see below). If there is any doubt it is safer to investigate. The author has observed a few examples of an unusual form of differential cyanosis in some severely asphyxiated newborn babies (see p. 115, Differential cyanosis).

CARDIAC MALFORMATIONS CAUSING CYANOSIS

TRANSPOSITION OF THE GREAT ARTERIES

This gross cardiac malformation, surprisingly enough, is the commonest example of congenital heart disease presenting with cyanosis in the newborn. Cyanosis is usually severe and cardiac enlargement may be detected within 48 hours of birth by the striking pulsation palpable beneath the xiphisternum. The heart action is dynamic. On auscultation the heart sounds are loud, there is accentuation of the second sound in the pulmonary area which should be split, thus distinguishing this condition from a persistent truncus arteriosus or a severe pulmonary stenosis, in both of which P_2 is single. Murmurs, which are not diagnostic, are due to associated lesions such as ventricular septal defect or pulmonary stenosis. After the first 48 hours the x-ray picture often assumes a characteristic 'egg on its side' appearance. Typically, there is a narrow vascular pedicle in the postero-anterior view but this may be concealed by the thymic shadow in the early days. Unless there is associated pulmonary stenosis the lung vascularity is increased. The electrocardiogram will usually reveal right axis deviation and right ventricular hypertrophy significantly greater than is to be expected in the newborn period,

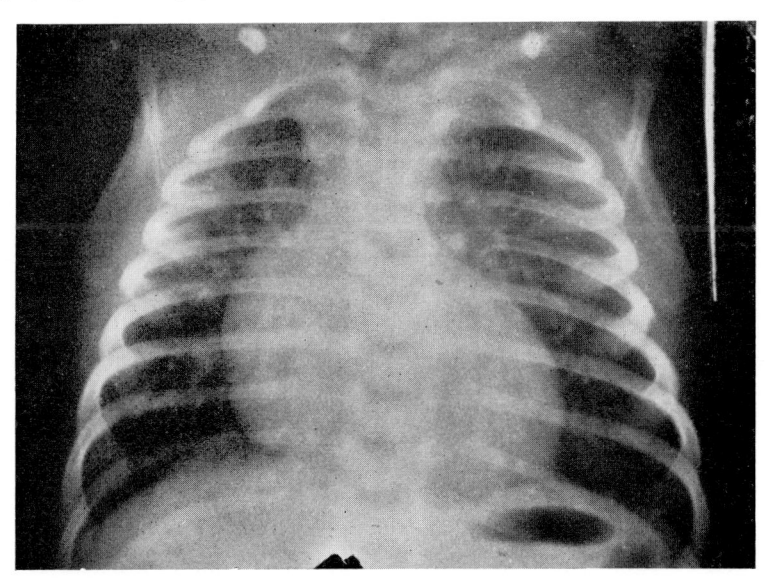

Fig. 3.6. Transposition of the great vessels: Large heart with 'egg-on-side' outline, narrow vascular pedicle and increased pulmonary vascularity.

often best shown by a persistence of a positive T wave in lead V_1 after the first 48 hours when it should become negative. There may also be ST and T changes in the left precordial leads as a result of myocardial ischaemia.

Until recently infants with transposition seldom survived more than a few months and many died within the first 6 weeks. Affected infants with the best chance of survival were those with a moderately large ventricular septal defect, but even in such cases survival to adult life was rare. Death was from heart failure. Anginal attacks from myocardial ischaemia were a frequent occurrence especially after feeds.

Early attempts at surgical treatment were disappointing. One of the more successful operations was Hanlon's atrial septostomy: the posterior aspects of the atria were approached through a right thoractomy and, after applying a curved clamp, the right atrium was opened and a portion of the atrial septum excised. Through this defect a proportion of the blood entering the left atrium could stream through to mix with the venous blood in the right atrium, thus increasing the oxygen saturation of the systemic blood leaving the right ventricle and, incidentally, improving the oxygenation of the coronary artery blood. If successful, this operation produced considerable improvement and increased the chances of long-term survival. Unfortunately, many of the babies were in severe cardiac failure at the time of the operation and the mortality could be as high as 40 per cent. More recently Rashkind has devised an ingenious technique for performing atrial septostomy with a special balloon catheter which may be introduced via the femoral vein. By this manoeuvre even the very ill infant may be dramatically improved and the overall mortality at this stage is below 20 per cent. With this procedure babies with transposition of the great arteries are enabled to survive in good health until they have grown to sufficient size to have a second operation carried out under cardio-pulmonary by-pass, which is designed to re-route the systemic and pulmonary venous return. This operation, designed by Mustard and modified by Aberdeen, has proved a great success. Its most troublesome complication is arrhythmia which accounts for some of the post-operative deaths. Improved techniques are likely to eliminate such complications in the future so that the operative mortality will soon be very low in the major cardiac centres. Thus, a congenital cardiac abnormality which was once regarded as having an almost hopeless prognosis, has quite suddenly become amenable to corrective surgery. Paradoxically those who are most severely ill before the initial Rashkind septostomy will be the best cases for a subsequent Mustard operation because they are less likely to have any other intracardiac abnormality, such as a ventricular septal defect. It is, therefore, mandatory that the malformation should be suspected and diagnosed as soon as possible after birth, and it is a safe rule to consider any baby with cyanotic heart disease to be suffering from transposition of the great arteries until proved otherwise.

The Hypoplastic Left Heart Syndrome

This useful term was coined by Lev in 1952 to include a group of anomalies in all of which there is an obstructive lesion of the left side of the heart. These anomalies are as follows:

Aortic valve atresia
Aortic valve atresia with mitral atresia
Aortic valve atresia with mitral hypoplasia
Mitral atresia
Mitral stenosis
Atresia of the transverse aortic arch
Hypoplasia of the aortic arch

Of these, some form of hypoplasia of the aortic arch is the most common, and this includes the so-called 'infantile type' of coarctation of the aorta.

The clinical features of this group as a whole are slight to moderate cyanosis, cardiac enlargement (often maximal at birth), congestive cardiac failure, possible engorgement of pulmonary vessels, relative hypertension in the right arm, a non-specific heart murmur, and an electrocardiogram showing obvious right ventricular hypertrophy.

Aortic atresia can usually be picked out from this group by the rapid onset of heart failure, usually after about 48 hours, with a large heart, apical gallop rhythm, and almost impalpable peripheral pulses.

In hypoplasia of the aortic arch the femoral pulses are often almost impalpable and in any event there is nearly always relative hypertension in the arms.

Table 3.2 may prove helpful in differentiating the various types of this left heart syndrome.

Treatment. At present the only lesion that has been amenable to successful surgical treatment (and that only rarely) has been hypoplasia of the aortic arch. Cases of mitral stenosis have been treated with valvotomy with temporary benefit. Otherwise supportive therapy with digitalis and diuretics is all that one can offer, and this has no effect on the outcome of severe examples such as aortic atresia.

Cor Biloculare or Triloculare

These anomalies are usually associated with multiple defects, and characterized by a large heart with pulmonary vascular engorgement, a systolic murmur, congestive cardiac failure and an electrocardiogram revealing right ventricular hypertrophy. Sometimes there is severe

TABLE 3.2
Chart for helping to differentiate the various types of the left heart syndrome (adapted from Noonan & Nadas, 1958)

Clinical entity	Usual length of survival	Cyanosis	X-ray findings	Remarks
Aortic valve atresia	Under 1 week	Moderate, generalized, appearing immediately after birth	Large globular heart, in a few hours from birth	Sudden onset of cardiac failure and rapid downhill course in first week of life
Mitral atresia	2–4 months	Mild, generalized, usually detected in second week	Moderate cardiac enlargement, narrow waist (occasional). Pulmonary vasculature may be diminished	Clinical picture rather like aortic atresia, but symptoms appear later. X-rays somewhat atypical for the group
Mitral stenosis	6–24 months	Variable, usually dating from birth. Constant in cases with V.S.D., but intermittent in others	Moderate cardiac enlargement, contour variable. Pulmonary vasculature sometimes diminished	Very poor gain in weight is constant. Dyspnoea always present, but paroxysms may occur. Typical presystolic mitral murmur occasionally
Aortic arch atresia	Under 1 month	There may be differential cyanosis, but moderate generalized, more common. Noted soon after birth	Moderate cardiac enlargement, sometimes pulmonary plethora	Clinical picture is surprisingly similar to aortic valve atresia, but symptoms appear somewhat later. Murmurs are present in only half
Hypoplasia of aortic arch	Half die by 6 weeks— some survive through childhood	Mild, generalized in most cases, appearing between 4 and 15 days usually. Differential cyanosis in only 10 per cent	Cardiac enlargement moderate to extreme. Frequently pulmonary plethora	Most common form of the syndrome. Relative hypertension in arms in most cases

pulmonary stenosis, in which case the lungs will be oligaemic. However, left axis deviation and left ventricular hypertrophy are sometimes found on the electrocardiogram in single ventricle, so that this lesion can be confused with tricuspid atresia. Angiocardiography will normally permit an accurate diagnosis to be made.

Severe Tetrad of Fallot and Pulmonary Atresia

It is only in those cases of the tetrad of Fallot where the degree of pulmonary stenosis is extreme that cyanosis is likely to appear in the newborn period. The classical tetrad of Fallot produces cyanosis beween 3 and 6 months but may have been discovered in the early weeks because of a precordial systolic murmur. The diagnostic signs are a small heart, a harsh systolic murmur at the left sternal border with a diminished pulmonary second sound, a radiograph showing a small boot-shaped heart with decreased pulmonary vasculature, and an electrocardiogram indicating right ventricular hypertrophy. The T wave in lead V_1 is normally upright for the first 24 hours and then becomes negative, but if it remains upright after 72 hours this constitutes abnormal right ventricular hypertrophy, and this sign may assist earlier recognition of the tetrad in the young infant. Radiographic evidence of a right-sided aorta is also a most useful diagnostic sign when present, and it occurs in 20 per cent of cases. The rare atypical case where there is overcirculation of the lungs (the 'acyanotic Fallot') presents a very difficult diagnostic problem.

If there is complete atresia of the pulmonary artery, cyanosis is very severe, cardiac enlargement appears early and there is usually no murmur. Murmurs indicating increased circulation through collateral channels such as a persistent ductus arteriosus or enlarged bronchial arteries may make their appearance later. In such cases, too, the x-ray appearance of the heart tends to become very characteristic and has been likened to a 'sitting duck' outline (see Fig. 3.9). Congestive failure does not occur in these cases. Angiocardiography is the most useful diagnostic procedure. Early surgical treatment to create a pulmonary-systemic anastomosis may be contemplated in severe examples of the tetrad of Fallot, but in pulmonary atresia it may be thought unlikely that surgery can improve upon the anastomotic channels that already exist. However, these naturally occurring anastomoses are quite haphazard and would be difficult to modify or eradicate should it prove possible at a later date to insert a prosthesis connecting the right ventricle with the pulmonary circulation. Such an operation combined with closure of the septal defect can give a result comparable to the so-called 'total correction' of Fallot's tetrad.

Tricuspid Atresia

The common type of tricuspid atresia is characterized by cyanosis associated with an electrocardiogram showing left axis deviation and left ventricular hypertrophy. However, this combination may be found in other anomalies such as single ventricle and persistent truncus arteriosus. In tricuspid atresia, however, the heart is normally quite small and may appear boot-shaped on the x-ray, and the pulmonary vasculature is normally decreased. Murmurs are not specific and depend very much on the type of associated lesion. Congestive failure does not occur unless tricuspid atresia is associated with transposition of the great arteries, but the clinical picture in such cases is more akin to that of transposition as previously described. Angiocardiography is necessary for accurate diagnosis.

It may be possible to improve some examples of this anomaly with a Potts procedure (anastomosis of the pulmonary artery to the aorta), or Waterston–Cooley procedure (anastomosis of right main branch of pulmonary artery to ascending aorta), provided the atrial septal defect is enlarged at the same time, or alternatively, the Glenn procedure of anastomosing the superior vena cava to the right main pulmonary artery. Without treatment, survival beyond a few months is unusual, the infant usually succumbing to anoxia during one of the 'blue spells' which are a characteristic feature of the malady.

Pulmonary Stenosis with Intact Ventricular Septum (Normal Aortic Root) and Reversed Interatrial Shunt

In this anomaly, sometimes referred to as the triad of Fallot, cardiac enlargement and cyanosis appear within a short time after birth and there is a harsh systolic murmur at the upper left sternal border and in the suprasternal notch. The x-ray confirms the cardiac enlargement and also reveals decreased pulmonary vasculature, while the electrocardiogram exhibits very obvious right ventricular hypertrophy and the P waves in leads I and II are often tall and peaked. The electrocardiogram differs from that found in the tetrad of Fallot by the presence of negative T waves, frequently of the ischaemic type, in the right precordial leads; there may also be RS–T elevation with a positive T wave in leads I and aVL. The gross cardiac enlargement also helps to distinguish this lesion from the tetrad. On the contrary, the presence of a right-sided aorta would be very much in favour of the latter. Wood draws attention to the association of other anomalies, especially arachnodactyly and hypertelorism, with this lesion. Selective angiocardiography is the best means of establishing the diagnosis, contrast medium being injected while the tip of the catheter is directed towards the outflow tract of the right ventricle. A jet of contrast medium will usually be seen passing through the stenosed pulmonary valve and entering the dilated pulmonary artery beyond. Simultaneous opacification of aorta and pulmonary artery immediately rules out the diagnosis. Complete pulmonary valve atresia with normal aortic root is a much more severe lesion, and can normally be distinguished by the absence of the harsh systolic murmur and its replacement by a soft continuous murmur (from the patent ductus which provides the pulmonary blood flow), but the angiocardiogram will demonstrate the atresia (see fig. 3.7). This is one of the conditions which may present as an acute emergency in the newborn period when a quick diagnosis by means of angiocardiography might enable a life-saving pulmonary valvotomy to be performed. In pulmonary stenosis valvotomy may produce dramatic improvement, but in severe cases the mortality for the operation is high. However, if no treatment is offered, the outlook is very poor.

PERSISTENT TRUNCUS ARTERIOSUS

By this is meant the rare anomaly in which there is a single trunk arising from both ventricles with the pulmonary arteries originating from it. If the lungs appear to be supplied by a patent ductus or by bronchial arteries the diagnosis is more likely to be pulmonary atresia (sometimes referred to as a 'pseudotruncus'). In the absence of heart failure cyanosis may be slight. The arterial pulse is often of water-hammer quality which may lead one to suspect a patent ductus arteriosus, particularly when, as is often the case, there is a basal diastolic murmur, but the very pure single second sound in the pulmonary area is a useful diagnostic point. Radiography shows an enlarged heart with prominence of the right ventricle which projects right forward in the lateral view from a somewhat posteriorly placed arterial trunk and forms a horizontal shelf. This, along with the single P_2, helps to distinguish the anomaly from transposition of the great vessels in which the aorta is typically placed in a very anterior position. As in transposition, the pulmonary vascularity is greatly increased. The electrocardiogram shows evidence of biventricular hypertrophy but there are often abnormalities of the P

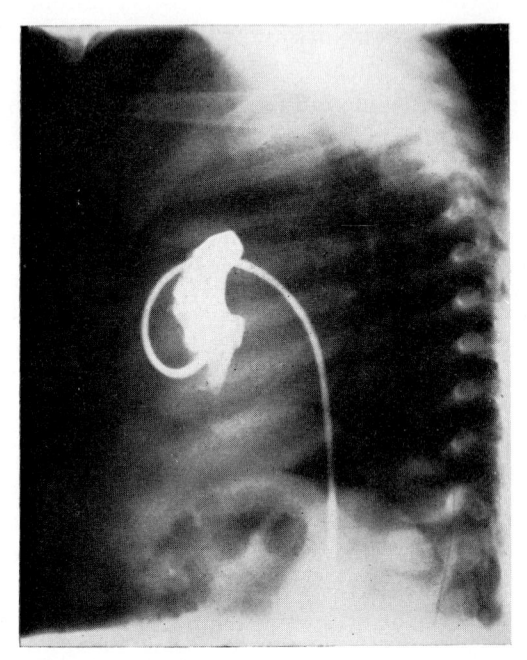

FIG. 3.7. Atresia of the pulmonary valve. Selective angiocardiography after the catheter has been introduced into the outflow tract of the right ventricle. Contrast medium cannot pass the completely atretic valve.

wave, and there may be left axis deviation. Angiocardiography may be used to clarify the diagnosis.

Total Anomalous Pulmonary Venous Drainage

The variety of this anomaly which is most likely to present with symptoms in the newborn period is that in which all the pulmonary veins drain via a common trunk into some branch of the portal system below the diaphragm (infracardiac type). The reason why this type produces early symptoms is that the long common trunk is almost certain to be narrowed at some place, causing obstruction with consequent pulmonary venous congestion or pulmonary oedema. In fact, the cardiac or supracardiac types can result in the same clinical picture if there is a constriction in the 'common pulmonary vein'. There is severe cyanosis and early congestive failure. Those babies in whom the anomalous drainage is into the portal system may have gastrointestinal disturbances,

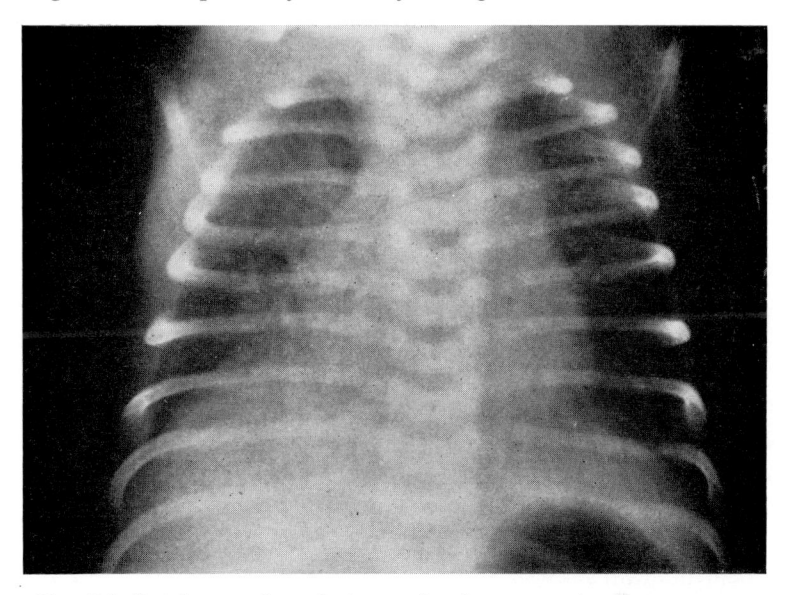

FIG. 3.8. Total anomalous drainage of pulmonary veins by a common trunk into the ductus venosus in a 6-day-old infant presenting with vomiting and diarrhoea, cyanosis and congestive cardiac failure. Note almost normal heart size.

especially diarrhoea. In one case in my experience there was vomiting of bright red blood from ruptured oesophageal varices, for in this case the anomalous pulmonary veins were draining into the left gastric vein. The x-ray picture may be very characteristic, there being a relatively small heart and a stippled ground-glass appearance of the lungs due to the venous engorgement. Sometimes a lateral view will show the horizontal 'Kerley's lines' of distended lymphatics. The electrocardiogram shows moderate right ventricular hypertrophy. Bearing in mind these peculiar features, a correct diagnosis can be made. Although the anomaly can be corrected surgically, successful treatment has been achieved rarely, and then only in cases where survival has gone beyond the first week or two (where the venous obstruction is less severe). Indeed, where venous obstruction is extreme and death has occurred within a few days of birth, postmortem has often revealed pulmonary lymphangiectasis (see p. 95).

Ebstein's Malformation

Ebstein's malformation of the tricuspid valve is another rare congenital malformation which is associated with cyanosis in infancy. The abnormality is a downward displacement of a deformed tricuspid valve, which results in a small inefficient right ventricle and a large dilated right atrial chamber (part of which is composed by the upper part of the right ventricle). In infancy the right ventricle can maintain only a relatively poor pulmonary blood flow because of the increased peripheral resistance in the pulmonary vessels at this age, and the blood in the dilated right atrium is at a higher pressure than that in the left atrium so that there is a reversed shunt through the foramen ovale (or an atrial septal defect if present). Clinically, there is a very gentle cardiac impulse, a widely split second sound, a tricuspid systolic murmur and a superficial tricuspid diastolic murmur. The x-ray is often very characteristic, showing an enlarged heart with a clear 'stencilled' outline, because of the lack of vigorous pulsation of the enlarged right heart, and hypoplasia of both great vessels. The lung fields appear oligaemic. The electrocardiogram shows a right bundle branch pattern with low voltage of the complexes over the right precordium. The combination of the unusual clinical features, the characteristic x-ray picture and the electrocardiogram is pathognomonic of Ebstein's malformation.

These patients are very prone to cardiac arrhythmias, especially paroxysmal tachycardia, and cardiac catheterization is dangerous for this reason. There is no treatment, but the outlook is not as bad as might be imagined, and many patients grow up to live an active life. In early infancy the disease may cause considerable feeding difficulties but later the child tends to progress quite well.

Acyanotic Lesions Producing Cyanosis from Left Ventricular Failure

Such lesions as patent ductus arteriosus, severe aortic stenosis, cor triatriatum and mitral stenosis, which might not be expected to cause cyanosis, may do so as a result of left ventricular failure.

It is also important to note that 'cyanotic attacks' are apt to occur in lesions with large left-to-right shunts such as patent ductus arteriosus and ventricular septal defect when transient shunt reversal occurs, for example, in the presence of respiratory distress and hypoxia.

Differential Cyanosis

Differential cyanosis occurs in two forms. The first type, where there is cyanosis of the lower limbs and the pelvic region, and absence of cyanosis in the remainder of the body, occurs in preductal coarctation of the aorta or absent aortic isthmus, the lower limbs being supplied with 'venous' blood via the ductus. The second type, where the head, trunk and upper limbs are cyanosed with pink lower extremities, occurs where there is coarctation of the aorta with transposition of the great arteries. In fact, differential cyanosis is quite rare because so often there is an intracardiac lesion which permits venous–arterial mixing before the blood reaches the coarctation, resulting in uniform cyanosis.

Prognosis in Cyanotic Congenital Heart Lesions

In general it must be admitted that the presence of cyanosis with a cardiac malformation in the young baby is indicative of a serious prognosis. Many of the lesions, as we have seen, are incompatible with life for more than a few weeks or months. Ebstein's malformation is a notable exception and often has quite a good prognosis. Patients with this disease have been known to survive to middle age and beyond with surprisingly little impairment of activity though sometimes subject to attacks of paroxysmal tachycardia. In recent years there has been some improvement in the prognosis of some of the severe cyanotic lesions. As we have seen the introduction of Rashkind's procedure of atrial septostomy is saving a great many babies with transposition of the great arteries who would otherwise have died in early infancy, and giving them a chance to have a Mustard operation later.

In cyanosed infants who survive beyond their second birthday the tetrad of Fallot is the most common lesion. The prognosis for these infants has undoubtedly been improved by surgical procedures but it is important to emphasize that this is a very serious malformation. Average cases become progressively more cyanosed and dyspnoeic after the first 6 months, but very few will have suffered from 'blue spells' in infancy and most will reach early childhood without serious difficulties. After the dangerous first 2 years have been passed the child adapts himself to anoxia, limits his own activities and adopts postural manoeuvres such as squatting to relieve severe dyspnoea. Providing any existing iron-deficiency anaemia is recognized and treated, they can often remain well until puberty, after which there would be a progressive decline until death occurred towards the end of the second decade. Severe cases who are subject to frequent 'blue spells' or cerebrovascular accidents may have died from anoxia or attempted surgical relief during their first year, whereas mild cases could remain free of cyanosis or disability for many years.

It is against this background that advances in surgical treatment have to be measured. At the present time 'total correction' can be attempted in all but the most severe cases, but the overall mortality in the best centres is still about 10 per cent. The type of surgical correction and optimal time for operation must vary with the severity of the malformation, and sometimes a two-stage procedure may be preferred. In the young infants with severe symptoms there is still a place for 'shunt' operations as a preliminary palliative procedure. Pulmonary atresia or the type of persistent truncus arteriosus in which pulmonary blood flow is achieved via collaterals can sometimes be considered for radical surgical treatment. For example, a homograft or a prosthesis may be inserted into the right ventricle to connect with the major vessels supplying the lungs, and if this proves surgically feasible the septal defect can be closed to give a result very nearly as satisfactory as a 'total correction' in Fallot's tetralogy. This advance in surgical technique has resulted in a changed outlook towards this severe type of lesion; hitherto one was happy to see large collateral channels developing as this would lead to survival with progressively diminishing cyanosis and increased exercise tolerance (the paradoxical situation in which pulmonary atresia could have a better prognosis than a severe tetrad of Fallot without treatment), but now the surgeon would prefer to try to create some anastomoses of his own choice which would be easier to close at the time of the major corrective operation than the multitudinous haphazard anastomoses which nature would provide. This implies the need for early investigation of all cyanotic congenital heart lesions.

Non-Cyanotic Congenital Heart Lesions

Congenital heart lesions which are not associated with cyanosis in the newborn period will usually be suspected because of the presence of a cardiac murmur, the onset of cardiac failure, the occurrence of respiratory difficulty, or the chance finding of cardiomegaly. Some may come to light because of the occurrence of feeding difficulties. It seems appropriate to consider them under these different headings.

Cardiac Murmurs in the Newborn

Although one might assume that the presence of a significant cardiac murmur in the newborn infant would be reliable evidence of heart disease, this is far from the case. The widely differing figures from various authors of the incidence of such murmurs (e.g. 0·5 per cent, Gyllensward, 1956; 0·94 per cent, Benson, Bonham-Carter & Smellie, 1961; 38 per cent, Creery, 1953) indicate that there is either considerable observer-error sometimes on auscultation or, more probably, that there is difficulty in deciding what constitutes a significant murmur. It is also a well-established fact that many murmurs in the newborn period are transient and do not indicate congenital heart disease, whereas gross congenital malformations may never exhibit significant murmurs. The presence of associated findings will, of course, give added significance to a cardiac murmur. It is essential to follow up neonates with cardiac murmurs for a long time, probably 2 or 3 years, before dismissing their murmurs as innocent.

Unfortunately, at this early period the timing of the murmur, its intensity, or its site cannot be relied upon to help in the diagnosis. However, some general remarks are appropriate.

In general the systolic murmurs associated with semilunar stenosis or ventricular septal defect appear earliest (those due to semilunar stenosis earliest of all), but even these may be delayed for a few days or even weeks. A harsh, easily audible murmur at the second left interspace means pulmonary stenosis, and at the second right interspace aortic stenosis. Ventricular septal defects are often accompanied by a harsh well-localized murmur at the lower left sternal border. A murmur which is louder in the back than in the front usually means coarctation of the aorta.

Continuous machinery murmurs are rarely heard in the newborn period. It has been stated that when such a murmur is heard it is almost never due to a patent ductus arteriosus but rather to some form of truncus arteriosus. This is rather overstating the case, for with careful

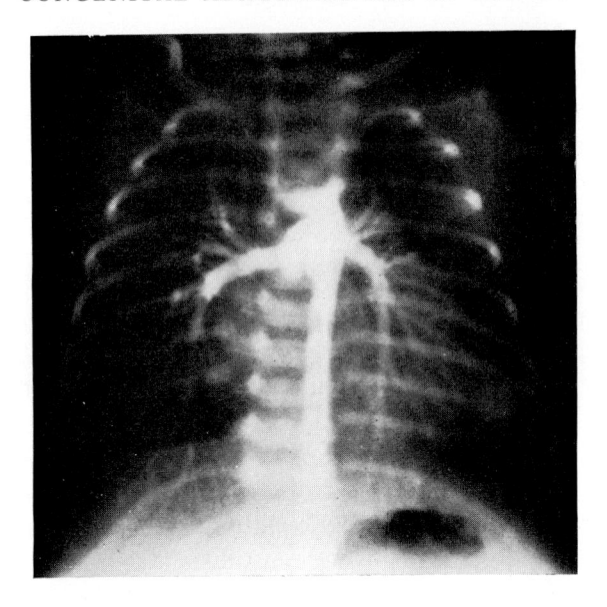

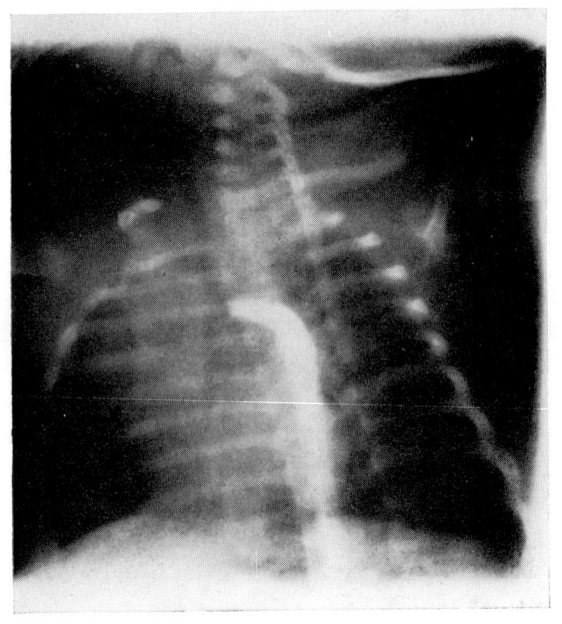

FIG. 3.9. Patent ductus arteriosus in a premature infant (birth weight 3 lb 15 oz) which closed spontaneously at the age of 9 weeks. A: retrograde aortogram via femoral artery at 4 weeks showing dye passing via the ductus into the pulmonary arteries. B: retrograde aortogram at 11 weeks. No dye entered the pulmonary arteries from the aorta.

auscultation the continuous character of a murmur due to a patent ductus arteriosus may be heard occasionally at this age and sometimes the machinery quality is quite obvious. In doubtful cases the injection of mephentermine sulphate (Mephine: John Wyeth and Brother) in a dose of 1 mg/kg body weight has proved useful for bringing out the typical continuous murmur by increasing the velocity of flow across the duct. Apart from producing slight pallor and sweating this manoeuvre has no ill effects. Transient machinery murmurs have been noted in asphyxiated newborns, and special mention must be made of the occurrence of a very characteristic machinery murmur in some very small premature infants usually following the occurrence of severe respiratory distress. With the aid of retrograde aortography I have shown that this is due to a patent ductus arteriosus capable of spontaneous closure. In one case closure occurred 9 weeks after birth (aortograms before and after closure are shown: Fig 3.9). Such murmurs are thus much more likely to be due to an unusual prolongation of a normal physiological state rather than a true congenital anomaly.

The Pulse

Certain characteristics of the pulse may lead to diagnosis of congenital heart disease. Absent or weak peripheral pulses in all four limbs have already been mentioned as a feature of aortic valve atresia. Absence of the femoral pulses with strong brachial pulses is diagnostic of coarctation of the aorta. For this reason it is important to make it a routine practice to palpate for the femoral pulses.

One of the most valuable physical signs in the newborn infant is the presence of a collapsing pulse. This denotes patent ductus arteriosus in nearly all cases, though, of course, a similar type of pulse may be found in persistent truncus arteriosus. It is rarely due to aortic incompetence in infancy.

A slow pulse, around 60 per minute, will suggest heart block, but in general, cardiac arrhythmia in the infant is best detected on auscultation followed by electrocardiography.

Cardiac Failure

Congestive cardiac failure in the newborn is much more frequent than is commonly realized. According to Keith, of all children with a congenital heart lesion who are destined to develop heart failure, approximately 20 per cent will go into failure in the first week of life. Very often heart failure is not recognized as such and the rapid respirations and pulmonary rales are attributed to pulmonary infection. This is excusable when heart failure is predominantly left-sided, but this is rare in infancy. The hepatic enlargement followed by peripheral oedema in right-sided heart failure should clearly indicate the true state of affairs. Oedema occurs first in the face, as a rule. Babies with congestive cardiac failure often exhibit a troublesome ineffectual cough, and they may seem unusually pale, and sweat a great deal particularly about the face and head.

Apart from the relatively rare occurrence of myocarditis and of an arrhythmia, such as paroxysmal tachycardia or auricular flutter, heart failure in the newborn is likely to be due to a severe congenital anomaly and the following lesions must be considered (in order of frequency).

(1) Hypoplastic left heart syndrome; (2) transposition of the great arteries; (3) coarctation of the aorta; (4) patent ductus arteriosus; (5) severe pulmonary stenosis, or pulmonary atresia with normal aortic root; (6) endocardial fibroelastosis.

Keith, Rowe and Vlad provide some very useful tables listing the important causes of heart failure in infancy and their relative frequency at different ages. It may be useful to remember that in the first week the most common cause of heart failure is aortic atresia, from 1 week to 1 month it is coarctation of the aorta, from 1 to 2 months it is transposition of the great arteries, from 2 to 3 months it is endocardial fibroelastosis.

It is important to recognize uncomplicated coarctation of the aorta, patent ductus arteriosus, severe pulmonary stenosis and pulmonary atresia with normal aortic root, for in all these lesions surgery may be urgently required and can be dramatically successful.

A careful routine examination which includes palpation for the femoral pulses should reveal all cases of uncomplicated coarctation of the aorta, especially when a murmur is heard loudest at the back and blood-pressure estimations reveal an appreciable difference between the right arm and the right leg. An x-ray will show significant cardiac enlargement and pulmonary congestion. An electrocardiogram will show right ventricular hypertrophy or combined ventricular hypertrophy.

Patent ductus arteriosus will not always produce a continuous murmur at this age, but when a prolonged and rather uneven systolic murmur is heard down the left sternal edge and the peripheral pulses are of water-hammer type, this is the most likely diagnosis. The x-ray in this condition shows generalized cardiac enlargement and pulmonary congestion. These infants are very liable to attacks of cyanosis especially when the left ventricle is failing. The diagnosis can be established by retrograde aortography or venous cine-angiography, but if the heart is failing in spite of adequate digitalis therapy ligation of the ductus is urgently required, and under these circumstances immediate thoracotomy is justified.

Severe pulmonary stenosis is characterized by pure right-sided failure with clear lung fields. Cyanosis is often deep and does not disappear with digitalis therapy. The murmur may not be as loud as expected. The x-ray shows a large heart with clear lung fields and the electrocardiogram shows severe right ventricular hypertrophy and right-sided ventricular 'strain' with tall pointed P pulmonale. If in addition there is a pulsating liver the diagnosis is virtually certain. In the small infant, once heart failure has appeared, surgery offers the only hope, and it will usually consist of a Brock type valvotomy. Pulmonary atresia with normal aortic root produces a similar clinical picture with absence of the harsh systolic murmur. Diagnosis is best made with emergency angiocardiography, for immediate valvotomy might prove life-saving.

Primary endocardial fibroelastosis and other endomyocardial diseases such as that produced by an anomalous left coronary artery arising from the pulmonary artery, calcification of the coronary arteries, and glycogen storage disease of the heart and skeletal muscles are characterized by increasing cardiomegaly and heart failure outside the neonatal period and need only be mentioned as rare diagnostic possibilities because they may all present with feeding difficulties at this time and perchance an x-ray or electrocardiogram may lead to diagnosis before heart failure supervenes. Some of the infants appear to suffer from anginal attacks during feeding. Certain individual characteristics of the electrocardiogram are helpful in the diagnosis and the reader is referred to more detailed accounts of these and other features in the text-books.

Cardiomegaly as a Presenting Sign

Sometimes a baby is found to have an enlarged heart without any other signs of heart disease. This is usually a radiological finding, but cardiac enlargement may be recognized by increased pulsation below the xiphisternum. Cardiomegaly may be a transient occurrence in the newborn baby during the first 24 hours when the transition from intra-uterine existence to an independent air-breathing existence is taking place. At such a time cardiomegaly may be exaggerated by an over-generous 'placental transfusion'. In such instances congenital heart disease may be mistakenly suspected. Possible congenital abnormalities responsible for cardiomegaly (in the absence of other signs) include endocardial fibroelastosis (E.F.E.), glycogen storage disease (Pompe's disease), and anomalous origin of the left coronary artery from the pulmonary artery. E.F.E. and Pompe's disease are characterized by an E.C.G. showing left ventricular dominance and, possibly left ventricular strain. E.F.E. is also characterized by extreme sensitivity to digitalis, but a good response to small doses when cardiac failure supervenes, and in most cases a positive skin test and C.F.T. to mumps antigen. The anomalous left coronary artery will usually have an E.C.G. with a pattern suggesting anterior myocardial infarction.

An unusual cause of cardiomegaly is diverticulum of the left atrium, a condition which is characterized by recurrent embolism.

Respiratory Difficulty as a Presenting Symptom

Respiratory difficulty characterized by rapid laboured breathing, often with expiratory grunt, chin-tug, xiphisternal retraction and intercostal recession may be an early indication of heart failure, especially when this is predominantly left-sided. It may also indicate a cardiac anomaly with a pronounced left-to-right shunt resulting in pulmonary engorgement. In the acyanotic infant this is most likely to be either a patent ductus arteriosus, a ventricular septal defect, or combined atrial and ventricular septal defects as in the atrioventricular canal defects. In the cyanotic infant this type of breathing is seen in transposition of the great arteries and persistent truncus arteriosus, because in both these conditions there is engorgement of the pulmonary vessels. In all these instances it is thought that the vascular engorgement leading to rigidity of the lungs is responsible for the reduced pulmonary compliance which interferes with normal expansion.

Laryngeal stridor, especially when associated with dysphagia, may be the result of compression of the larynx and the oesophagus by a vascular ring due to anomalies of the aortic arch. Careful fluoroscopy and radiography following an opaque meal may be necessary to detect the anomalous vessels.

CERTAIN GROSS OUTWARDLY VISIBLE ANOMALIES

Ectopia cordis. This is a rare malformation in which the heart protrudes outside the chest through a split sternum. (It has also been described in two other forms, one in which the heart protrudes through the diaphragm into the abdominal cavity, and the other where it protrudes into the neck.) These infants rarely survive for more than a few days.

Diverticulum of the left ventricle. In this rare anomaly a diverticulum of the left ventricle protrudes through a defect in the diaphragm into the epigastrium. A pulsating mass is visible and palpable in the upper part of the abdomen. Successful excision of such a diverticulum has been performed. In one case seen recently there appeared to be very little disturbance caused by the anomaly except that pressure upon the pulsatile swelling produced alarming slowing of the heart rate.

DEXTROCARDIA

Dextrocardia implies that the heart is in the right hemithorax with the apex pointing to the right, and it must be clearly distinguished from dextrorotation of the heart. The electrocardiogram is quite characteristic in mirror image dextrocardia: lead I is the mirror image of the normal tracing with inverted P and T waves, and these waves are upright in aVR. Dextrocardia may exist with or without situs inversus. In dextrocardia with situs inversus the heart is quite commonly normal, but the condition may be associated with bronchiectasis and sinusitis (Kartagener's syndrome). Isolated dextrocardia, on the contrary, is frequently associated with structural defects which determine its prognosis, which is often poor.

Problems in differential diagnosis may be created by such conditions as left-sided diaphragmatic hernia or eventration which displace the heart into the right chest.

Laevocardia with situs inversus is nearly always associated with severe cardiac malformations, so that the majority of patients die during infancy. Absence of the spleen may also occur, and be indicated by the finding of Howell–Jolly bodies in some of the red blood cells; this associated anomaly lowers these patients' resistance to certain bacterial infections.

Cardiac Arrhythmias in the Newborn

An unusually slow heart rate, usually around 60 per minute, suggests complete atrioventricular block. This may be detected *in utero* and it is then possible that one may be misled into thinking there is foetal distress and so hasten the delivery. The diagnosis is confirmed by electrocardiogram. This will exclude bradycardia from hyperpotassaemia resulting from severe respiratory distress, in which the electrocardiogram is completely disorganized.

Congenital heart block is commonly asymptomatic but attacks of syncope may occur. The peripheral pulse is of the water-hammer type due to the large stroke volume and peripheral vasodilatation, and the systolic pressure is raised. Irregular jugular venous pulsations may be seen with occasional 'cannon waves' when the atrium contracts against a closed tricuspid valve. The intensity of the first sound varies and isolated atrial sounds may be audible down the left sternal border. A systolic murmur may also be audible down the left sternal border and there may be an apical mid-diastolic murmur, but these do not indicate the presence of a ventricular septal defect. Septal defects are, in fact, rarely present in association with congenital heart block. The prognosis for uncomplicated heart block is good.

Supraventricular tachycardia is characterized by a regular rapid heart rate, over 180 per minute, which can be confirmed by electrocardiography. Most infants with this arrhythmia have no associated heart lesion and a good prognosis, though prolonged tachycardia may lead to heart failure requiring prompt treatment. Infants with incipient failure may appear acutely ill with pyrexia, ashen grey colour and restlessness. Cardiac function returns to normal after the attack, and although there may be repeated attacks the prognosis is good provided there is no structural anomaly of the heart. Some children who have repeated attacks show the Wolff–Parkinson–White syndrome probably due to the presence of anomalous conducting fibres between the right atrium and ventricles. On the electrocardiogram there is a widened QRS complex encroaching on the P–R interval which is thereby shortened, the P–S interval being normal. This is not usually associated with cardiac disease but may sometimes be found in endocardial fibroelastosis.

Paroxysmal nodal or *ventricular tachycardia* is rare in infants and children.

An irregular pulse at a normal rate is usually due to frequent ventricular extrasystoles which are of no consequence, but sometimes the electrocardiogram will reveal atrial flutter with varying degrees of atrioventricular block. The latter is more serious since cardiac failure may supervene and require treatment. Atrial flutter is not frequent in children but may complicate myocarditis of any cause. It can be recognized on the electrocardiogram by the rapid and regular 'f' waves, producing a 'saw-tooth' appearance. The prognosis will depend upon the underlying lesion.

The treatment of cardiac arrhythmias is considered under the section on treatment of heart failure.

Interpretation of the Electrocardiogram in the Newborn

The normal electrocardiogram in the newborn reveals an axis greater than 90° and chest leads characteristic of right ventricular hypertrophy. The T waves in all chest leads are upright for 24 to 72 hours: after 72 hours T in leads V_1 and V_2 is inverted, while T in V_5 and V_6 remains upright. The presence of left ventricular hypertrophy or even the normal degree of adult left heart dominance is abnormal at this age, and is a definite indication of heart disease. Tricuspid atresia, aortic stenosis and 'primary myocardial disease' show this type of electrocardiogram. To assess what represents an abnormal degree of right ventricular hypertrophy is more difficult, but the following are regarded as indications of this:

(1) Pure R in V_1, preferably greater than 10 mm.
(2) qR in V_1 of any length.
(3) R of greater than 17 mm in RS pattern.
(4) Upright T in V_1 beyond 72 hours.
(5) Right axis deviation greater than 135°.

Most conditions with abnormal right ventricular hypertrophy at this age belong to the cyanotic group.

The electrocardiogram tends to be very characteristic in endocardial cushion defects, whose clinical manifestations vary from a simple ostium primum atrial septal defect to persistent common atrioventricular canal. The basic pattern consists of left axis deviation in the limb leads with a partial or complete right bundle branch block pattern in the precordial leads and right, left or combined ventricular hypertrophy.

THE TREATMENT OF CONGENITAL HEART DISEASE IN THE VERY YOUNG INFANT

Treatment of Heart Failure

The principles of treatment of heart failure in the infant are the same as for the older patient.

Position. It may be advantageous to have the infant placed in a semi-upright position, and devising methods of supporting the sick infant in such a position by means of special chairs, splints or slings may tax one's ingenuity. However, in most cases it would seem to be sufficient to raise the head end of the mattress with padding or to elevate the head of the cot on blocks.

Oxygen. By placing the infant in a small oxygen tent the oxygen in the inspired air may be raised to 35–40 per cent. If higher concentrations are needed oxygen must be administered by means of a funnel or face mask. The passage of oxygen through a Wolff's bottle containing 20–30 per cent ethyl alcohol for 10 minutes every half-hour may help to relieve pulmonary oedema by reducing the surface tension of the froth in the alveoli, but other methods of treating pulmonary oedema have tended to supersede this technique.

Digitalis. Digitalis therapy is fundamental in the management of cardiac failure whatever the cause (with the possible exception of anaemia or cardiac tamponade). Experience suggests that digoxin is the drug of choice and this can be conveniently administered orally in a dilute preparation, Lanoxin (Burroughs Wellcome), which allows for a wide margin of safety. There are intravenous or intramuscular preparations for emergency use, the dose for parenteral administration being approximately two-thirds of the oral dose. For children up to 2 years digitalization is usually achieved with an oral dose of 0·06 to 0·08 mg/kg body weight during the first 24 hours. It is probably best to give half of this dose initially and divide the remainder equally into 6- or 8-hourly doses. Thereafter daily maintenance therapy approximates to one-quarter of the digitalizing dose and this may be administered in two divided doses. Individual requirements, and the liability to toxicity, vary quite considerably so that it is impossible to lay down a rigid dosage schedule.

Signs of digitalis toxicity in infants are not as obvious as in adults and frequent electrocardiographic observation may be necessary during the establishment of digitalis therapy. Perhaps the most frequent symptoms are vomiting, first- and second-degree heart block and supraventricular arrhythmia. Toxicity is most likely to occur in situations which lead to potassium depletion so that periodic estimation of serum electrolytes is also recommended during treatment. Severe toxicity is often quickly relieved by the administration of potassium salts.

Diuretics. Diuretics are required only when digitalis therapy in proper dosage fails to produce the expected improvement in the infant's condition. Happily this is rarely the case, but even so one should not hesitate to use diuretics when necessary. There is now a wide range of diuretics available; as well as the well-tried mercurial diuretics, there are, for example, chlorthiazide, ethacrynic acid and frusemide, and the three last-named have the advantage that they can be administered orally. It is important to avoid potassium depletion and hyponatraemia when using these drugs, so that periodic checks on serum electrolyte levels are necessary. Potassium supplements are required when there is prolonged administration of chlorthiazide or frusemide. The following are recommended doses.

Mercurials, I.M., 0–1 month: 0·1 ml (maximum 0·25 ml)
               1 month–2 years: 0·2 ml (maximum 0·5 ml)

Chlorthiazide, Oral, 0–1 year: 125 mg per day.
               1–2 years: 250 mg per day.
               Single daily dose: do not give more than 5 consecutive days' therapy per week.

Ethacrynic acid, Oral, 0–1 year: 2·5 mg/kg per day.
               1–2 years: 25 mg per day.
    Once daily.

Frusemide, Oral, 0–1 year: 2 mg/kg per day.
               1–2 years: 20 mg per day.
    Once daily, or on alternate days
    I.V. or I.M.: Half the oral dose; in emergency situations, such as pulmonary oedema, repeated I.V. doses at intervals of 4–6 hours may be required until desired therapeutic effect is achieved.

Antibiotic therapy. Since cardiac failure may be precipitated by infection it is generally considered advisable to administer a broad spectrum antibiotic for 5 to 10 days. Sometimes it is not easy to be sure whether the physical signs indicate heart failure or pneumonia and then antibiotic therapy is obligatory.

Morphine. Morphine is one of the most valuable drugs for the relief of symptoms in congenital heart disease. In heart failure it is the best of sedatives. It is remarkably effective for the relief of severe 'blue spells' in Fallot's tetralogy where the drug possibly acts by overcoming infundibular spasm. Anginal attacks which are a feature of anomalous coronary artery and possibly also of transposition of the great arteries are quickly relieved by morphine. The recommended dose is 0·2 mg/kg body weight.

Propranolol. In recent years a group of drugs have been developed which produce blockage of the β-adrenergic fibres. The safest and best of these is propranolol. Its use in paediatric cardiology is confined to the prevention of 'blue spells' in Fallot's tetralogy and the control of certain arrhythmias. The drug may produce severe bradycardia which is 'exercise-resistant' and must be used with caution, especially when there is incipient heart failure. The oral dose is 0·5 mg/kg for infants up to one year and 5 mg t.d.s. for children of 1–7 years, but it is advisable to start with half the dose for 2 days. It may be given intravenously at a rate of 1 mg per minute until the maximum dose, as already mentioned, is given.

The Treatment of Specific Causes of Heart Failure

Emergency surgery may be necessary for certain remediable conditions such as patent ductus arteriosus and coarctation of the aorta when heart failure has intervened. However, it is always necessary to institute medical treatment first and if the immediate response is good it is advisable to use this opportunity to carry out any diagnostic procedures which may be necessary to establish a definite diagnosis before surgery is carried out.

The treatment of cardiac arrhythmias. When arrhythmias result in cardiac failure it is imperative to use appropriate drugs to bring them under control. Sedation with such drugs as chloral or barbiturates may be enough to cut short an attack of supraventricular tachycardia, but when the attack is prolonged it is better to use digitalis, which is the most effective drug. It is contra-indicated in paroxysmal ventricular tachycardia but this is so rare in infants that digitalis may be prescribed without hesitation if an electrocardiogram cannot be obtained.

Quinidine is useful in ventricular tachycardia, but in auricular tachycardia and flutter it is usually less effective than digitalis. The dosage schedule is as follows:

Statim	3 mg/kg body weight
2 hours	6 mg/kg body weight
4 hours	9 mg/kg body weight
6 hours	12 mg/kg body weight

Then repeat this dose 2-hourly until normal rhythm is restored, after which a maintenance dose of 3 mg/kg three times a day is given for 24 hours.

A careful watch is kept on the pulse and daily electrocardiograms should be taken in the early stages.

Procaine amide hydrochloride (Pronestyl-Squibb) has proved effective for both forms of paroxysmal tachycardia. It is rapidly absorbed by mouth, and may be given intramuscularly or intravenously in an emergency. Suggested doses for infants are as follows:

Oral	10 mg/kg 6-hourly.
Intramuscular	5 mg/kg 2–4 hourly.
Intravenous	5 mg/kg. Do not give more rapidly than 1·0 mg per minute.

Acetyl methyl choline (Mecholyl: Savory & Moore). This is a dangerous drug and should only be used as a last resort. It is given by subcutaneous injection. Temporary asystole follows and it may be necessary to administer 0·03 mg atropine. The dose of mecholyl is 0·1 mg/kg body weight. If this is ineffective double the dose is administered 30 minutes later, and this dose may be doubled again if necessary after a further 30 minutes.

Propanolol. As already stated, this drug has proved useful in the control of arrhythmias, especially supraventricular paroxysmal tachycardia, and may be tried in resistant cases. It is also useful as preventive treatment where there is a tendency to repeated attacks of tachycardia. The dose has already been mentioned, but for long-term use one should employ the smallest possible effective dose.

Auricular flutter is best treated with digitalis which converts the flutter to auricular fibrillation before normal rhythm is restored. In resistant cases quinidine may be tried.

SELECTED REFERENCES

FORSHALL ISABELLA (1961) Duplication of the digestive tract. Simpson Smith Memorial Lecture at the Institute of Child Health, London
BENSON P.F., BONHAM CARTER R.E. & SMELLIE JEAN M. (1961) Transient and intermittent systolic murmurs in newborn infants. *Lancet* **1,** 627
CREERY R.D.G. (1953) Cardiac murmurs in newborn. *Ulster Med. J.* **22,** 73
GYLLENSWARD A. (1956) Incidence and significance of heart murmurs in newborn infants. *Acta Paediat. Stockh.* **45,** 63
KEITH J.D. (1956) Congestive heart failure: review article. *Pediatrics* **18,** 491
KEITH J.D., ROWE R.D. & VLAD P. 2nd Edition 1967 *Heart Disease in Infancy and Childhood.* New York: Macmillan
KJELLBERG S.R., MANNHEIMER E., RUDHE U. & JONSSON B. (1955) *Diagnosis of Congenital Heart Disease.* Chicago: Year Book Publishers
LANDING B.H. (1957) Anomalies of the respiratory tract. *Pediat. Clin. N. Amer.* February issue, p. 73. Philadelphia and London: W. B. Saunders
LAURENCE K.M. (1959) Congenital pulmonary lymphangiectasis. *Journal of Clinical Pathology* **12,** 62
MURPHY D.P. (1947) *Congenital Malformation. A study of Parental Characteristics with Special Reference to the Reproductive Process*, 2nd edn. Philadelphia: Lippincott
NADAS A.S. (1957) *Pediatric Cardiology.* Philadelphia: W. B. Saunders
NOONAN JACQUELINE A. & NADAS A.S. (1958) The hypoplastic left heart syndrome. *Pediat. Clin. N. Amer.* November issue, p. 1029
POTTER EDITH L. (1952) *Pathology of the Foetus and the Newborn.* Chicago: Year Book Publications Inc.
RASHKIND W.J. & MILLER W.W. (1966) J.A.M.A. **196,** 991
SCHNITKER M.A. (1952) *Congenital Anomalies of the Heart and Great Vessels.* New York: Oxford University Press
TAUSSIG HELEN (1960) *Congenital Malformations of the Heart.* New York: The Commonwealth Fund
WATSON H. (1968) *Pediatric Cardiology.* St. Louis, C. V. Morsby Co.
ZIEGLER R.F. (1951) *Electrocardiographic Studies in Normal Infants and Children.* Springfield, Illinois: Charles C. Thomas
ZIEGLER R.F. (1956) The importance of positive T waves in the right precordial electrocardiogram during the first year of life. *Amer. Heart J.* **52,** 533

4

Abnormalities of the Ear, Nose and Throat

H.S.SHARP

COMMON OTOLARYNGOLOGICAL ANOMALIES

The development of the ear, nose and larynx is highly complicated and it is not surprising that anomalies are fairly common. Many conditions are correctable by surgery and it is essential that treatment should be instituted as soon as possible by an otolaryngologist experienced in paediatric pathology. The child must be given every opportunity to adjust to life and to overcome educational problems as they arise.

THE EAR

Embryology

In the developing embryo five branchial arches separated by four branchial grooves appear in the ventro-lateral wall of each side of the primitive pharynx. Each arch is lined externally by ectoderm and internally by entoderm, and each contains a core of mesoderm in which a cartilaginous framework develops which in certain of the arches becomes ossified. In the external grooves the ectoderm is indented inwards, whilst in the internal grooves the entoderm is depressed outwards to meet the ectoderm. The thin membrane forming the floor of the grooves consists of a layer of ectoderm meeting entoderm without the interposition of any mesoderm. In man this membrane does not break down to form branchial or gill clefts.

The first and second inner grooves become the Eustachian tube, tympanic cavity and tympanic antrum. The septum becomes the tympanic membrane. The first outer groove becomes the external

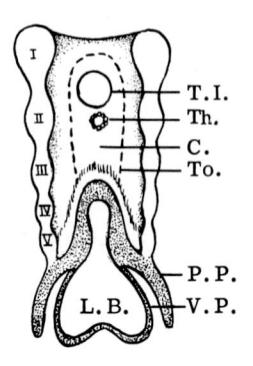

FIG. 4.1. Floor of the embryonic pharynx.
T.I.   Tuberculum impar   P.P.   parietal pleura
Th.   thyroid   V.P.   visceral pleura
C   copula   L.B.   lung buds
To.   tongue   I–V   branchial arches

DEVELOPMENT OF MIDDLE AND EXTERNAL EAR

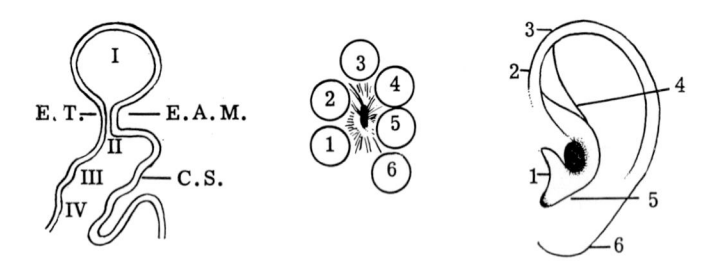

FIG. 4.2. Development of middle and external ear.
I–IV   Branchial grooves   1   tragus
E.T.   eustachian tube   2   crus helix
E.A.M.   external auditory meatus   3   helix
C.S.   cervical sinus   4   anti-helix
                                        5   anti-tragus
                                        6   lobule

auditory meatus. The remaining external grooves should normally disappear but they may persist as cysts.

The malleus and incus are derived from the mesoderm of the first arch. The stapes is derived from the mesoderm of the second arch. The inner ear is developed from the ectoderm in the region of the primitive hindbrain. An invagination of this ectoderm leads to the auditory pit which later becomes the auditory vesicle, from which the membrane labyrinth is formed.

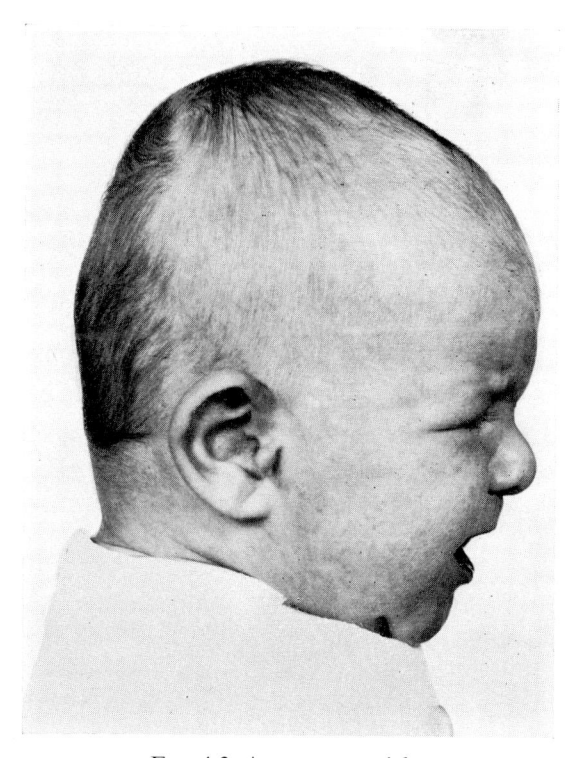

FIG. 4.3. Accessory auricles

ABNORMALITIES OF THE EXTERNAL EAR

Abnormalities of the Auricle
Variations in the shape of the auricle are many. The appendage may be completely absent (anotia), smaller than normal (microtia), larger than normal (macrotia) or displaced (melotia). The grosser irregularities can be corrected in later life by plastic surgery or replaced by a prosthesis. Accessory auricles are quite common and are easily removed in later life, but need no immediate treatment in infancy. Those with a narrow

pedicle are easily removed by tying a ligature around the base soon after birth.

Bat ears should be corrected after the age of 6 years if they cause embarrassment.

Malformed auricles may be associated with renal abnormalities (see

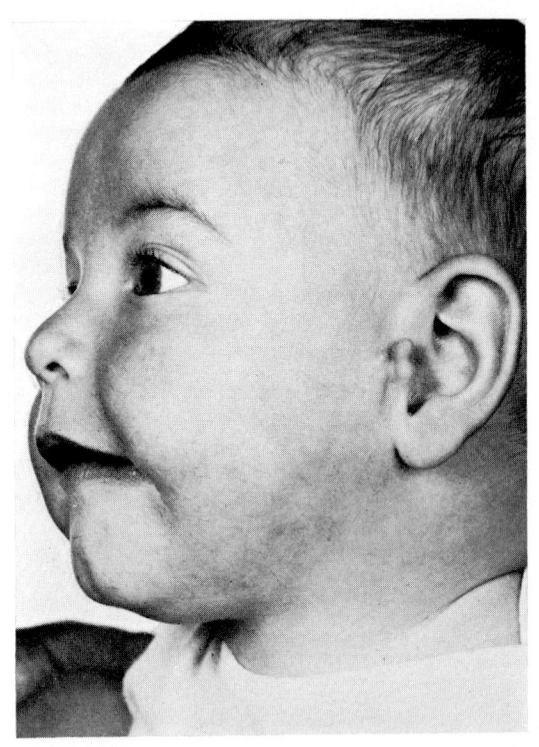

FIG. 4.4. Pre-auricular fistula with accessory auricles

Potter's syndrome) with various dyscephalies and the Treacher-Collins syndrome.

Treacher-Collins syndrome
This was first described by Treacher-Collins in 1900 and later by Franceschetti and Zwahlen. The principal features are laterally sloping palpebral fissures, hypoplasia of the facial bones, microstomia, high palate, abnormal position and malocclusion of the teeth, and malformations of the ear. The auricle is usually low in position. Atresia of the

external auditory meatus is relatively common. The ear deformities require surgical treatment on their own merits (*vide infra*).

The Treacher-Collins syndrome is due to a dominant mutant gene which has a variable manifestation.

Congenital Aural Fistula

This condition is due to persistence of some part of the first branchial cleft. Ninety per cent are found opening close to the anterior border of the ascending limb of the helix. Most of the remainder open on a line extending from the lower border of the crus helix to the angle of the mouth. The condition presents as a small pin-point hole in a depression. If infection develops along the track, these fistulae require excision. The track is often deep and complete removal must be aimed at in order to obtain a lasting cure.

Collaural fistulas have a second opening in the neck between the angle of the mandible and the sternomastoid muscle.

Atresia of the External Auditory Canal
This condition arises from a failure of development of the first branchial groove with an ectopic development of mesoderm between the outer ectoderm lining and the inner entoderm. Sometimes this mesoderm ossifies and produces a bony wall in the situation of the tympanic membrane. There is nearly always some degree of deformed pinna, or the pinna may be absent. Often the ossicles in the middle ear groove show signs of maldevelopment, the first arch derivatives (malleus and incus) being more commonly affected than the second arch derivatives (stapes). The auditory vesicle may develop normally, however, and hence while there is a severe conductive deafness in such cases (80 db loss) common perception by bone conduction may be only moderately reduced, except in the Treacher-Collins syndrome. Usually the condition is unilateral, the other meatus being normal. On the affected side there is no meatal opening. Provided the unaffected ear is normal, no immediate steps in treatment are called for during infancy, as hearing and speech development will not be retarded. At the age of 3 to 4 years a reconstruction operation will be needed to restore the meatal opening and to reform the pinna.

If, however, both auditory meati are absent, then the hearing loss is severe, and operation on the meati is called for earlier. The author prefers to do these cases at 18 months.

A pre-operative assessment of hearing should always be carried out and special radiological views of both temporal bones are sometimes of value. The operation consists of exposing the middle-ear groove, removing any rudimentary ossicles and coring out a passage between the

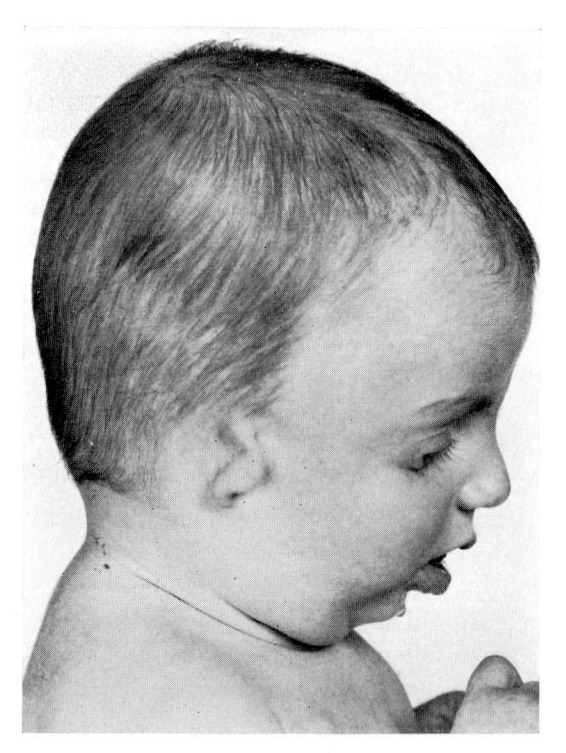

Fig. 4.5. Absent auditory meatus with malformed pinnae, with micrognathia (Treacher-Collins syndrome)

middle ear and the covering skin at the site of the external meatus. A tympanoplasty graft is placed in position and the newly created external meatus is lined by carefully fashioned, nearly full thickness skin grafts. Plastic procedures to reconstruct a pinna if it is absent, or to refashion a grossly deformed existing pinna, are carried out when the child is older. In many, quite reasonable hearing has followed operation. In others, a hearing aid with an insert into the newly reconstructed meatus is needed.

The severer abnormalities of the auricle, meatus, middle and inner ears often found combined in the Treacher-Collins syndrome do not give good results following surgical exploration.

CONGENITAL DEAFNESS

It should be realized that in most children deafness is not congenital, but acquired. It is then usually conductive in type. This subject, however, does not concern us here.

Congenital Perceptive Deafness

Congenital perceptive deafness is, by comparison, relatively rare. In most cases the cause remains unknown but heredity plays a role since there is a higher incidence of deafness in a family with other deaf-born individuals. Similarly, there is a greater risk of deafness in children born of a consanguineous marriage than in the normal population.

Large-scale population surveys have shown that the majority of instances of congenital deafness are now due to autosomal recessive genes. Maternal rubella is an important cause of congenital deafness only after an epidemic of rubella. Probably several different autosomal recessive genes are concerned; one which may be distinguished is that causing congenital deafness in association with retinitis pigmentosa.

The empirical risk to the relatives of congenitally deaf index patients, excluding those with a known environmental cause of the deafness, and those where the deafness is part of a recognized syndrome, is:

Brothers and sisters of index patients, both parents unaffected and not blood relatives	1 in 6
Brothers and sisters of index patients, both parents unaffected and blood relatives	1 in 4
Brothers and sisters of index patients, one parent affected	1 in 2
Brothers and sisters of index patients, both parents affected	2 in 3
Children of index patients, if index patient married to an unaffected individual	1 in 20
Children of index patients, if index patient married to a congenitally deaf individual	1 in 4

Deafness may be inherited as an isolated defect or as part of a syndrome.

Waardenburg's syndrome consists of malformation of the inner angles of the eyelids, congenital perceptive deafness, different coloured eyes and a white forelock. It is due to a dominant gene which has a variable manifestation (see p. 357).

Pendred's syndrome: sporadic goitre is sometimes associated with deaf mutism in Pendred's syndrome, due to a recessive mutant gene. The physical and mental development of the children is normal but pathological changes are evident in the middle ear (see p. 372).

Alport's syndrome: hereditary nephritis, ophthalmic defects and perceptive deafness (see p. 372).

Cardio-auditory syndrome of Jervell and Lange-Nielson: liability to fainting attacks or sudden death, abnormality of the electrocardiograph and perceptive deafness; a recessive condition.

Cockayne's syndrome: perceptive deafness associated with retinal atrophy and dwarfism: a recessive condition.

Usher's syndrome: retinitis pigmentosa and perceptive deafness.

Hunter-Hurler syndrome (the sex-linked form only): mucopolysaccharide metabolic defect with perceptive deafness (see p. 376).

Cogan's syndrome: Interstitial keratitis with perceptive deafness: not a genetically determined syndrome.

Wildervanck's syndrome: (cervico-oculo-acoustic syndrome) a combination of the Klippel–Feil deformity, Duane's syndrome and perceptive deafness: genetics uncertain, possibly X-linked dominant, lethal in males.

Perceptive deafness may also be associated with Marfan's syndrome (p. 362), Klippel–Feil's syndrome (p. 367), Moebius syndrome (p. 382), Endemic cretinism, Duane's syndrome (congenital abnormality of horizontally acting rectus muscles of the eye), Chondrodystrophy (p. 359), Von Recklinghausen's syndrome (p. 311), leucodystrophy, Schilder's syndrome and Djerine-Sottas syndrome.

Perceptive deafness has also been recorded in chromosomal abnormalities.

Prenatal and perinatal environmental factors may also cause perceptive deafness; *Rubella* was first reported as a cause of congenital deafness in Australia in 1945. Jackson & Fisch (1958) in Britain showed that 30·4 per cent of children whose mothers had rubella during the first 16 weeks of pregnancy were found to have some degree of deafness when tested at the age of 4. Other virus infections may have similar effects.

Hyperbilirubinaemia due to rhesus incompatibility or to prematurity; drugs, e.g. thalidomide taken in pregnancy; congenital syphilis; birth injuries and perinatal anoxia are other environmental factors which may produce deafness.

Thyroid dysfunction has also been described as a possible cause of congenital deafness. In cases of endemic goitre the incidence of congenital deafness is 20 per thousand (the normal incidence of congenital deafness is 0·3 per thousand of the population). The aetiology is considered to be environmental and not genetic and the pathology is in the middle ear where the ossicles are enlarged and distorted, and the lining is grossly thickened. In the inner ear a hyaline ridge develops between the organ of Corti and the membrane of Corti.

Congenital Conductive Deafness

This may be due to meatal atresia as described earlier or to isolated defects in the tympanic membrane or ossicular chain—e.g. stapes footplate fixation and incudo-stapedial joint separation.

Otosclerosis is transmitted by an autosomal dominant gene with variable manifestation but the deafness rarely begins before the age of ten. A familial association of osteogenesis imperfecta, blue sclerotics and otosclerosis is known as:

Van de Hoeve's syndrome: this also is a dominant condition.

Detection of Deafness

All children at risk should be screened for deafness at the earliest possible opportunity. A complete examination of the ears, nose and throat should be done when deafness is suspected, and after this an attempt must be made to assess the child's hearing. The mother's opinion as to the ability of her child to hear is, in the author's opinion, most valuable. It is rare for a mother to be wrong and if she is sure of the presence of deafness, this is almost always found. Not only will she remark on her child's auditory shortcomings, but will frequently have noticed also how active is his ocular sense.

Mental deficiency, and other central nervous abnormalities, may co-exist with the deafness. When these are present as well, the whole problem becomes more involved, but in any infant suspected of mental deficiency it is important to be as sure as possible that deafness is not the actual cause of apparent retardation or lack of speech.

Hearing Tests in Children

It has been found possible to test most normal children by pure tone audiometry at the age of 3 years or more. In intelligent and co-operative children this age limit may be reduced to $2\frac{1}{2}$ years. The audiometrician should be trained in all the accepted procedures of audiometry and should have special experience in testing small children. Various techniques of play audiometry have been described.

At an earlier age one must rely on observing behaviour—that is the reaction to sound in a *free field*. From the age of 5 or 6 months onwards the normal hearing child will turn the head to sounds, but before this age testing is extremely difficult because of the lack of a reliable response. More objective tests of hearing are desirable. At present there is no single reliable objective test in clinical practice although in research departments electroencephalographic and other physiological responses are used.

It is most important that all these tests be carried out in a quiet test situation.

THE NOSE

Embryology

The development of the nose depends on the co-ordinated development of many complicated structures.

The suggestion has been made that choanal atresia is due to persistence of the buccopharyngeal membrane which normally disappears when the embryo is about 24 days old or the bucconasal membrane which normally disappears at about 36 days. Craig and Simpson, however, find these theories untenable and they have suggested that during the upgrowth and enlargement of the nasal fossae, congenital adhesions form in the very narrow area of the posterior choanae. These persist and as they may contain mesoderm they may be either membranous or bony.

In the developing embryo a median septum grows down from the median nasal process and from the base of the skull. This contains a core of cartilage in and around which the bones of the septum are formed. A part of this persists as the cartilage of the septum. The septum grows into a groove formed between the four prevomerine processes of the premaxilla. These prevomerine processes each have a separate centre of ossification. If the site of growth is greater on one side than the other the tendency will be for the relatively soft septal cartilage to be displaced towards the side of the slower growth. This leads to a congenital deviation of the nasal septum.

Deviated Nasal Septum

This condition rarely produces a complete nasal obstruction in infancy and childhood. Whenever possible operative treatment should be postponed until the age of 10 or more years, when growth is nearing completion. Before this, unless surgical correction is very conservative, the operation may be followed by the development of deformity such as broadening of the nose or depression of the nasal tip.

Nasal Dermoid

Inclusion dermoids arising in the nose are not common but they do arise in relation to the midline. The cyst is liable to increase in size and may become infected. If it ruptures, a chronic sinus will form. Treatment consists of a complete surgical excision of the cyst.

Posterior Choanal Atresia

This results from failure of canalization of one or both nasal cavities. A bilateral atresia at birth is a surgical emergency, since the infant is quite unable to breathe through the nose, and feeding is impossible. The diagnosis of the bilateral case is a comparatively easy matter, since the infant asphyxiates if the mouth is held shut. It struggles continually to breathe through the nose, and may only manage to get air in through the mouth when it cries. A curious fluttering movement of the lips is characteristically seen. A malleable metal probe passed down the nostril will meet a firm obstruction, and cannot be felt in the nasopharynx by the observer's little finger.

Treatment consists in breaking through the obstruction with blunt-ended forceps and curved urethral dilators, sometimes combined with nibbling away the membrane and the posterior end of the septum, and then inserting polythene tubing from the front to the back of each nostril. Subsequently repeated dilatation using metal urethral bougies is necessary. This dilatation is very important and may have to be continued regularly for some years as stenosis tends to occur. Some cases in later life require a transpalatal operation to obtain permanent patency.

The unilateral case presents with persistent one-sided nasal discharge and obstruction. Investigation and treatment is the same as for the bilateral except that there is no need for immediate surgery, since one side of the nose is patent and normal. Feeding difficulty may be present in small infants but there is no obvious respiratory distress. However, the condition should later be treated surgically as outlined above.

In the period 1959–68, sixty-five cases of *posterior choanal atresia* were seen at The Hospital for Sick Children, Great Ormond Street. Of these thirty cases were male and thirty-five female. The condition was bilateral in thirty cases and unilateral in thirty-five cases. There were associated congenital anomalies present in twenty-eight cases. One case died while under observation. All cases were treated surgically and subsequent transpalatal operation was not needed.

Hereditary Haemorrhagic Telangiectasia

(Osler–Rendu–Weber disease)
This condition commonly presents with frequent and severe epistaxes.

LARYNX

Embryology

The hypobranchial eminence or copula is formed in the floor of the primitive pharynx between the ventral ends of the second, third and fourth arches. The primitive larynx, bronchi and lungs develop from the floor of the embryonic pharynx in the third week. The tracheo-bronchial groove appears behind the copula and it gives rise to the tracheobronchial tube and lung buds. The cephalic end of the groove is the first rudiment of the larynx. The boundaries of the primitive laryngeal inlet are derived from the sixth branchial arch. The laryngeal cartilages are derived from the fourth arch (thyroid cartilage) and the sixth arch (epiglottis, arytaenoid cartilages, cricoid cartilage) and they appear about the sixth week. The laryngeal inlet is at first a vertical slit but this shape is altered when the arytaenoids develop and change into a T-shaped opening. The walls of this opening adhere to each other soon after its appearance and the aperture becomes occluded. The lumen is re-established in the third foetal month. Failure of recanalization of this primitive laryngeal cleft may result in a laryngeal web.

Laryngeal Stridor

The age incidence and the character of the stridor are not particularly helpful in making a diagnosis. In almost every case the direct inspection of the larynx and trachea by a laryngologist experienced in paediatric pathology is advisable.

Coincident micrognathia is sometimes associated with stridor. The obstruction in these cases is not laryngeal in origin but due to the tongue falling back, and if the tongue can be kept forward it will cease. Sometimes the obstruction is so severe that tracheostomy is called for.

A few words on the actual performance of a tracheostomy on very young infants may be helpful. It is by no means an easy procedure. Except in the direct emergency, the operation should be done under general anaesthesia. A suckling bronchoscope, or suitable-sized endotracheal anaesthetic tube, should always be passed into the trachea before the operation is started. If this precaution is taken, the airway is secure, and the operation can be done without undue haste. The actual approach to the trachea, which in infants is very soft, is simplified, since there is a tube already in it, and if a bronchoscope is used the terminal illumination can be employed to outline the trachea. The opening into the trachea should be as low as possible, remembering always that the innominate vessels protrude up into the root of the neck in the very young.

'Congenital Laryngeal Stridor', 'Laryngomalacia', 'Infantile Larynx'

The common congenital anomaly of the so-called 'infantile larynx' has been shown to account for 40 per cent of cases of laryngeal stridor in infants and children. In this condition the large arytenoids prolapse forward with each inspiration into the glottic opening. The aryepiglottic folds are lax and the epiglottis is narrowed and folded backwards. Once the diagnosis is established by direct laryngoscopy the parents may be reassured that the child will outgrow the stridor as the larynx develops. A warning must be given to treat respiratory infections with special care.

Laryngeal Webs

Most commonly these are seen as a membrane across the anterior half or two-thirds of the cords but may also occur in the supraglottic and subglottic regions. In cases where the airway is insufficient a tracheostomy must be done and when the child is older the web excised through a laryngo-fissure approach and a graft inserted.

Laryngeal Atresia

The newborn infant with this condition cannot survive without an immediate tracheostomy, and prompt diagnosis is essential. Those responsible for resuscitation of the newborn should be trained in the use of the infant laryngoscope. No time should be wasted before examining the larynx when a baby is seen to be making powerful respiratory movements without any air exchange.

Congenital Cysts and Laryngoceles

Cysts occasionally occur in relation to the aryepiglottic folds, false cords, or laryngeal ventricles. A tracheostomy may be necessary as an emergency procedure and the cyst is de-capped and aspirated endocystically. Because these cysts tend to reform, this endocystic procedure may need to be repeated several times.

Hemi-Larynx

This consists of a cleft in the posterior wall of the larynx between the arytaenoids. Rarely this may prove fatal as a result of laryngeal spillover.

Congenital Subglottic Stenosis

Thickening of the subglottic tissues and sometimes of the true cords may cause severe respiratory obstruction and necessitate tracheostomy. Decannulation is particularly difficult in these cases.

Tracheal stenosis due to deficiency of the tracheal cartilaginous rings is rare; it gives rise to inspiratory and expiratory stridor, unlike the conditions localized to the glottis, which produce only an inspiratory stridor. Similarly, narrowing of the trachea by tracheal webs and by aberrant blood vessels also produces an inspiratory and expiratory stridor.

Haemangioma

A haemangioma of the larynx or trachea may be present at birth. When this tumour is localized to a sessile or pedunculated growth severe respiratory distress may result. Emergency tracheostomy becomes necessary. These tumours tend to grow smaller and become increasingly avascular after the first year of life, but they may necessitate excision through a laryngofissure after a preliminary short course of radiotherapy.

Congenital Laryngeal Nerve Paralysis

This may be bilateral or unilateral, partial or complete. The bilateral cases are always associated with other neurological lesions. The left-sided unilateral cases are commonly associated with cardiovascular anomalies.

SELECTED REFERENCES

Birch D.A. (1961) Laryngeal stridor in infants and children. *J. Laryng.* **75,** 833

Collins E. Treacher- (1900) Case with symmetrical congenital notches in the outer part of each lower lid and defective development of the malar bones. *Trans. Ophth. Soc. U.K.* **20,** 190

Craig D.H. & Simpson N.M. (1959) Posterior choanal atresia. *J. Laryng.* **73,** 603

Crooks J. (1954) Non-inflammatory laryngeal stridor in infants. *Arch. Dis. Childh.* **29,** 12

Fearon B. & Dickson J. (1968) Bilateral choanal atresia in the newborn. *Laryngoscope* **78,** 1487

Fisch L. (1959) Deafness as part of an hereditary syndrome. *J. Laryng.* **73,** 355

Fisch L. & Norman A.P. (1961) Hyperbilirubinaemia and perceptive deafness. *Brit. med. J.* **2,** 142

Franceschetti A. (1944) Un syndrome nouveau: la dysostose madibulo-faciale. *Bull. Schweiz. Akad. Med. Wiss.* **1,** 60

Fraser G. (1964) Profound childhood deafness. *J. med. Genet.* **1**, 118
Gill N.W. (1969) Congenital atresia of the ear. *J. Laryng.* **83**, 551
Hall J.G. (1962) A histological investigation of the auditory pathways in neonatal asphyxia. *Acta Otol.* **54**, 369
Hollinger P.A. (1961) Anomalies of the larynx, trachea, bronchi and oesophagus. *J. Laryng.* **75**, 1
Hough J.V.D. (1969) Inaudo-stapedial joint separation; etiology, treatment and significance. *Laryngoscope* **69**, 644
Jackson & Fisch L. (1958) Deafness following maternal rubella. *Arch. Dis. Childh.* **2**, 1241
Jervell A. & Lange Nielsen F. (1957) Congenital deaf-mutism, functional heart disease with prolongation of the Q–T interval and sudden death. *Amer. Heart J.* **54**, 59
Livingstone G. & Delahunty J.E. (1968) Malformation of the ear associated with congenital ophthalmic and other conditions. *J. Laryng.* **82**, 495
Stevenson A.C. & Cheeseman E.A. (1956) Hereditary deaf-mutism. *Ann. Hum. Genet.* **20**, 177
Waardenburg P.J. (1951) New syndrome combining developmental anomalies of eyelids etc. *Amer. J. Hum. Genet.* **3**, 195
Wilson T.G. (1962) *Diseases of the Ear, Nose and Throat in Children*, 2nd edn. London: Heinemann.

5

Abnormalities of the Eyes and Associated Structures

C.A.BROWN

METHODS OF EXAMINATION

The eyes of a newly-born infant are not easy to examine in detail without special methods. The essentials are:

(i) a darkened room,
(ii) dilated pupils,
(iii) a magnifying lens,
a focusing torch and
an ophthalmoscope,
(iv) relaxed eyelids of the infant.

The room is darkened but a complete blackout is unnecessary. The pupils are dilated with drops of homatropine 1 per cent or phenylephrine 10 per cent instilled half an hour beforehand. A binocular loupe (magnifying $\times 2\frac{1}{2}$) or a monocular loupe ($\times 10$) are necessary for details in the anterior segment of the eye. Direct illumination can be obtained from a torch that will focus to a narrow beam, a hand slit-lamp or an ophthalmoscope with the head detached. In most cases good relaxation of the eyelids is obtained when the infant sucks a feeding-bottle. Standing above the head, the examiner separates the lids by thumb and forefinger, or the assistant may retract the lower lid. A speculum or separate lid-retractors are rarely necessary. If the eyes roll up during examination, the baby should be lifted on the nurse's shoulder for a few seconds and the righting reflex brings the eyes central again. If further details are required or if a good view is not obtained, a general anaesthetic should be given, a speculum inserted, and fixation forceps used to rotate the globe. If slit-lamp microscopy is indicated, this can be done under heavy sedation (e.g. rectal 'avertin').

Results of Examination

External anomalies of the eyes, lids or lacrimal apparatus are easily seen on routine inspection. Magnification is required for details in the anterior segment—e.g. anomalies of the iris and lens. Finally, ophthalmoscopic examination of the fundi and media is carried out through dilated pupils. The pupillary area is examined with a $+12$ dioptre lens in the ophthalmoscope, when anomalies of the pupil and lens will be seen, and the fundus is examined with a plain lens in the ophthalmoscope, when anomalies of disc, retina and choroid can be detected. Intermediate plus lenses are used for anomalies in the vitreous, e.g. hyaloid artery, and minus lenses are often required to counteract the temporary myopia of small premature infants.

EYELIDS

Certain abnormalities of the eyelids, well described by Duke-Elder, occur during intra-uterine development.

Epicanthus

This is an abnormal fold of skin at the inner end of the upper lid which crosses the inner canthus obliquely and is lost in the skin on the side of the nose (Fig. 5.1). It is usually bilateral, though perhaps unequal, and is associated with a flat broad bridge of the nose. The fold covers part of the sclera on the inner side of the cornea, and the eye appears to be nearer the inner canthus than it really is, giving the illusion of a convergent squint, especially when the eye is adducted (Fig. 5.1). Epicanthus often occurs in infants who are otherwise normal, and tends to disappear as the bridge of the nose develops. It may, however, be associated with other ocular anomalies such as ptosis and blepharophimosis, or other general defects like brachycephaly.

Simple epicanthus is often inherited as a dominant characteristic but other types of inheritance are also found. Sex incidence is equal and consanguinity sometimes is present.

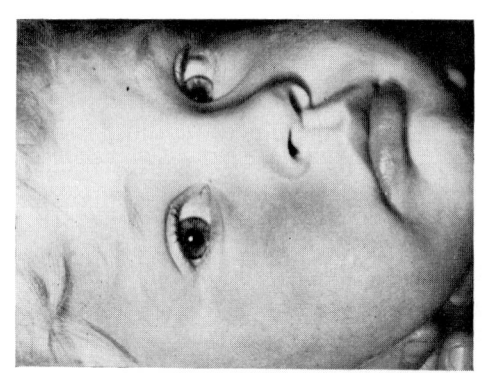

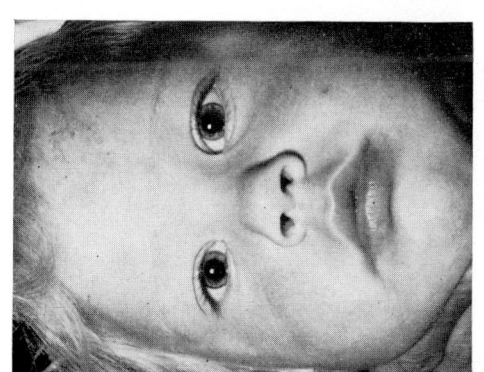

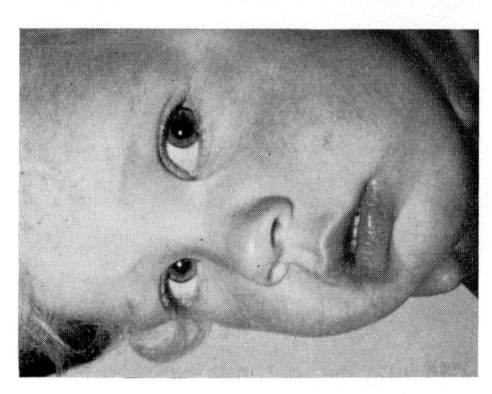

FIG. 5.1. Bilateral epicanthus showing the illusion of a convergent squint.

Epicanthus with ptosis is a dominant affection which is commoner in males than females. In Down's syndrome (mongolism) there is the characteristic slant of the palpebral fissures upwards and outwards. It is frequently associated with epicanthus and the highest point of the upper lid is at its mid-point and not, as it is normally in Western races, at the junction of the inner one-third and outer two-thirds.

Treatment. The simple form disappears with growth and no treatment is required. In epicanthus with ptosis the child's appearance can be improved by operations on the upper lid and the inner canthus after the age of 3 years.

BLEPHAROPHIMOSIS

Blepharophimosis is a congenital shortening of the palpebral aperture, both horizontally and vertically. It is very rare as an isolated defect and usually occurs in association with epicanthus (which may be 'epicanthus inversus'—see Fig. 5.2) and ptosis or with dwarfism or mongolism. It is inherited as a dominant affection.

Treatment is similar to that for epicanthus with ptosis (see above).

CRYPTOPHTHALMOS

Cryptophthalmos is a very rare condition where there is congenital absence of the eyelids. The cornea and conjunctiva are replaced by skin, and under it is a grossly disorganized globe. Occasionally the upper lids only or the lower lids only are absent. The condition has been recorded in several sibships.

Treatment. In total cryptophthalmos nothing can be done. If only one eyelid on each side is absent, an immediate attempt—in the first days of life—should be made to cover the cornea.

ANKYLOBLEPHARON

Ankyloblepharon is a condition where the lid-margins are fused in part of their length. The union is usually at the inner or outer canthus but rarely there may be a band-shaped adhesion or adhesions of the lid-margins away from the canthi (filiform type). It may be associated

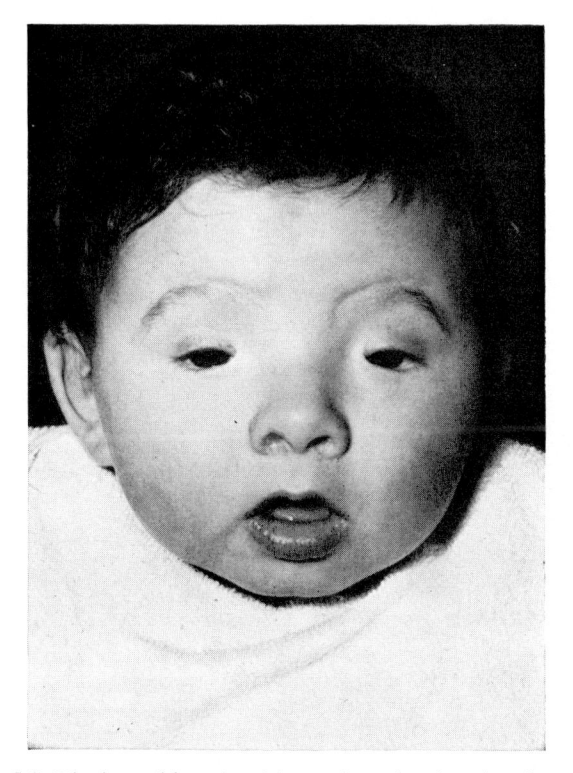

FIG. 5.2. Blepharophimosis with ptosis and epicanthus inversus.

with microphthalmos or anophthalmos. Some cases have been described in sibs, and a genetic cause is most likely.

Treatment. The bands can be simply divided and excised.

Entropion

Entropion of the lower lids occurs in infants in association with epiblepharon, which is an abnormal skin fold which crosses the lower lid horizontally and causes its inversion. The inversion is increased on looking down and decreased on looking up. The lashes rub on the cornea and may cause some irritation, but as they are soft in infants they rarely

152 CONGENITAL ABNORMALITIES IN INFANCY

cause ulceration. It is probably due to an abnormal insertion of strands of the orbicularis or the inferior rectus into the skin (Fig. 5.3).

Strapping down the lid is usually sufficient treatment, as the condition undergoes spontaneous cure in most cases by the age of 1 year. Occasionally a skin-muscle operation is required.

Coloboma

Coloboma, or notch, of the lid (Fig. 5.4) may occur as an isolated

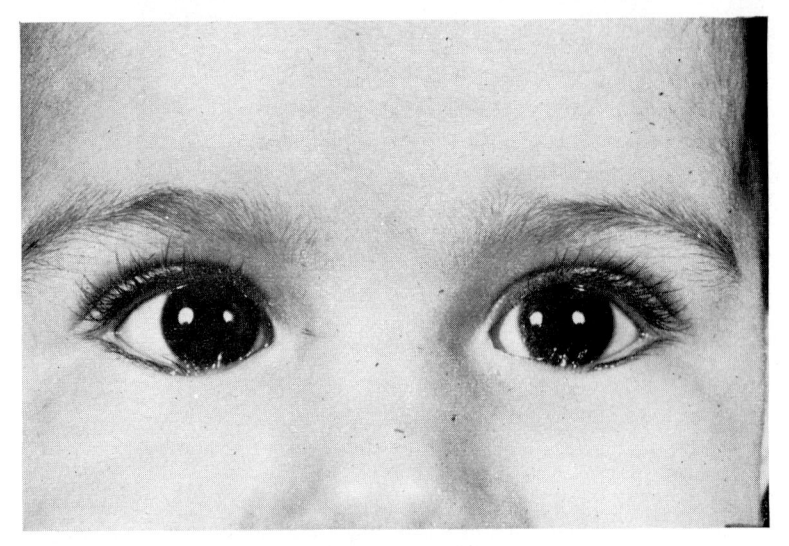

FIG. 5.3. Entropion.

ocular defect or in association with other defects in the eye or elsewhere in the body. In the upper lid it is usually in the inner half, and in the lower lid in the outer. The ocular defects include dermoids (often limbal and opposite the coloboma), corneal opacities and coloboma of iris, and general malformations include harelip and cleft palate and mandibulo-facial dysostosis (coloboma at outer end of lower lids, palpebral fissures sloping down and out, hypoplasia of the malar bones and macrostomia).

Treatment. Plastic repair of the defect should be carried out. The operation is urgent if the cornea is exposed.

Ptosis

Congenital ptosis occurs as a congenital defect of one or both upper eyelids, the unilateral type being the commoner. It may be associated with a weakness of the superior rectus muscle on the same side. This simple form is the commonest type and accounts for 77 per cent of all

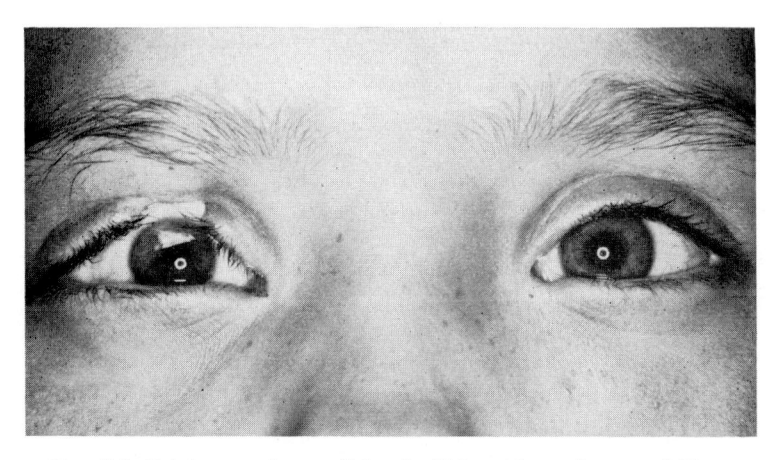

Fig. 5.4. Coloboma of upper lid and of iris, with persistance of fibrovascular tissue in the pupil.

cases. It shows a dominant transmission and equal sex incidence in most cases, and is due to faulty development of the levator palpebrae superioris between the third and fourth month *in utero*. In a second type additional deformities of the lids may be present, especially epicanthus and blepharophimosis. Again, according to Berke, the transmission is dominant and males are more commonly affected (3·5 per cent of all cases).

In a third type ptosis is complicated by varying degrees of external ophthalmoplegia. This may be peripheral or central (nuclear) in origin, and is transmitted as a dominant or recessive characteristic (9–12 per cent of all cases).

Ptosis also occurs rarely in congenital paralysis of the sympathetic and in jaw-winking (q.v.).

In bilateral cases the young child contracts the frontalis in an effort to raise the upper lids, and in a severe case will also throw his head back in an effort to uncover the pupils. The drooping upper lids are smooth and devoid of the normal lid folds. The true amount of ptosis can be shown by fixing the eyebrow with the thumb when the frontalis is relaxed.

Treatment is surgical. The best operation is a shortening (resection) of the levator muscle itself, either by a conjunctival (Blaskowic) or skin (Everbusch) approach. This is not usually attempted before the age of 3 years because of the chance of spontaneous improvement up to that time and the technical difficulty of the operation in an infant. In a severe bilateral case in an infant, ptosis spectacles should be provided till then.

Jaw-winking

Jaw-winking (the Marcus Gunn phenomenon) is an interesting paradoxical movement present from birth where the upper lid is elevated as the mouth is opened and the infant sucks. It is unilateral and is associated with ptosis on the same side. An abnormal connection between the nerve-supplies of the upper lid and jaw may exist or there may be a reflex contraction of smooth muscle in the levator initiated by jaw movements. In mild cases no treatment is required but in the severe forms the operation of division of the levator and elevation of the lid by other means (e.g. fascial strips) can be performed.

Distichiasis

Distichiasis is a very rare anomaly where a double row of lashes is present on upper and lower lids on both sides. The posterior row are finer and are in the line of the Meibomian duct orifices.

The defect may be familial, with dominant transmission. If the lashes cause irritation they should be removed by electrolysis, or by excision of the lash-bearing area followed by a mucous-membrane graft to fill the defect.

Angiomata

These are congenital tumours of blood vessels or lymphatics. They are often present at birth and tend to grow in the first few weeks and months after birth. After that, spontaneous regression may occur, so that by the age of 2 years they may be much smaller. They occur in the eyelids, conjunctiva and orbit as two main types—haemangioma and lymphangioma. In the lid and conjunctiva (Fig. 5.5) they may be disfiguring and in the posterior part of the orbit they cause proptosis.

Treatment
Nothing need be done before the age of 2 except in desperate cases.

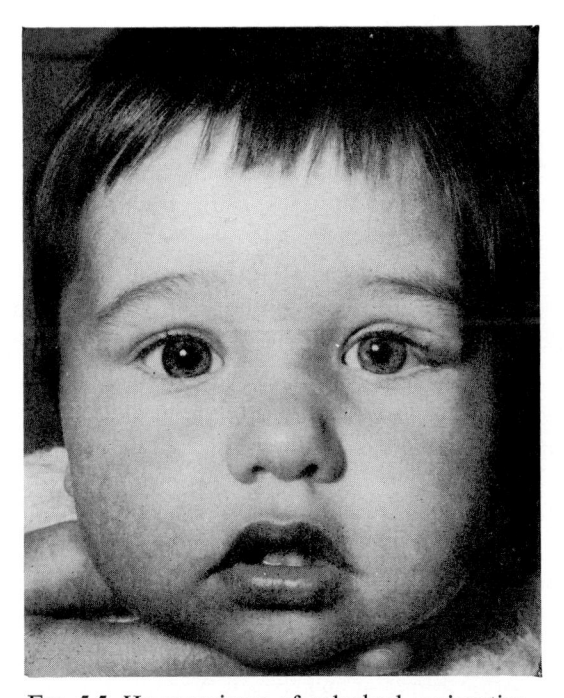

FIG. 5.5. Haemangioma of palpebral conjunctiva.

Small accessible tumours should be excised or treated by radiotherapy. Larger tumours may be treated by surgery or by radiotherapy.

GLOBE

CYCLOPIA

This monstrosity occurs when a single median eye exists or varying degrees of fusion of the two eyes has taken place. There has been suppression of the midline structures very early on in development. There may be a complete eye, with a single cornea, sclera, lens or retina, or there may be varying degrees of fusion of two eyes. Colobomata are common. There are gross deformities of the skull and brain and the monster is not viable.

Anophthalmos

Anophthalmos, where no development of the eyes has occurred, is rare, and is usually associated with abnormalities of the brain. According to Mann, three types occur—(1) primary anophthalmos, where there is failure of development of the primary optic vesicle; (2) secondary anophthalmos, where there is failure of development of the whole fore-brain and the absence of the eyes results from that; (3) degenerative anophthalmos, where the optic vesicle, after its formation, degenerates and disappears. In many cases of apparent anophthalmos, a small rudimentary eye may be found microscopically at the apex of the orbit and so should be classified as microphthalmos. The cause is probably genetic, with recessive transmission. A recessive sex-linked pedigree of anophthalmos has been described where mental deficiency was present in 50 per cent of cases.

Microphthalmos

This is present when the globe has failed to develop to its normal size, being usually about two-thirds of normal (Fig. 5.6). In extreme cases there may be only a vestigial remnant. The eye is abnormal in other respects and is often blind or nearly so. Accompanying ocular defects include corneal opacities, cataract, vitreous haze, and chorio-retinal inflammation and degeneration. The condition may be unilateral or bilateral. If it is unilateral, the other eye is usually defective.

Causes

(a) *Inflammatory.* There are two well-recognized intra-uterine causes —maternal rubella in the first 3 months of pregnancy and maternal toxoplasmosis transmitted to the foetus early in pregnancy. The role of other maternal illnesses early in pregnancy or other physico-chemical or nutritional factors is so far undetermined.

(b) *Genetic.* Microphthalmos frequently occurs as an inherited anomaly associated with other ocular defects, especially coloboma of iris and choroid (q.v.). According to Sorsby, transmission may be dominant, with variations in the severity of the affection. Thus minor degrees may have coloboma of choroid only, and severe degrees will have bilateral microphthalmos with colobomata of iris and choroid. A few cases may be of the recessive sex-linked type associated with corneal opacities,

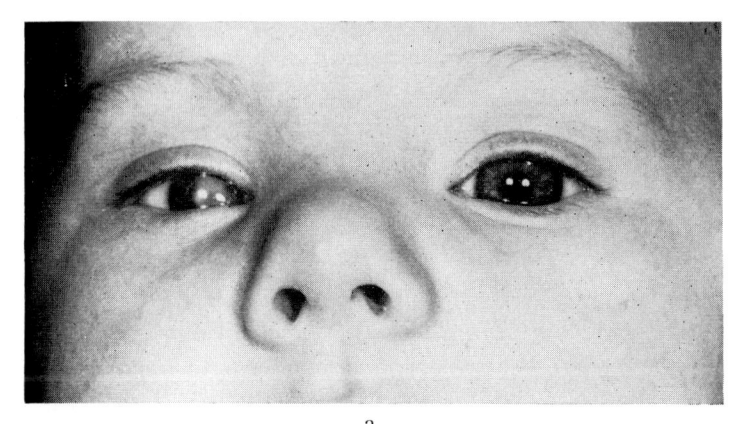

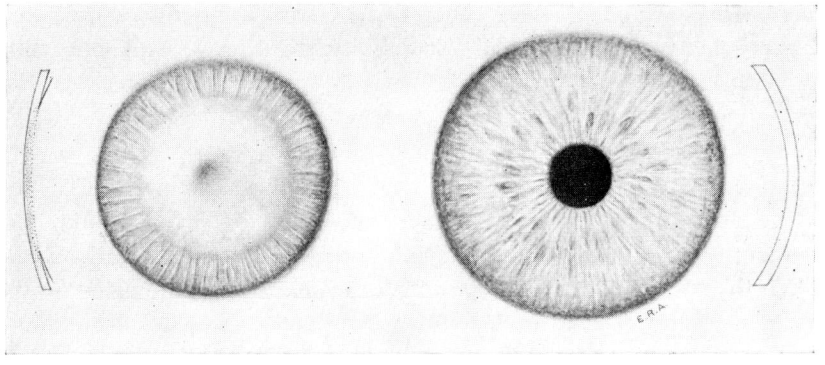

Fig. 5.6 (a and b). Unilateral congenital corneal opacities and microphthalmos.

cataract and mental deficiency, but the exact mode of inheritance of many is not clear. It has also been described in association with myopia and retinitis pigmentosa, glaucoma and cataract. In other cases it must be admitted that the cause is unknown.

(c) *Retrolental fibroplasia* is also a cause of microphthalmos. In the severe form there are small, shrunken eyes with the appearance of enophthalmos, shallow anterior chambers, atrophic irides, and bilateral retrolental membranes. This is not, of course, a congenital abnormality but an acquired disease in premature infants due to excessive concentrations of oxygen in the infant's incubator.

Treatment
If the defect is unsightly, enucleation and replacement by an artificial eye should be carried out. An implant buried in Tenon's capsule gives a better-fitting eye with a small range of movement. Enucleation in infancy tends to inhibit orbital growth and so operation should be deferred till 5 or 7 years of age.

Coloboma of Iris and Choroid and Retina

During the early weeks of intra-uterine development the foetal fissure is open on the under-surface of the optic vesicle. This closes by the sixth week (14 mm stage). When normal closure fails to occur, a coloboma will result. This may be due to a variety of causes, such as genetic defects, with dominant transmission, infections (including rubella, toxoplasmosis) and possibly other factors such as toxins, anoxia and physico-chemical, mechanical or radiational causes, still not fully understood.

Clinical Appearances (Fig. 5.7)
The defect is usually partial, involving choroid and retina, but it may extend forwards to involve the iris and the ciliary body, and, less frequently, back to involve the disc. It is bilateral in over half the cases. When the iris is involved, the pupil is pear-shaped and the defect in the iris passes downwards and slightly inwards. When the choroid and retina only are involved, there is a large ectatic area of chorio-retinal atrophy in the lower part of the fundus. This passes down and slightly outwards and has a white background (bare sclera), sharp edges, often with clumps of pigment on them, and a rounded upper border. Usually this border is below the disc but occasionally the disc is included in the defect. The anterior part of the defect usually spreads to the periphery of the fundus but occasionally both ends are visible or there may be several islands along the line of the fissure. The coloboma is often deeply excavated (ectatic) and a few retinal or choroidal vessels may be seen on its surface.

A varying degree of visual defect is always present, and nystagmus and squint are common. Other ocular abnormalities are frequently

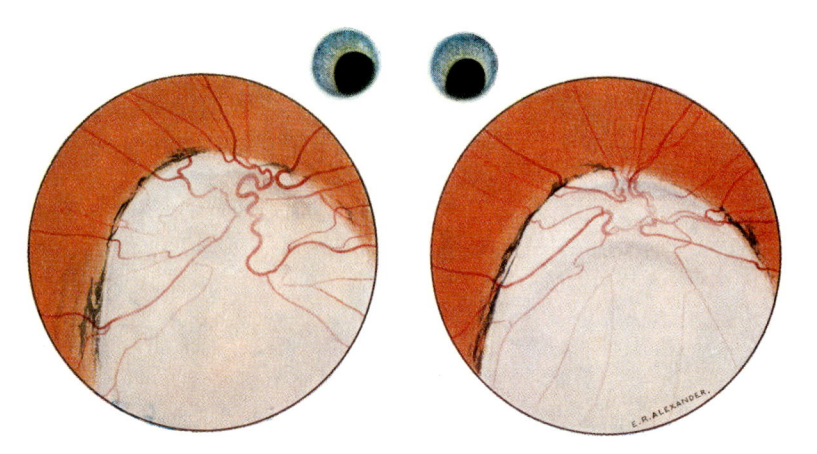

FIG. 5.7. Coloboma of iris, choroid and retina, involving the disk.

facing p. 158

present—microphthalmos, corneal opacities, cataract, hyaloid remnants, macular and optic nerve defects, and high myopia. Varying degrees of microphthalmos and colobomata have been described in different members of the same family. According to Sorsby, congenital malformations elsewhere in the body may also exist, e.g. heart, brain, kidney.

Treatment
The defect cannot be repaired and the only possible treatment (not often carried out, or rarely done before the age of 10) is the fitting of an opaque contact lens with an artificial iris painted on it, leaving a clear central pupil.

Coloboma of the Disc

This may occur in two forms:

(a) *As part of a coloboma of choroid and retina*, when the defect includes the disc. It is possible to identify the pale disc enclosed by the white coloboma of the choroid (Fig. 5.7). In extreme cases there may be thinning of the wall of the coloboma, which becomes ectatic and projects backwards to form a retrobulbar cyst. The upper retinal vessels reach the fundus normally, but the lower either skirt the edge of the coloboma to reach normal retina, or they may run separate from the nerve to pierce the coloboma or enter round its edge.

(b) *As an isolated coloboma of the optic nerve*. This is a rare condition and may be of varying degree from a small crater in the disc to a deep excavation much larger than the disc, pushing the nerve to one side. Except in the smallest defects, the visual acuity is seriously affected.

The causation is similar to that of coloboma of the choroid (q.v.)

(c) *Crater-like holes* in the disc are essentially small colobomata of the optic nerve. The hole dips down towards the vaginal sheath of the nerve, being within the dural sheath. There is often, but not always, a scotoma associated with the hole in the corresponding area of the visual field.

Dermoids

(a) *Limbal*. These occur as solid tumours of a pink-white colour astride the limbus, half on sclera and half on cornea, usually in the lower outer segment (Fig. 5.8). Sometimes they are purely *corneal* (7 per cent) or *scleral* (13 per cent). Usually no other malformation is present but they may be present opposite a coloboma of the lid.

(b) *Conjunctival.* A frequent situation is on the globe between the recti muscles, usually between superior and external. They are a yellowish-white colour, oval in shape, and tend to grow after birth. The tumour is adherent to the underlying sclera, which may be thinner than normal.

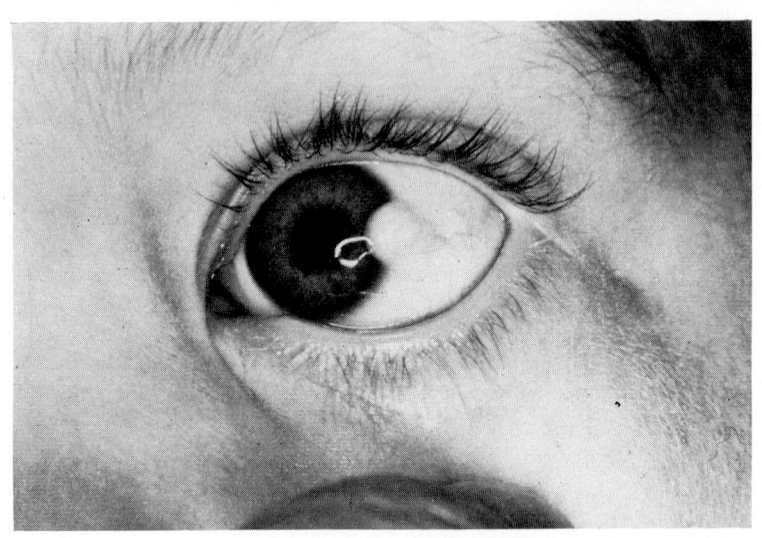

Fig. 5.8. Limbal Dermoid.

Sometimes they are subconjunctival and are then known as dermolipomata. Microscopically they are typical of dermoids elsewhere in the body—fibro-fatty tumours with keratinized epithelium on the surface, and containing hair follicles, sebaceous and sweat glands.

The cause of the developmental defect is unknown. The existence of a coloboma of the lid is perhaps a developmental fault secondary to the presence of the dermoid on the globe.

Treatment
If they are cosmetically noticeable or if they cause irritation, they should be removed. Limbal dermoids can be shaved off, but care must be taken as the underlying cornea may be already thin. A corneal scar will be left at the site of the tumour which can be tattooed if noticeable.

CORNEA

MICROCORNEA

This occurs when the anterior segment of eye, though normal, is small, and the cornea is less than 11 mm in diameter. The eye is not very hypermetropic and vision is good. A familial tendency has been noted and glaucoma is a frequent complication in adult life. It must be distinguished from *microphthalmos* where there are other associated deformities and vision is always defective.

There is no treatment except for the complication of glaucoma.

Megalocornea

This is a condition where both corneae are abnormally large (over 13 mm in diameter) (Fig. 5.9). It is inherited as a sex-linked recessive, or

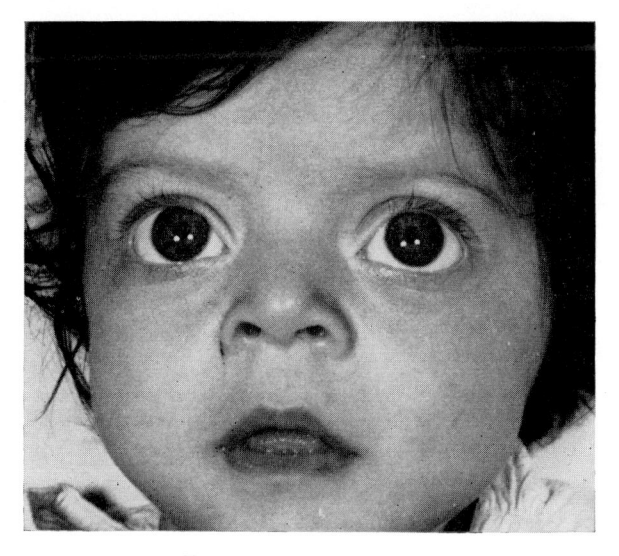

Fig. 5.9. Megalocornea.

more rarely, as a dominant characteristic. Males are more commonly affected, but it does occur in females after consanguineous marriages. The zonule tends to be weak, so that subluxation of the lens often occurs in adult life, with the further possible complications of cataract and secondary glaucoma. The primary lesion may be an abnormally large ciliary ring and the large cornea would then be a secondary feature.

Differential Diagnosis

It must be carefully distinguished from congenital glaucoma (buphthalmos). In megalocornea the ocular tension is normal, the cornea is clear and the disc is normal, whereas in congenital glaucoma the tension is raised, the cornea is often cloudy and the disc may be cupped.

Treatment is required only if cataract or glaucoma develops in adult life, when operation may be necessary.

Congenital Corneal Opacities

Corneal opacities may be present at birth in one or both eyes (Fig. 5.6). They may be partial or total. If total, no details of the iris can be seen. Many other ocular abnormalities are usually present, which may include microphthalmos, anterior and posterior synechiae, coloboma of iris and choroid, iris atrophy, cataract and retinal defects.

In severe cases the whole of the anterior segment is disorganized and the tissues are fused together to form an *anterior staphyloma.*

The *cause* may be an intra-uterine inflammation (e.g. syphilis) or other intra-uterine toxic, physico-chemical or mechanical disturbance, birth trauma (e.g. forceps), or occasionally a genetic defect. Pressure of forceps during delivery may cause a split in Descemet's membrane and a localized opacity in the substance of the cornea. This often clears up completely, although the split in Descemet's membrane will always be visible on the slit-lamp.

Treatment

If the cause might have been intra-uterine inflammation and if the anterior chamber is present, it is worth trying the effect of hydrocortisone drops or ointment q.i.d. for a few months, as they may help to produce some clearing of the opacity.

Embryotoxon

This is a ring of opacity round the periphery of the deeper layers of the cornea. It is caused by an adhesion of the capsulo-pupillary lamina to the cornea and is associated with a poorly developed iris. It is often genetically determined. It may occur in cases of megalocornea and blue sclerotics. Sometimes the opacity reaches the centre of the cornea, two such cases having been seen in sisters.

Hyaline Membrane

This is a rare anomaly of the posterior corneal surface in which a thin membrane stretches round the anterior chamber, mainly in the periphery, where it is only partly adherent to the posterior corneal surface, and is associated with a poorly developed iris.

There is no treatment for either of these conditions.

IRIS

Coloboma

This is of two types:

(a) *Typical* coloboma occurs down and in, and is always associated with coloboma of the choroid, as part of failure of closure of the foetal fissure (see above and Fig. 5.7).

(b) *Simple* coloboma involves the iris only (Fig. 5.4). The pupil is often pear-shaped and the cleft may point in any direction. There may be a slit, notch or hole in the iris or there may be partial or total aniridia. It is usually unilateral. A persistent pupillary membrane is often present and there may be a coloboma or opacity of the lens.

If the foetal fissure has closed normally, a coloboma of the iris, which is later in development, cannot be due to faulty closure of the fissure. The cause may either be a primary ectodermal defect at the rim of the optic cup with secondary failure of the mesoderm, or growth of the rim may be inhibited by the presence of abnormal vascularized strands of the fibro-vascular sheath of the lens. The latter cause is more likely for sporadic cases and the former for hereditary cases, when the deformity is transmitted as a dominant characteristic. There is a close relationship of these cases to aniridia (see below).

Treatment
A contact lens can be tried (see coloboma of iris and choroid).

Aniridia

In aniridia no iris is visible on ordinary examination but a stump is always present on gonioscopic examination. The condition is bilateral and is a hereditary defect of the dominant type. There is a close link with simple coloboma of the iris, and according to Sorsby, many pedigrees have been reported which contain both defects in different members of the same family.

The cause is failure of ectodermal development at the 70–80 mm stage (3 months) when ectoderm should grow forwards to form the rim of the optic cup (to become the ectodermal layer of the iris).

Clinically the infant with aniridia suffers from extreme photophobia, defective vision (from faulty macular development) and nystagmus. Other ocular defects such as congenital lens opacities (anterior or posterior capsular) or microphakia may also be present, and occasionally there are corneal opacities. Glaucoma may develop in later childhood or adult life. The only treatment is for photophobia (dark glasses or opaque contact lenses with an artificial pupil) and surgical treatment for glaucoma if it develops.

ABNORMAL PUPILS

Slit-shaped Pupils

This is a rare developmental defect in which the pupils may be slit-shaped or triangular. White strands may be present at either end of the slit, these being thought to be remains of an abnormal primary vitreous. There is often an associated congenital lens opacity, but the posterior segment of the globe is normal. A familial tendency has been observed.

Polycoria

True polycoria, where more than one true pupil is present, is very rare indeed.

False polycoria is less rare. Round or slit-like gaps are present in the iris, usually near the pupil border. These are due to patches of iris atrophy, either developmental or inflammatory in origin. Other ocular defects may be present, such as corneal opacities and capsular cataract. A bilateral congenital dialysis at the root of the iris also occurs; here a familial incidence has been reported.

Ectopic Pupils

An abnormal situation of the pupil may occur in one or both eyes.

Normally the pupil is slightly down and in from the centre of the iris, but it may be grossly displaced in any one direction, with or without abnormal strands of tissue associated with the displacement, and in most cases with subluxation of the lens. A hereditary tendency (dominant or recessive) is often found.

Ectropion of the Pigment Layer

This is an exaggeration of the normal pigment border of the pupil. There may be grape-like clusters of pigment (flocculi) round the pupil margin and projecting into the anterior chamber, common in animals but rare in man.

Iris Cysts

As congenital lesions these are rare and their cause is obscure. Unpigmented cysts may be derived from the surface epithelium, being an ingrowth from the surface similar to the developing lens, and pigmented cysts from the neural epithelium, including flocculi referred to above, these being dilatations of the marginal sinus at the anterior end of the primary optic vesicle.

No treatment is advisable for any of the abnormal pupils. Small iris cysts can be left alone, but if they are large and causing secondary glaucoma, they should be removed.

LENS

Coloboma

This may occur along with a typical coloboma of the choroid and iris as an anomaly of closure of the foetal fissure when the defect is in the usual situation downwards. More frequently it is seen as a defect (notch in, or flattening of, the edge of the lens) in any position round the circumference. There is usually an associated defect of the zonule, which indeed may be the primary lesion. There may also be a simple coloboma of the iris with a persistent pupillary membrane, when the cause is probably a persistence of capsulo-pupillary vessels in that area. Some cases are genetically determined, and in these an association with dislocation of the lens has been recorded, both conditions occurring in different members of the same family.

There is no treatment.

Ectopia Lentis

Congenital subluxation or dislocation of the lens is due to weakness or absence of a segment of the zonular fibres. The dislocation is usually upwards, the lower zonular fibres being the weak part (in the line of the foetal fissure). The edge of the lens may be seen in the pupil, showing a dark ring on ophthalmoscopic examination, so that two views of the fundus can be obtained, phakic and aphakic. If the dislocation is slight (subluxation) the only feature will be a tremulous iris (iridodonesis) on ocular movement in the subluxated area.

Ectopia lentis may occur as an isolated hereditary defect of the zonule (often with dominant transmission) perhaps associated with ectopic pupils, but more commonly it is seen as part of arachnodactyly (Marfan's syndrome). This is a widespread mesodermal anomaly in the body in which transmission is again dominant and ectopia lentis occurs in 55–60 per cent of cases. Miosis and high myopia are frequent features, and there may be megalocornea, coloboma of the lens and divergent squint.

It also occurs in homocystinuria. This is an inborn error of metabolism characterized by ectopia lentis, high myopia, mental retardation, fair complexion with malar flush, hepatosplenomegaly and genu valgum.

Treatment
If vision is good and ocular tension is normal, no treatment is required. If vision is defective, either from monocular diplopia or the development of cataract in the dislocated lens, surgical removal of the lens by discission or extraction (always difficult procedures in these cases), should be attempted. If the lens becomes dislocated into the anterior chamber, secondary glaucoma will develop and its immediate extraction is necessary.

Spherophakia

This is a rare condition in which the lens is small and spherical and the zonule is weak round the entire circumference of the lens. The latter, therefore, becomes more spherical, making the eye highly myopic, and the zonule will be clearly seen when the pupil is dilated. Complications are subluxation of the lens and 'inverse glaucoma' (glaucoma precipitated by miotics instead of mydriatics). It is a hereditary disease with recessive transmission, and there may be consanguinity. It may be associated with brachydactyly and brachycephaly (Marchesani's syndrome). There is no treatment unless complications develop.

ANTERIOR AND POSTERIOR LENTICONUS

These are rare conditions in which there is a localized conical elevation in the centre of the lens on its anterior or posterior surface. The posterior type is the commoner of the two. The ophthalmoscopic appearance is of an oily droplet in the centre of the pupil. There may be a persistent hyaloid artery associated with the posterior type. It may be due to a congenital weakness of the capsule but the exact cause is unknown. No treatment is of any value.

CONGENITAL CATARACT

This term includes cataract, whether total or partial, that is present at birth or develops soon after. Cataract which develops in adolescence or early adult life, such as coronary cataract, although developmental in origin, is excluded. On the other hand, other types of cataract which may develop soon after birth but which are not strictly congenital, are mentioned, as the differential diagnosis is important.

The classification of congenital cataract is not easy. Many authors classify them according to the appearance of the cataract (e.g. nuclear, sutural, posterior polar) but here an attempt is made to classify them according to cause.

There will, of course, be some overlapping of the groups, as more than one cause gives rise to the same type of cataract, and there is a group in which no cause is known. The main types are developmental, hereditary, nutritional (including lamellar), following maternal infection (especially rubella), and postnatal (in premature infants or in galactosaemia). In addition cataract occurs in certain syndromes—including Down's syndrome, oxycephaly. Lowe's syndrome, punctate epiphyseal dysplasia, and certain skin conditions.

An understanding of the embryology of the lens is important in placing the opacities in time of development. The central (embryonic) nucleus is earliest in development, being formed in the first 3 months by the original lens fibres. The foetal nucleus is formed round it from the third to ninth month by cells growing from the equator in onion-like layers under the anterior and posterior capsules. After birth the infantile nucleus develops outside the foetal nucleus and outside that again the adult nucleus. The cortex is a very thin layer at birth and gradually increases in thickness through life.

The 'sutures' are the zones of junction of the lens fibres as they join at anterior and posterior poles of the developing lens. Hence the anterior Y and the posterior inverted Y are formed in the whole thickness of the foetal nucleus.

DEVELOPMENTAL CATARACT

(a) POLAR

(i) Anterior Polar
This white opacity is localized in the centre of the capsule at the anterior pole. A persistent pupillary membrane is often attached to it. It may be inflammatory in origin, when it occurs before or after birth and is due to damage to the lens from foetal keratitis or a perforated corneal ulcer postnatally. On the other hand it may be a developmental defect due to a persistent pupillary membrane abnormally adherent to the lens. It also occurs in aniridia. In a few cases it occurs as a hereditary defect with dominant or rarely recessive transmission. The foetal nucleus is clear and so it is a late intra-uterine development. If it is a large opacity, it will impair vision and surgical removal may be attempted.

(ii) Posterior Polar
This is a localized opacity in the centre of the posterior pole of the lens. There are usually remnants of the hyaloid artery attached to it in spiral form. It is usually an isolated defect of the hyaloid system but a few cases are hereditary with dominant transmission. The latter may be later in onset (childhood or early adult life) and progressive and then will require operation.

(iii) Fibrous Tissue Cataract
This may result from a posterior polar cataract when vascular mesoderm

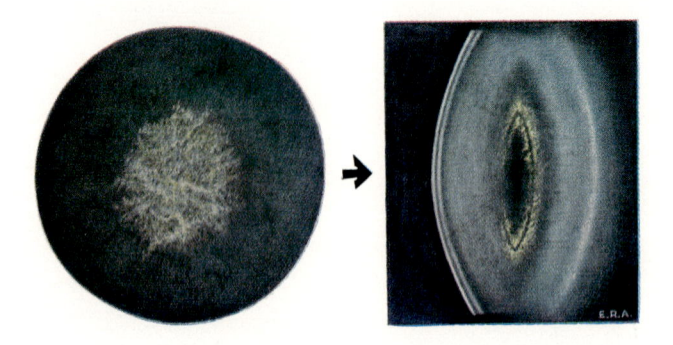

Fig. 5.10. Hereditary nuclear cataract, showing the numerous white dots in the foetal nucleus.

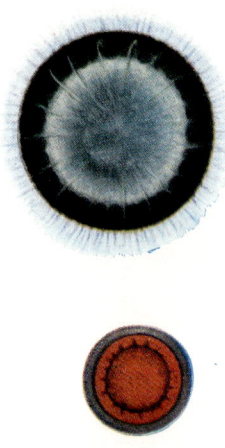

Fig. 5.11. Lamellar cataract showing the appearance in direct illumination and with ophthalmoscope.

facing p. 169

spreads through the lens capsule into the lens substance. The lens substance gradually degenerates and shrinks, leaving the pupil filled by a dense white membrane.

(b) Sutural Cataract

This is composed of many minute white dots along the lines of the anterior and posterior 'Y'. In babies these suture-lines lie very near the surface of the lens, as the cortex is thin and most of the lens composed of embryonic and foetal nucleus. Occasionally sutural cataracts are hereditarily determined with dominant transmission, having been observed in three generations.

The opacities are slight and do not interfere with vision.

HEREDITARY CATARACT

Some cataracts are genetically determined and are (usually) of dominant transmission. They are present in the early months of life, are bilateral and do not alter much with time, although they may get a little denser. The exception is the hereditary type of the posterior polar cataract, which is often progressive.

Nuclear Cataract (Cataracta Centralis Pulverulenta)

Nuclear cataract (Fig. 5.10) occurs as a central nuclear opacity consisting of large numbers of minute white granular dots in the embryonic or foetal nucleus. This is the same as the 'Coppock' cataract which occurred in the Coppock family originally described by Nettleship & Ogilvie in 1906 and which showed a strong familial tendency with dominant transmission. It remains unchanged through life and does not interfere with vision to any serious extent.

Anterior and posterior polar, sutural and lamellar cataracts are occasionally hereditary.

CATARACTS DUE TO NUTRITIONAL DISTURBANCES

Lamellar (Zonular) Cataract

This is the commonest type of congenital cataract (Fig. 5.11). It is bilateral and develops just before or just after birth. It consists of hundreds of small white dots in one of the central zones of the lens, in part of the foetal or infantile nucleus. The most central lens fibres are usually clear (embryonic nucleus) as is the most peripheral part of the lens (cortex), so that the lamellar cataract appears as a disc of opacity in the centre of the dilated pupil. There may be loops of opacity passing into the clear cortex, or there may be sectors where the opacity is absent. The density of the opacity varies greatly from case to case, from a faint haze only (with normal vision) to a dense opacity (with a gross visual defect). The smaller the size of the disc, the earlier it developed (if it is less than 6 mm in diameter, it developed before birth; if over 6 mm, it developed after birth). The eye is usually normal in all other respects.

Causes

There are many different causes.

(a) *Anoxia* plays a part in some cases. Experimental cataracts have been produced in newly-born rats by depriving the pregnant rat of oxygen. Lamellar cataracts have been seen to develop postnatally in premature infants who suffered from prenatal or postnatal anoxia (Brown, 1963; Hull, 1969). In some the lens itself becomes oedematous before going opaque. Further work is required to confirm this factor.

(b) *Calcium deficiency* was previously thought to be an important factor in their aetiology, either before or after birth, leading to infantile tetany and convulsions. These cases are now rare in this country and in a recent series of congenital cataracts Hull (1969) found no cases of tetany.

(c) There may be a link with aminoacid disturbance. Hyperaminoaciduria has been found in 16 out of 34 cases of congenital cataract described by Franceschetti, and this is also a factor in Lowe's syndrome.

(d) Some are due to toxic causes acting before or after birth.

Treatment

If the opacity is only slight and the fundus can be seen through it, then reasonably good vision can be expected and no operation is required. If the opacity is dense, permitting only a poor red reflex through it (but a normal view of the fundus through the periphery of the lens) vision will be defective and operation will probably be necessary. When there is any doubt, operation should be deferred till the age of 5 or 6 when more accurate subjective tests are possible. Cataract extraction usually gives good results in these cases—the best results for any single group of congenital cataracts. The modern technique is removal of the soft lens matter by an aspiration–irrigation technique, with or without a preliminary discission one week before. Either a single two-way syringe (Fuchs or Fink) or two separate syringes can be used.

CATARACTS DUE TO MATERNAL INFECTIONS

Rubella

Maternal rubella in the first 16 weeks of pregnancy may cause various congenital abnormalities in the infant, as Gregg first showed in 1941.

Cataract is more likely after infections in the first 6 weeks, when the lens vesicle is being formed and is separating from the surface ectoderm (14 mm stage or 6 weeks). The risk of cataract if maternal infection occurs in the first 4 weeks is as high as 50 per cent in some epidemics. Heart defects are more likely after infections between the fifth and ninth weeks and deafness between the eighth and twelfth weeks. Thus combinations of cataract and heart defects or heart defects and deafness are common, but cataract with deafness is rare. Cataract alone is rare, but heart defects alone or deafness alone are common. Cataract is 117 times commoner after maternal rubella than among the controls. It is thought to be due to a direct invasion of the lens by a virus which can be grown from the lens for up to 2 years after birth.

Clinical Features
The infant is small and undernourished and of low normal birthweight (17·7 per cent were under 2·5 kg compared with 4·3 per cent in the control series).

Ocular Signs
The eyes tend to be microphthalmic and the anterior chambers shallow. The cataract is usually a dense white nuclear opacity filling a small pupil. It is usually present at birth but has been seen to develop in the second month after birth. The pupil is most resistant to dilatation with mydriatics but after their instillation some peripheral clear lens giving a red reflex may be seen. If the cataract is unilateral, which it is in 25 per cent of cases, fine pigmentary degeneration of the retina, including the macula, will usually be present in the other eye.

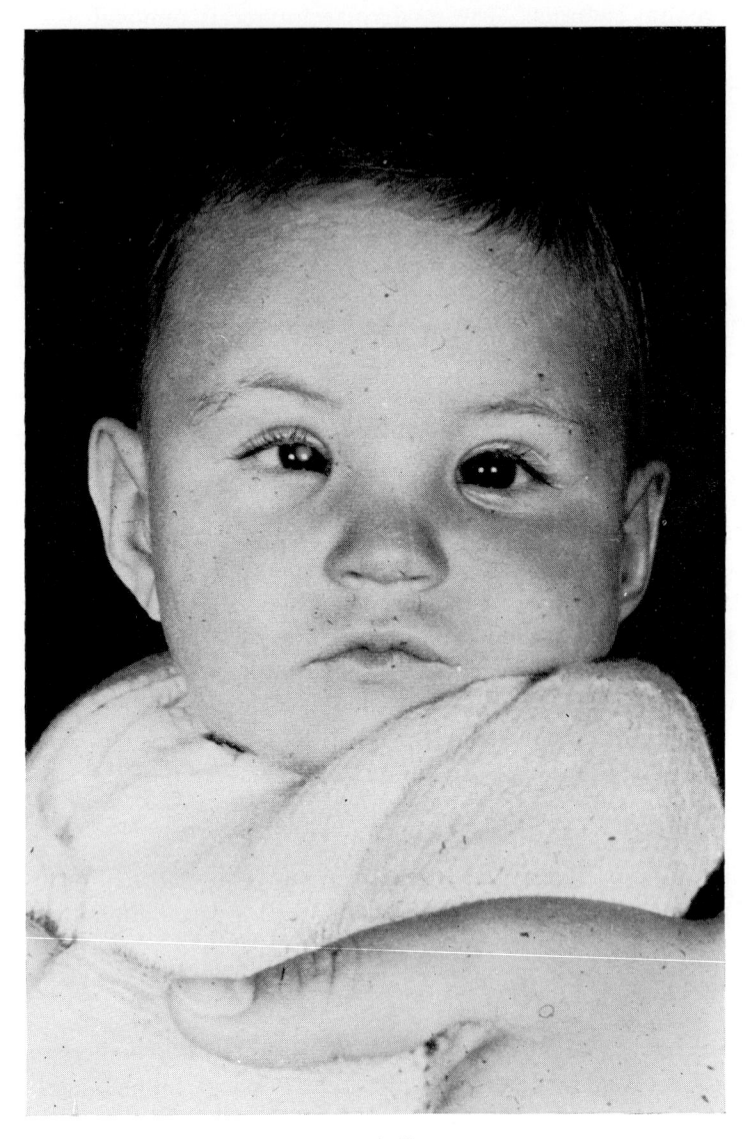

FIG. 5.12. Rubella cataract.

Occasionally spontaneous absorption of the lens matter occurs during the first or second year leading to a 'membranous' cataract.

Section of the cataractous lens shows degeneration and vacuolation of lens fibres and necrosis of the nuclei. The 'membrane' is a thin sheet of tissue in the pupil composed mostly of lens capsule.

Treatment

If the cataracts are dense and bilateral, early operation (usually between 6 and 9 months of age) is advisable to stimulate the development of vision. The general condition of the infant is usually poor and operation may have to be deferred for a few months on general grounds. Rubella cataracts tend to be more difficult to clear by operation than other types. There is also a risk of post-operative uveitis from release of live virus from the lens into the anterior chamber.

Monocular cataract does not do well after operation and an amblyopic eye is almost invariably present despite successful surgery. It is, therefore, best left alone.

Prophylactic Treatment

It is desirable that girls should have rubella before marriage, but unfortunately they do not always contract it when exposed to it. A more certain way is by inhalation of droplets produced by atomization of throat washings from patients with the disease. Passive immunization of pregnant women exposed to rubella can be given by using rubella gamma globulin from convalescent serum and active immunization should be available soon.

OTHER INFECTIONS IN PREGNANCY

Cataracts also occur in *toxoplasmosis* and *congenital syphilis*. In these cases they are complications of severe ocular inflammation—i.e. secondary cataracts. Severe uveitis may have occurred before birth and the baby is born with microphthalmos and cataract in one or both eyes and with a small irregular pupil or pupils showing posterior synechiae. In toxoplasmosis the active uveitis may take place postnatally and the cataract, often unilateral, will then develop postnatally.

In congenital syphilis cataract is a rare complication and is a sign of severe iridocyclitis, although in rare cases it may be present without other ocular signs.

The role of virus infections in pregnancy other than the above is, according to Manson, so far undetermined.

POSTNATAL CATARACTS

(a) *In Premature Infants*

A small group of cataracts occurs in premature infants. McDonald (1962) found eleven cases of cataract in a series of 1128 children who weighed 1·8 kg or less at birth, an incidence of 1 per cent compared with an incidence of one case among 2906 children of all birth weights. Lamellar cataracts have been seen to develop postnatally in premature infants who suffered from prenatal or postnatal anoxia (Brown, 1963; Hull, 1969). The eyes are normal at birth but bilateral swollen cataracts develop between the third week and third month postnatally. Anoxia may well play a part in the formation of these cataracts and may be linked with generalized oedema of the premature infant.

(b) *Galactosaemia*

Cataract is a common feature and occurs in at least 75 per cent of cases. The eyes are normal at birth but in the untreated case cataracts will develop any time between the third week and sixth month. The opacities are bilateral and nuclear in type, appearing as refractile discs in the foetal nucleus, which resemble large oil droplets. They are more like an early nuclear senile cataract than a lamellar cataract, being smaller in diameter and more translucent than the usual lamellar type. In the later stages they become more opaque, and cortical opacities develop near the surface of the lens. When the infant is treated by withdrawal of lactose from the diet, the cataracts often regress and even complete clearing has been seen.

CATARACT IN CERTAIN SYNDROMES

Cataract occurs in:
- (1) Down's syndrome (mongolism)
- (2) Oxycephaly
- (3) Lowe's syndrome (cerebro-oculo-renal dystrophy with amino-aciduria, congenital glaucoma and cataract) (see p. 372).

(4) Punctate epiphyseal dysplasia

It also occurs in certain cases of mental retardation inherited as a recessive characteristic and often associated with other abnormalities. It occurs in the following congenital skin diseases:

(1) Congenital ectodermal dysplasia
(2) Schaffer's syndrome
(3) Congenital ichthyosis
(4) Incontinentia pigmenti
(5) Rothmund's syndrome

Down's Syndrome (Mongolism)

In this condition a ring of pinpoint white spots near the periphery of the iris (Brushfield's spots) may occur. They are also found in normal eyes.

Cataract is present in about 50 per cent of all mongols. There are three main types:

(i) Arcuate lens opacities in the foetal nucleus, which accounts for one-sixth of the cases and is the type peculiar to mongolism.

(ii) Sutural opacities in the anterior Y of the foetal nucleus.

(iii) Flake opacities in the juvenile and adult nucleus, which is the commonest type. Other types also occur which are not typical of mongolism—disc-shaped, lamellar, and anterior and posterior polar cataract. The opacities are not often present at birth, being found at that stage in only 8 per cent of 165 mongols; then they are central and perinuclear (see Fig. 5.13). Most do not develop till adolescence or early adult life. They are nearly all very slow in progressing, they rarely become dense and surgery is not often required.

RETINA AND CHOROID

Coloboma of the Retina and Choroid

This has already been described.

'Coloboma' of the Macula

This is occasionally a developmental defect, but much more commonly it is due to intra-uterine inflammation and then should not be classed as a coloboma.

Familial Development Defect

This has been described a few times. Sorsby recorded a typical pedigree where a mother and five out of seven children all had bilateral macular colobomata and anomalies of hands and feet (absent nails, stunting of phalanges and a tendency to doubling of the terminal phalanx of the thumb). At both maculae there were white oval ectatic areas where the

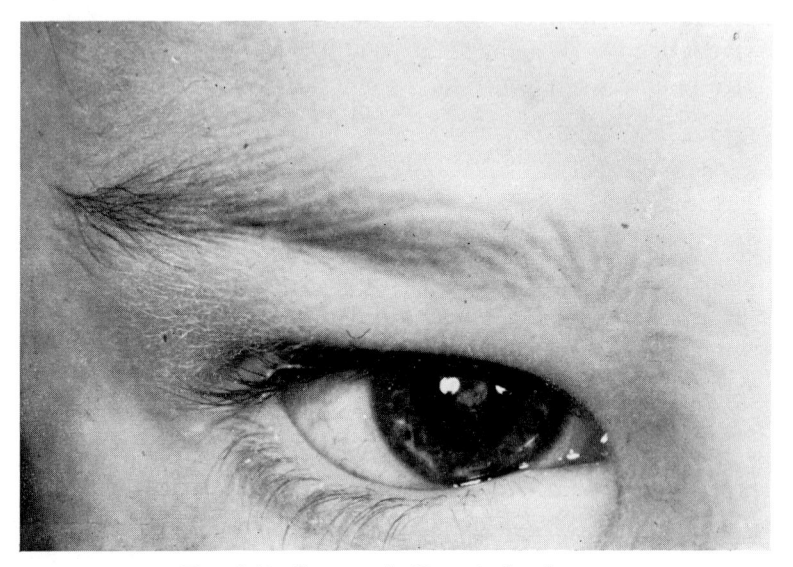

FIG. 5.13. Cataract in Down's Syndrome.

choroid and retina were absent, with some pigment round the edges of the lesions.

RETINAL SEPTUM

This is a rare anomaly where a fold of retina stretches forward from the disc across the vitreous to the periphery of the fundus, where it is attached to the ora and strands may pass to the lens. It may occur in any meridian but usually the majority are on the temporal side. It is associated with an anomaly of the hyaloid system, as a persistent hyaloid artery is present on the apex of the fold. It probably develops at the 13 mm stage, when the foetal cleft is closing. There is no treatment.

OPAQUE NERVE-FIBRES

These are due to abnormal myelination of the retinal nerve-fibres near the disc. Normally medullation stops just behind the lamina cribrosa, but in these cases it starts again on the edge of the disc. Myelination is not fully developed at birth and so this condition does not develop till a few weeks later. The ophthalmoscopic picture is of a large white patch with feather edges above and/or below the disc and perhaps arching towards the macula. The retinal vessels are partly or wholly buried in it. Vision is unaffected.

Intra-uterine Chorioretinitis

This may occur at the macula only or be disseminated through the fundus.

(a) *Macular*
The ophthalmoscopic picture is exactly like that of a developmental defect described above and such cases were previously wrongly classified as congenital macular colobomata. It is now known that the majority are due to intra-uterine infection from toxoplasmosis, but some may be due to other inflammatory causes not yet confirmed or so far unknown.

(b) *Disseminated*
There may be widespread lesions of varying clinical appearances in the fundi. Toxoplasmosis can cause peripheral lesions as well as macular defects and the allied cytomegalic inclusion disease also causes widespread chorioretinitis, mainly peripheral There is ample proof that maternal rubella and syphilis can cause chorioretinitis in the foetus, and there is some evidence that the viruses of poliomyelitis and smallpox can interfere with the development of the foetus and damage the eyes. The role of other viruses, including influenza, measles, herpes zoster, epidemic hepatitis and vaccinia, is so far undetermined. Reports of ocular damage from these infections are sporadic and more evidence is required before any conclusions can be drawn. Other possible causes are maternal tropical diseases such as malaria due to plasmodium falciparum. The different types will now be considered.

(i) Toxoplasmosis

This is an infection with the protozoan parasite toxoplasma. The infection is widespread through the animal kindgom and affects 25–75 per cent of human beings without clinical signs.
Ocular changes. The main feature is a bilateral chorioretinitis which

affects chiefly the macula (80 per cent) and other parts of the fundus (20 per cent). The disease may be active before birth or in the early weeks or months of postnatal life. In the *active postnatal* phase the vitreous is very hazy, being packed with inflammatory cells, and no fundus details can be seen. As it slowly clears, an area or areas of cotton-wool exudate become dimly visible, and later large areas of chorioretinal atrophy become clearly defined at the macula and elsewhere. The *chronic* phase (Fig. 5.14) may be present at birth or may develop postnatally as above. The areas of atrophy are often excavated, with varying degrees of pigmentation round the edges. The disc may be involved in the inflammation, causing secondary optic atrophy.

Other ocular changes include microphthalmos (often unilateral), iridocyclitis, secondary cataract, papilloedema and optic atrophy (from hydrocephalus or chorioretinitis), nystagmus and squint.

The *diagnosis* is confirmed by serological tests on mother and child.

Treatment in the active phase can be attempted with pyrimethamine, sulphadiazine and prednisolone systemically but no encouraging results have so far been reported in congenital cases.

(ii) Cytomegalic Inclusion Disease

This is a virus disease which gives a clinical picture similar in some ways to toxoplasmosis. The virus is found in the salivary glands of normal adult animals and also in those of 12–32 per cent of children dying from other causes. In adults the infection is usually subclinical and like toxoplasmosis is widespread in the community. It is most severe in babies, when it is generally fatal.

Clinical features. The infant is usually premature. There may be hepatosplenomegaly, anaemia, thrombocytopenia, hydrocephalus, mental retardation, cerebral calcification, chorioretinitis and optic atrophy. The chorioretinitis may be acute or chronic, and is active at any time between 6 weeks and 6 months of postnatal life. The lesions are small, multiple and mainly peripheral in the fundi. A generalized atrophy of choroid, retina or optic nerve may follow.

Diagnosis. The typical inclusion bodies are found in the epithelium of the renal tubules, bronchi and salivary glands. They should be looked for in the urine, and have been seen in the aqueous. Specific antibodies are found in the serum.

No treatment is known at present.

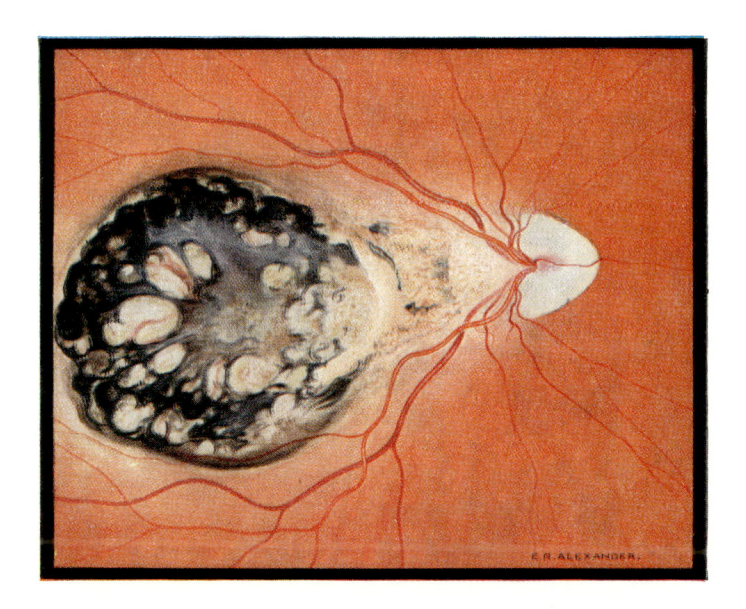

FIG. 5.14. Toxoplasmosis showing chorioretinitis at the macula and involving the disk.

facing p. 178

(iii) Congenital Syphilis

In countries where adequate antenatal care and modern methods of treatment are available, this is now a rare disease. The ocular features are those of a widespread bilateral chorioretinitis. The acute phase, which is rarely seen, resembles acute toxoplasmic chorioretinitis.

The chronic disease is of two types: (1) the pepper-and-salt type, which consists of fine pigmentation and tiny spots of chorioretinal atrophy spread through the fundi; (2) the disseminated type, which consists of larger patches of pigmentation and atrophy, irregular in size and shape, scattered through the fundi. Signs of iridocyclitis, with posterior synechiae, are frequently present. In a severe case microphthalmos and secondary cataract may also occur. The mother's blood Wasserman reaction will be positive.

Treatment is that of syphilis. In addition acute chorioretinitis should be treated with systemic steroids, and acute iridocyclitis with local atropine and steroid drops. In the chronic stage no treatment will improve the established eye lesions.

(iv) Tuberculosis

In a few cases of chorioretinitis seen in babies the cause may be tuberculosis acquired in the early weeks of postnatal life.

(v) Rubella

Maternal rubella in the first 3 months of pregnancy frequently causes cataract and retinopathy in the infant. The retinopathy is most clearly seen in the second eye in cases of unilateral cataract but is also present behind bilateral cataracts in a large proportion of cases, estimated at from 15 per cent to 60 per cent.

The ophthalmoscopic picture is of small roughly circular grey or black spots of pigment scattered over the posterior poles, especially at the macular areas. The diameter of the spots does not exceed the diameter of a main retinal vessel. The disc and retinal vessels are normal.

Fortunately vision is not affected in most cases. The electroretinogram is usually normal.

(vi) Pseudoglioma

If the intraocular inflammation has been severe, the baby may be born with one eye totally disorganized and in which the vitreous is filled with organized inflammatory tissue. The other eye may be normal or show some signs of uveitis. The cause may be one of the five diseases described above. Another cause is incontinentia pigmentii (p. 318). In this rare skin disease, ocular complications occur in 28 per cent of cases. The writer has observed one case developing postnatally, the eyes being virtually normal at birth and blind by 3 months. The cause was a gross neovascularization of retina and choroid, starting round the discs and posterior poles, spreading into the vitreous, and causing dense vitreous opacities.

The main clinical features are (1) microphthalmos; (2) chronic iridocyclitis, with posterior synechiae; (3) a white mass or membrane visible on direct illumination behind the lens (if there is no cataract); (4) little or no red reflex with the ophthalmoscope; (5) sometimes a secondary cataract.

Differential diagnosis. There are three other common causes of a white mass behind the lens.

1. *Retinoblastoma* is a malignant tumour of the retina usually arising in the first few months or years of life, although a few may be present at birth. It is bilateral in 20–30 per cent of cases. Most cases are sporadic but a few are hereditary with dominant or irregular dominant transmission. The first sign is a white or yellow reflex in the pupil (so-called 'cat's eye' phenomenon). In an advanced case the whitish-yellow mass will be seen by direct illumination through the pupil. In any retinal detachment in an infant one must suspect retinoblastoma. There may be a small tumour in the other eye, which must always be carefully examined under full mydriasis.

Treatment is enucleation for an extensive tumour and radiotherapy for a small localized tumour in the second eye.

2. *Persistent fibrovascular sheath* of the lens is an abnormality of the primitive vascular system.

3. *Retrolental fibroplasia* is a postnatal disease of premature infants which is due to an excessive concentration of oxygen administered after birth.

In a severe case there is bilateral microphthalmos, shallow anterior chambers, atrophic irides, anterior and posterior synechiae and smooth white retrolental membranes. When the cause was known and the oxygen concentration had been rigidly restricted to less than 35 per cent, the disease was virtually eliminated. More recently higher concentrations of oxygen have been given and cases of retrolental fibroplasia are again occurring. To avoid blindness in these babies it is essential that the blood oxygen and carbon dioxide levels should be monitored every few hours when over 35 per cent oxygen is being given.

3. ABIOTROPHIES

These are genetically determined defects that occur postnatally, and are only briefly mentioned here.

(a) *Choroideraemia* is a rare condition in which the choroid is absent in both eyes. The striking ophthalmoscopic picture is a white fundus background in all areas except the macula, where the red choroidal circulation fades irregularly into the surrounding white. The disc and retinal vessels are normal. It is a genetic defect with intermediate X-chromosomal transmission. The males are affected and the heterozygous females show minimal fundus changes of fine pigmentation.

The onset of symptoms may be early in childhood or later (10–30 years).

The symptoms are progressive night-blindness and increasing concentric contraction of the visual field. Central vision is not affected till late adult life. There is no treatment.

(b) *The Lawrence–Moon–Biedl syndrome* consists of the association of obesity, hypogenitalism, mental deficiency, polydactyly and retinitis pigmentosa; the latter is usually of the classical type.

OPTIC NERVE

THE NORMAL DISC

It must be stressed that it is very difficult to decide whether a baby's discs are normal or not, as there is a wide variation in the colour of the discs in the first year of life. In the early months of life the discs are pale. This may at first be a *greyish* pallor, due to lack of myelination of the optic nerves. Myelination proceeds in the foetus from the chiasma forwards, starting there at 24 weeks and stopping just behind the lamina cribrosa at birth, but full development of the myelination there may be delayed till a few weeks after birth. With myelination the discs show a *whitish* pallor which is the usual colour in a young infant. As capillaries ramify in the nerve head this in turn is gradually replaced by the normal pink colour. This occurs at 2 to 4 months of age in the full-term infant and somewhat later in the premature infant.

Optic Atrophy

The wide variation in the colour of normal discs makes the diagnosis of optic atrophy a difficult one. If marked pallor of the discs persists after 4 months and if the infant does not respond to the visual stimuli to which he should at that age, one should be suspicious that some visual handicap, either central or peripheral, is present. He may, however, be a late developer or may be deficient in understanding, in feeling or in motor power.

Causes of Optic Atrophy

Causes of Optic Atrophy
Optic atrophy may be present at birth but in some cases it does not develop till a few weeks or months after birth. The differential diagnosis is important and so both congenital and postnatal types are included here.

The older classification of optic atrophy was primary and secondary, but it is better to group the cases according to cause.

(1) *Consecutive atrophy* may be *post-inflammatory*, as in toxoplasmosis, where it is associated with chorioretinitis or *degenerative*, as in Tay–Sach's disease.

(2) *Pressure atrophy* may occur from (a) increased intraocular pressure, as in buphthalmos or (b) increased intracranial pressure, as in cerebral haemorrhage, subdural haematoma, hydrocephalus or oxycephaly. In (b) papilloedema may precede optic atrophy. If this occurs, the disc edges may remain blurred, but more frequently they later become clearly defined and all trace of previous swelling disappears.

(3) *Traumatic atrophy* may be due to birth trauma causing haemorrhage into the optic nerve or nerve-sheaths.

(4) *Anoxic atrophy* may occur as part of a general anoxia in the first week of life. Premature infants are more liable to haemorrhage at birth and to anoxia in the first few days of life, and so an increased incidence of optic atrophy from these causes is found among premature infants compared with those born at full-term.

(5) *Genetically determined atrophy*. (a) Congenital optic atrophy may

be inherited as a *dominant* characteristic. It is present at birth or appears in early childhood. The discs are dead white, nystagmus is common, and the visual fields show concentric contraction. Once established, the defect is usually stationary. This disease must be carefully distinguished from the other familial optic atrophy, Leber's disease, where the onset is much later (at about the age of 20), the field defect is a bilateral central scotoma and there is an unusual type of inheritance with transmission through the sisters of affected men and not their sons or daughters.

(b) *Aplasia of the optic nerves and retina* also occurs as a rare hereditary disease with dominant or intermediate transmission.

In infancy and early childhood there is no gross abnormality in the fundi, both discs and retinae looking fairly normal, and yet a severe degree of blindness is present. In childhood and early adult life optic atrophy and pigmentary chorioretinal degeneration gradually develop, and cataract is a frequent complication.

Treatment is that of the cause. In most cases nothing can be done, but there are a few exceptions. In congenital glaucoma the ocular tension should be controlled by goniotomy. In hydrocephalus and oxycephaly the increased intracranial pressure should be relieved at an early stage before optic atrophy has developed.

ORBIT

Dermoid Cysts

Dermoid cysts in the orbit occur most frequently (60 per cent) in the upper outer quadrant, over 25 per cent in the upper inner quadrant, and the remainder in the other two quadrants.

They vary in size from a small pea to an orange. The skin is freely movable over them, and they are usually adherent to the underlying bone, in which there may be a gap. If they are cosmetically noticeable, they should be excised, but care must be taken if there is a communication with the dura.

Meningo-encephalocele

Meningo-encephalocele is a relatively rare defect in the bony walls of the orbit. The usual situation is at the upper inner corner, where a gap in the sutures between frontal, lacrimal and maxillary bones allows a herniation of meninges and brain substance into the orbit. The condition is often present at birth but may not become apparent till early childhood. The swelling is fluctuant and pulsatile: it increases on crying and can be reduced by pressure. The latter manoeuvre must be carefully carried out as it may induce slowing of the pulse, convulsions and even coma. More rarely the bony defect occurs towards the back of the orbit, when a pulsatile proptosis occurs. Treatment is excision of the hernial sac and repair of the defect in the bone.

THE VASCULAR SYSTEM

THE NORMAL EYE

Premature Infants

In premature infants there are several differences in the eyes at birth and in the early weeks of life from those of full-term infants.

(i) In the infant born before 32 weeks' gestation a *pupillary membrane* is nearly always present. It is also present in about half of those born between 32 and 34 weeks' gestation. It consists of a fine network of obliterated vessels filling the pupil. These are the remnants of the anterior part of the hyaloid system.

It is best seen with a $+12$ D lens in the ophthalmoscope if the pupil is dilated with 1 per cent homatropine drops and the infant is examined in a semi-darkened room. It usually disappears in the first week in all except the smallest premature babies (under 32 weeks' gestation). In an infant born at 28 weeks, it may persist for 6 weeks.

(ii) The *hyaloid artery* is nearly always present in infants of under 34 weeks' gestation (or under 1·8 kg birth weight) and sometimes in those 34–36 weeks (1·8–2·2 kg). It is always an obliterated vessel and appears as a fine black thread, either straight or wavy, running forward from the disc into the vitreous. In the premature infant of under 32 weeks' gestation it will reach the back of the lens on the inner nasal side of the centre of the pupil. In those of 32–34 weeks it is probable that the posterior half only will be present, and will appear as a thin line tapering to a fine point in front of the disc. It gradually shrinks towards the disc and disappears before the infant reaches his full-term date.

(iii) The *media* in the small premature infant are hazy and the eye is usually myopic, so that the anterior part of the hyaloid artery is seen with a +10 D lens and the posterior part and the disc may require a −10 D lens in the ophthalmoscope. These changes gradually recede and disappear well before the infant reaches his full-term date. The haze is probably due to immaturity of the vitreous and the presence of the hyaloid system, while the myopia may be due to the spherical lens of the premature infant, although this cause has not yet been confirmed.

(iv) In the small premature infant the *fundus* has a poorly pigmented choroid, especially round the disc and at the posterior pole, where the choroidal pigment and vascular choroidal network have not yet developed. The retinal vessels are thin and at 28–30 weeks have grown little more than half-way from the disc to the ora serrata. In the periphery of the fundus there is a wide band of a greyish-white colour where the choroid and retina are not yet vascularized. The macula is immature and vision is very poor.

(v) The disc starts by being pale, grey–white at first, white at the full-term date and pink in a further 2 to 4 months.

The Full-term Infant

The eye at birth is now much more like the adult eye. In the white races the iris is a homogeneous blue colour and does not develop its delicate meshwork or change to brown for several months. The colour change may be delayed for a year. In the coloured races the iris is blue–grey at birth but within a day or two has become brown. This rapid pigmentation occurs in the eye just as it does in the skin.

All trace of the hyaloid system has gone and the media are clear. The disc is white at first and becomes pink in 2 to 4 months. The retinal vessels have almost reached the ora serrata and the peripheral grey–white band is now very narrow. In the coloured races the fundus background is a uniform steely grey instead of red, owing to the dense choroidal pigmentation, while the disc and retinal vessels show up clearly as pink and red against the great background. *Retinal haemorrhages* are frequently present at birth in premature and full-term babies, but usually clear up in a few days. The incidence has been variously estimated as from 2·6 per cent to 42 per cent, the higher percentage being found if babies are examined in the first 2 days of life. They probably occur from pressure on the head during delivery, as none are found after Caesarian section.

CONGENITAL ANOMALIES OF THE VASCULAR SYSTEM

(i) Persistent Pupillary Membrane

Strands of this membrane are very common in normal eyes of babies and young people, and tend to disappear in old age. It forms a delicate white network of varying size in the pupil, stretching from the lesser circle of the iris (beyond the pupillary margin) either tangentially across the pupil to another sector of the iris, or to the lens capsule, to which it may be attached by a white plaque. There may also be clusters of tiny brown pigment stars (epicapsular stars) on the lens capsule in the pupillary area.

(ii) Persistent Hyaloid Artery

This is a fairly common congenital anomaly. The artery persists in the whole or part of its course from disc to lens and appears as a thin line or thick cord which gently undulates with movement of the eye. It is usually obliterated but occasionally is patent and contains blood. More frequently the posterior half alone persists, being attached to the disc with a free anterior end. If the complete artery persists, the anterior end may be associated with a posterior capsular lens opacity and in a few cases there is extensive fibrosis in the substance of the lens (see 'Persistent fibrovascular sheath' below).

(iii) Hyaloid Cyst

Very rarely the posterior end of the hyaloid artery forms a cyst, which appears as a round or flask-shaped pearly white or translucent structure lying in the vitreous in front of and attached to the disc. It has been mistaken for a cysticercus, which gives a similar appearance.

(iv) Glial Remnants

Glial remnants on the disc are white plaques or membranes on the disc covering its edge or stretching as a veil between retinal vessels on or adjacent to it. They are mesodermal remnants of the hyaloid system. This congenital fibrosis with blurred disc edges and flat disc must be distinguished from the true swelling of papilloedema.

(v) Persistent Fibrovascular Sheath of the Lens

The posterior vascular sheath of the lens may persist as a dense smooth white membrane behind the lens, which itself is usually clear but may be invaded by fibrous tissue. It is unilateral and the other eye is normal. The differential diagnosis is very important as it may be mistaken for a retinoblastoma or a pseudoglioma or retrolental fibroplasia (see 'pseudoglioma' above).

Complications frequently occur. These include secondary glaucoma and spontaneous absorption of the lens. There is no treatment for any of these anomalies except that if the eye is painful and blind, it should be removed.

SQUINT

There are two broad groups of squints in babies and children—*congenital* (incomitant) squints which are present from birth or develop in the first year or 18 months, and *concomitant*, the common type, which develop between the ages of 2 and 5 or perhaps later. Here, only congenital squints are considered. These are at first obviously incomitant or paralytic, there being a definite paresis of one or more extra-ocular muscles in certain directions of gaze, but with the passage of time they may be converted into the concomitant type.

The *clinical features* are of an alternating squint, usually convergent but sometimes vertical and rarely divergent, with good vision in each eye and no significant refractive error. Abnormal head postures to overcome diplopia develop between 18 months and 2 years and suppression of the image of the squinting eye occurs when the eyes move in the direction of the weak muscle.

Aetiology. Congenital squints are due to two main causes—developmental defects and birth trauma. Squints may also be secondary to other ocular or systemic disease which may be present before birth (e.g. congenital cataract, chorioretinitis) or acquired postnatally, but these are not considered in this section.

The *development defect* may be due to abnormalities in the extra-ocular muscles themselves (absence, abnormal insertion or fibrosis of the muscle) or to defects in the neural pathways (e.g. maldevelopment of a nucleus in the midbrain). Occasionally these defects of muscle are genetically determined but often the cause is unknown.

Birth trauma may cause damage to the neural pathways or directly to the extra-ocular muscle. It may cause intracranial haemorrhage in the nucleus or along the intracranial course of the nerve supplying the muscle or direct haemorrhage may occur into the muscle or muscle-sheath. The nerve may also be torn by birth trauma in any part of its intracranial course. The third, fourth or the sixth nerve may be involved, the sixth being most prone to injury. These injuries are more likely in full-term babies after prolonged labour or from the pressure of forceps, or in premature infants from their increased liability to brain damage from haemorrhage. An increased incidence of squints among premature infants has been frequently reported and this is probably due to the increased incidence of congenital squints resulting from birth trauma.

There is also an increased incidence of squint in cases of cerebral palsy.

Types of Congenital Squint
(a) *Paresis of external recti.* This common type may be due to a developmental defect of the muscles, resulting from overdevelopment of the internal recti and underdevelopment of the external in the early months *in utero*. It is rarely due to a faulty development of the sixth nerve nucleus. It may also be due to birth trauma to the sixth nerve nucleus or the sixth nerve in its long intracranial course or damage to the muscle itself. The condition may be unilateral or bilateral.

Clinically the infant has an alternating convergent squint with inability to abduct one or both eyes beyond the midline. There is no significant refractive error and the fundi and media are normal.

Treatment is along the usual lines for squints—the correction of any gross refractive error, the occlusion of the fixing eye to keep the squint alternating, and surgical correction when indicated. This should be early, between 1 and 2 years, if the angle of squint is large and constant. In the smaller and variable degrees, operation can be deferred till after the age of 2 years, as some spontaneous improvement can be expected up to that date.

(b) *Duane's retraction syndrome.* This is a congenital abnormality of the external rectus itself where the muscle is replaced by inelastic fibrous tissue. The internal rectus may also be abnormally large and inelastic.

The main clinical features are:
  (i) Paralysis of abduction on one (usually the left) or both sides.
  (ii) Narrowing of the palpebral fissure on adduction of the affected eye and widening on attempted abduction.

(iii) A variable limitation of adduction on the affected side.

(iv) Updrift of the affected eye on attempted abduction.

(v) Head-turn to the affected side to maintain binocular vision.

Some cases may be developmental defects and some may be due to birth injury (haemorrhage into the muscle). A hereditary type has been reported which was transmitted by an irregular dominant autosomal gene with incomplete penetrance.

Treatment. Operation should be performed to straighten the eyes in the primary position (with the head straight). This should also help to improve the abnormal head posture. The usual operations are recessions of both internal recti in stages, and operation on one or more vertical muscles if a vertical deviation is present.

(c) *Anomalies of the vertically-acting muscles*. (i) A *paresis of the superior oblique* is associated with an overaction of the inferior oblique on the same side so that the affected eye is at a higher level than the other, the effect being most obvious on adduction. Ocular torticollis may develop as a compensatory head posture after the age of 18 months to 2 years. (There is often an apparent weakness of the contralateral superior rectus, and some authorities attribute the primary defect to this.)

(ii) A *paresis of the superior rectus* on one or both sides is often associated with ptosis.

(iii) The *superior oblique sheath syndrome* is caused by an abnormal contraction of the sheath of the superior oblique so that when the affected eye is adducted, it is held at a lower level than the other eye. Thus there is an apparent paresis of the inferior oblique on the same side.

(d) *Congenital paralysis of the third nerve* also occurs but is rare.

Treatment of vertical squints is surgical. Operation may be required on more than one muscle and should be carried out in stages.

CONGENITAL GLAUCOMA (BUPHTHALMOS)

This disease is due to an abnormal persistence of mesodermal tissue in the angle of the anterior chamber. This should normally be absorbed by the seventh month *in utero* but may persist as a congenital anomaly. It also occurs in the Sturge–Weber syndrome and in Lowe's syndrome and has been reported as a complication of maternal rubella. Gonioscopy shows that there may also be a high insertion of the iris on the trabeculum. As a result of inadequate drainage of the aqueous through the canal of Schlemm, the intra-ocular tension rises, and the eye, being distensible in infancy, gradually enlarges. Hence is derived the term buphthalmos, or ox-eye. The disease is bilateral in 80 per cent of cases. If the disease does not develop till childhood, it is termed juvenile glaucoma and no enlargement of the eye-ball occurs.

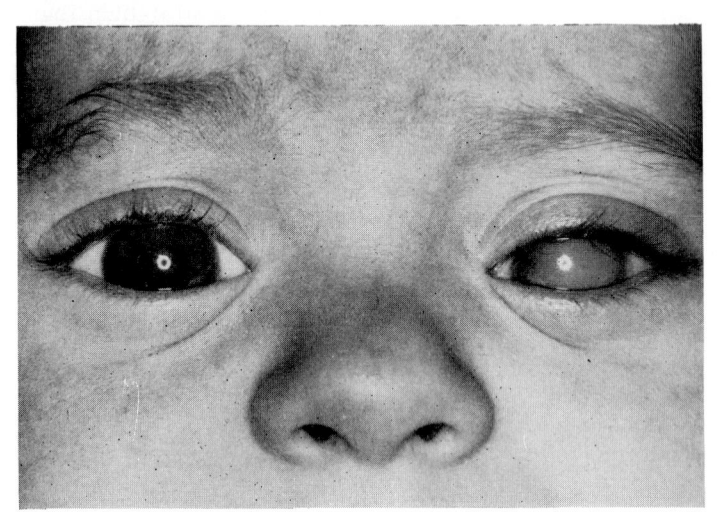

Fig. 5.15. Congenital glaucoma, showing enlargement of globes and corneal haze.

Clinical features (Fig. 5.15). The disease is probably present at birth, but the onset of symptoms is usually in the first few years of life, often in the first year. Occasionally a unilateral case, with gross changes in the anterior segment of the eye, may be present at birth. The earliest symptom is photophobia, and buphthalmos should be suspected in any infant who develops this without apparent cause. The eyes become irritable, watering and slightly red. As the intra-ocular tension rises, the corneal diameters gradually enlarge, the corneae become hazy and the discs become cupped. In the untreated case blindness ensues from pressure atrophy of the optic nerves.

Treatment. The operation of choice is goniotomy at an early stage in the disease. The indications for this are an intra-ocular tension of over 30 mm Schiotz as recorded by the tonometer, an increasing corneal diameter and/or cupping of the disc. An increased tension alone is not a sufficient indication for operation. Spontaneous arrest does occur in a few cases and so early cases, especially in babies of under 6 months, should first be treated with miotic drops and diamox tablets until definite deterioration is observed.

LACRIMAL APPARATUS

Lacrimal Gland

(i) Congenital Absence of Tears

This is very rare, but has been reported either with or without fifth nerve paralysis or more extensive cranial-nerve involvement. Usually there is chronic conjunctivitis and there may be kerato-conjunctivitis sicca. The cause is thought to be a congenital defect of the secretory nerves of the lacrimal gland.

Treatment. Drops of methyl cellulose ½ per cent solution should be used four times a day as artificial tears.

(ii) Congenital Lacrimal Fistula

Congenital lacrimal fistula which opens through the outer end of the upper lid is rare. It causes excoriation of the skin round the orifice. The fistula should be transplanted into the conjunctival sac or excised along with the associated part of the lacrimal gland.

Lacrimal Drainage Channels

Absence or Congenital Occlusion

Absence or congenital occlusion of the lacrimal puncta is a fairly rare anomaly. It has been recorded as a familial defect. There may be no sign of the puncta but usually there is a small dimple at the site. Epiphora is the only symptom. A fine sharp point (e.g. a sterilized pin) should be forced vertically through the site of the lower punctum, after which it should be possible to dilate and syringe the passages in the usual way. Otherwise the canaliculus should be located by an incision across its expected site and then dilated.

Congenital Obstruction of the Nasolacrimal Duct

Congenital obstruction of the nasolacrimal duct is a common defect. The duct should canalize between the eighth and ninth month in *utero* but may remain blocked by epithelial cells or by a membrane at its lower end. Watering of the eye occurs when tears are first formed at the age of 3 or 4 weeks, and secondary infection of the conjunctiva and lacrimal sac (mucocele) usually follows. In the latter case there is a painless swelling of the lacrimal sac, pressure on which causes regurgitation of muco-pus into the eye. In rare cases a mucocele of the lacrimal sac, either reducible or irreducible, may be present at birth. A lacrimal abscess may also develop in the first few days of life.

Treatment of the blocked duct is with drops of the appropriate antibiotic (determined by conjunctival culture) preceded by drops of adrenaline 1:1000, four to six times a day. If this fails, probing of the duct under general anaesthetic is required. This is not usually necessary before the age of 4 months but a large congenital mucocele is an indication for probing in the first 2 weeks of life.

A lacrimal abscess requires systemic treatment with antibiotics and incision, followed later, if watering persists, by probing of the duct.

CONGENITAL MYOPIA

Four types of congenital myopia are recognized.

(1) One type is associated with other congenital ocular defects, including colobomata, posterior staphylomata, albinism, mongolism, arachnodactyly, or growth anomalies of the pituitary or gonads.

(2) A second type is due to progressive degenerative myopia of very early onset. This is a genetically determined disease which is not usually detected till between the ages of 3 and 6 years, but may in exceptional cases develop in the first year of life. There is usually a strong family history of myopia. This group carries a grave prognosis with regard to sight, as chorioretinal degeneration, macular haemorrhages or retinal detachments may occur in adult life.

(3) A third type occurs in premature babies as a complication of retrolental fibroplasia. The condition may be bilateral, but frequently one eye is myopic with no other changes or only minor signs like traction of the disc towards the temporal side, while the other eye has

advanced retrolental fibroplasia. The myopia varies from 2·5 dioptres to 20 dioptres and is non-progressive during childhood. Some visual defect is usually present, probably due to macular damage, but vision may be good enough for ordinary school.

(4) A fourth type occurs in small premature babies of under 3 lb (1·5 kg) who do not fit into any of the first three groups. It is frequently a temporary feature and usually clears up in the first 3 or 4 months. Whether it be a curvature or index myopia is so far undetermined, but the spherical lens of the immature eye may be a factor. In those cases where the myopia persists into childhood, it may be due to a persistence of the immaturity of the eye; or some other factor, so far unknown, may be responsible.

Treatment. Regular examination of the eyes should be carried out by an ophthalmic surgeon every 6 to 9 months during infancy and childhood. Glasses should be worn constantly and care must be taken to give the weakest correction consistent with good vision. In high degrees of myopia contact lenses give better acuity and field, and can usually be fitted about the age of 8 to 10 years, or earlier if the child is cooperative. General measures should include fresh air and exercise and a good diet, with plenty of milk, fruit and vegetables. Close work is allowed in the normal way, with special attention to good light and the correct working distance, and education should be at ordinary school if at all possible.

SYNDROMES

Certain syndromes with a skeletal, metabolic or other basis have diverse manifestations in different parts of the body and their general features are discussed elsewhere. Some have specific ocular changes which may be of great value in clinching the diagnosis and these will now be mentioned. Only those syndromes which are manifest at or soon after birth are included here.

(a) *Skeletal*
   (i) Oxycephaly (Tower-skull) includes oxycephaly proper and acrocephalosyndactyly (Apert's Syndrome). The ocular abnormalities which are present in the severe form of the disease, include proptosis, divergent squint, papilloedema, optic atrophy and rarely, cataract.

They are progressive from birth to 5 years and stabilize about the age of 7. The proptosis and divergent squint are mechanical effects resulting from the shallowness of the orbits, which are too small to hold normally sized eyes. The proptosis may be so extreme that the lids are behind the equator of the globes. The increased intracranial pressure causes papilloedema, which in turn leads to optic atrophy and varying degrees of visual failure. This is rarely total blindness but partial loss of sight occurs in about half the cases. The condition is genetically determined. Most cases are sporadic but, it has been recorded in sibships and over two or three generations.

Treatment must be early to be of any value. Surgical removal of part of the bones of the vault of the skull by various methods gives the best chance of checking the progress of the disease and of preventing visual damage from optic atrophy.

(ii) *Cranio-facial dysostosis* (Crouzon's disease) is allied to Apert's syndrome but in addition there are several facial anomalies. The ocular changes are similar to those of oxycephaly (see (i) above). The syndrome is genetically determined with dominant transmission.

(iii) *Mandibulo-facial dysostosis* (Franceschetti & Klein) is a rare congenital anomaly where the main features are facial. The ocular features are the abnormal palpebral apertures, which slope down and out ('anti-mongoloid') and the coloboma at the outer end of both lower lids. The syndrome is hereditary, being transmitted as an irregular dominant.

(iv) *Hypertelorism* (Greig) is a condition in which there is an abnormally wide separation of the eyes. It is due to a widening of the nasal bridge, which itself is often depressed, and an enlargement of the lesser wing of the spheroid, so that the eyes tend to look in opposite directions in an animal-like fashion. A divergent squint is nearly always present but the eyes are otherwise normal and mentality is unaffected.

(b) *Mesodermal*

(i) *Marfan's syndrome* (arachnodactyly). The ocular changes are described above.

(ii) *Fragilitas ossium* is caused by a developmental defect of the mesodermal tissues. It consists of fragility of bone (60 per cent of cases), otosclerosis (24 per cent) and, almost constantly, blue sclerotics. The cause of the blue colour has in some cases been shown to be due to abnormal thinness of the sclera, causing the uveal pigment to shine through, but in other cases there appears to be an abnormal translucency of the sclera without variation in thickness. It is inherited as a dominant defect.

(c) *Ectodermal*
Congenital ectodermal dysplasia has already been mentioned in the section on cataract.

(d) *Neuro-ectodermal*
   (i) *Down's syndrome* (*mongolism*). The ocular features are described earlier.
   (ii) *Lawrence–Moon–Biedl syndrome.* The ocular features are described earlier.
   (iii) *Stürge–Weber syndrome* (*encephalo-facial angiomatosis*) consists of a capillary angioma of the fronto-parietal region, mucous membranes of eye and mouth, meningeal angioma, choroidal angioma, and unilateral congenital or juvenile glaucoma. The lesions are unilateral and are all related to the distribution of the trigeminal nerve.

   Unilateral congenital or juvenile glaucoma occurs in a fair proportion of cases. It may be associated with tortuosity of the retinal veins. There may therefore be a relationship with Lindau's syndrome (angiomatosis of retina and cerebellum). Glaucoma must be controlled by miotics or a drainage operation. The latter is usually necessary in children and young adults.

   (iv) *Neurofibromatosis* (Von Recklinghausen's disease) consists of multiple congenital tumours of the peripheral nerves and '*café au lait*' spots in the skin.

   The tumours are neurofibromata which may involve the eyelids, especially the upper, the orbit, and the eye (optic nerve, retina or uveal tract). The tumours are frequently present at birth but may not develop till childhood, puberty or later. In the orbit the tumour may cause proptosis, and if the uveal tract is involved, there may be congenital or juvenile glaucoma. There is a hereditary tendency with irregular dominant transmission.

   Excision of the tumour should be attempted if it is large and unsightly but complete removal is often difficult. Haemorrhage is often severe and in infants it has proved fatal.

(e) *Metabolic*
   (i) *Anomalies of mucopoly saccharide metabolism.* 1. Gargoylism

(dysostosis multiplex; lipochondrodysplasia; Hurler's disease) consists of widespread skeletal changes and lipid infiltration of many tissues throughout the body. The grotesque appearance develops in the first few months of life but some features may be present at birth.

The main ocular features are wide-set eyes and diffuse cloudiness of the corneae due to infiltration with deposits of mucopolysaccharides. These are often present in the first year of life and cause considerable visual defect. They consist of hundreds of minute white opacities scattered through the substance of the corneae. Superficially the haze resembles that of congenital glaucoma and indeed this disease may coexist, increased intra-ocular tension having been found in a number of cases. In one such case in the writer's experience the response to blind goniotomy was disappointing, there being only a temporary improvement in ocular tension.

2. *Familial lipoid degenerations.* Two of this group of diseases affect infants—Niemann–Pick's disease (lipid histiocytosis) and Tay–Sach's disease (amaurotic family idiocy).

Niemann–Pick's disease is a disease of infants at birth or in the early days or weeks of life. The fundus picture is similar to Tay–Sach's, there being a very pale disc (dense white in Tay–Sach's, a waxy yellow–white in Niemann–Pick's), attenuated arteries, and an area of oedema at the macula with a central brown-red spot.

The differences are that Tay–Sach's disease is of later onset, usually at about 5 months, and that the lipid degeneration affects the ganglion cells of the nervous system, including the retina, whereas Niemann–Pick's disease also affects other layers of the nervous system and retina and infiltrates the uveal tract and sclera.

There is no treatment and in both cases the disease terminates in blindness, paralysis, idiocy and death in a matter of months.

(ii) *Anomalies of aminoacid metabolism.* Cystinosis (Fanconi's syndrome) is an abnormality of aminoacid metabolism. It is probably inherited as a recessive defect. The ocular feature is the deposition of cystine crystals in the cornea and conjunctiva, and their detection is a valuable method of confirming the diagnosis. The crystals are sparse in the early stages of the disease (the first 6 months of life) and are so small that they require the slit-lamp for their detection. In babies sedation with rectal chloral hydrate enables this examination to be carried out. They appear as beautiful minute white scintillating dots under the corneal epithelium and in the conjunctiva. Later they pack the substance of the cornea and can be see with a loupe.

There is no treatment for the eye lesions.

(iii) *Anomalies of carbohydrate metabolism. Galactosaemia* is discussed and the ocular feature, cataract, is described above.

(iv) *Anomalies of pigmentation. Albinism.* As there is no pigment in the iris, this transmits light. The pupils appear pink or red as the light is reflected from the choroidal circulation back through them. The iris itself is a very pale grey in direct light and appears slightly pink in reflected light. The choroid and retina are similarly lacking in pigment, so that the choroidal and retinal vessels are seen sharply defined against the white sclera, the uniform red background of the fundus being absent.

Clinically there is extreme photophobia, defective vision (often with considerable myopia and astigmatism), and nystagmus. The defective vision is due to deficiency of pigment in the retinal epithelium or to a poorly developed macula.

Treatment includes correction of the large refractive error and the provision of dark glasses with side-pieces.

SELECTED REFERENCES

BROWN C.A. (1963) Postnatal cataracts in premature infants. *Trans. Ophth. Soc. U.K.* **83**, 493

BURNS R.P. (1959) Cytomegalic inclusion disease uveitis. *A.M.A. Arch. Ophthal.* **61**, 376

CARSON N.A.J., CUSWORTH D.C., DENT C.E., FIELD C.M.B., NEIL D.W. & WESTALL R.G. (1964) Homocystinuria. *Arch. Dis. Childh.* **38**, 425

DUKE-ELDER S. (1952) Developmental anomalies of the lids and orbit. *Textbook of Ophthalmology*, vol. 5. London: Henry Kimpton

FRANCOIS J. (1959) *Les Cataractes Congenitales.* Paris: Mason et Cie

FRANCOIS J. (1961) *Heredity in Ophthalmology.* St. Louis: C.V. Mosby Co.

GREGG N.M. (1941) Congenital cataract following German measles in the mother. *Trans. Ophth. Soc. Aust.* **3**, 35–46

HUDSON J.R. (1954) Clinical aspects of toxoplasmosis. *Proc. Roy. Soc. Med.* **47**, 484–8

HULL D. (1969) Cataracts associated with metabolic disorders in infancy. *Proc. Roy. Soc. Med.* **62**, 694

LIEBMAN S.D. (1955) Postnatal development of lamellar cataracts in premature infants. *Arch. Ophthal. Chicago* **54**, 257–8

LISTER A. (1959) Some aspects of congenital glaucoma. *Trans. Ophth. Soc. U.K.* **79**, 163–79

MCDONALD A. (1962) Neurological and ophthalmic disorders in children of a very low birthweight. *Brit. Med. J.* **i**, 895

MANN I. (1957) *Developmental Abnormalities of the Eye.* London: *Brit. med. J.* publication

Manson M.M., Logan W.P.D. & Loy R.M. (1960) Rubella and other virus infections during pregnancy. *Ministry of Health Reports on Public Health and Medical Subjects, No.* **101**. H.M.S.O.

Nettleship E. & Ogilvie F.M. (1906) A peculiar form of hereditary congenital cataract. *Trans. Ophth. Soc. U.K.* **26**, 191–206

Shaffer R.N. (1955) Symposium on congenital glaucoma. *Trans. Amer. Acad. Ophthal. & Otol.* **59**, 297–308

Sorsby A. (1951a) *Genetics in Ophthalmology*. London: Butterworth

Sorsby A. (1951b) 'Denetically determined anomalies' in *Systemic Ophthalmology*. London: Butterworth

Sorsby A. (1960) Retinal aplasia as a clinical entity. *Brit. med. J.* **i**, 293–7

6

Abnormalities of the Genito-urinary System

D.I.WILLIAMS

Urogenital abnormalities, as they are seen in infancy, may be conveniently discussed under two headings: those which are immediately evident to inspection in the newborn infant, affecting the external genitalia, urethra and bladder, and those involving only the internal urinary tract, hidden from view. In this second group the urethra and bladder may again be the site of the primary abnormalities, but the presenting symptoms and the problems of differential diagnosis are so different from the external abnormalities that they are more easily considered along with the renal and ureteric disorders.

EXTERNAL UROGENITAL ABNORMALITIES

The common external deformities present little in the way of diagnostic difficulty; once their appearance is familiar they are recognized with ease. For the most part they do not require any urgent surgical treatment, and there is therefore a tendency to shelve the problems they present until some weeks have elapsed. As will be pointed out later, this policy involves serious hazards in the intersex group of disorders, and in all cases it underestimates the agitation of the parents, to whom the deformity is equally evident: they often anticipate early operation and fear deficiencies in their child's sex life. It is wise, therefore, that a full assessment of the degree of the abnormality should be made very soon after birth, that the parents should be very fully informed as to the nature of the disorder, and that they should have an early opportunity for consultation with the surgeon who will, perhaps some years later, be called upon to perform the necessary reconstructive surgery.

The normal state of the external genitalia in the newborn differs a little from the more familiar appearance after the infant has begun to gain weight and develop a thick layer of subcutaneous fat. The penis is more prominent at first and may subsequently seem to shrink within the growing tissue; the scrotum is lax and may well be rather oedematous at first, particularly after a breech delivery. In the female the labia minora and clitoris may seem large since there is little fat in the labia majora, and often there is a mucoid vaginal secretion: slight uterine bleeding occurs in a proportion of infants during their first week due to the influence of maternal hormones.

Phimosis and the Need for Circumcision

The decision as to whether circumcision should be performed or not is seldom made on purely medical grounds; even when religious principles are not involved, parents and doctors often hold strong views based on their own experience or the local tradition, and emotional factors may play a more important part than scientific observations. No attempt will be made here to lay down firm recommendations, but certain clinical facts will be recorded, upon which a decision can be made.

The preputial sac is formed by an epithelial ingrowth from the surface of the penis; it is at first a solid lamella of epithelial cells and the cavity is ultimately formed by a split through this lamella. The process of splitting is normally incomplete at birth; separation will occur naturally during the course of the first year of life, but can be if necessary accomplished forcibly at any time, using a small probe. The white material which is released in the process consists largely of desquamated epithelial cells, and it is not entirely comparable with the smegma which accumulates in adults, nor has it the same tendency to produce inflammation in the preputial sac. Because of its natural adhesion to the glans the prepuce cannot be retracted at birth without inflicting a certain amount of trauma; this should not be taken to imply that phimosis, a stenosis of the preputial orifice, is present and it is not an indication for circumcision. True congenital phimosis is a comparatively rare condition, it can be recognized from the fact that it is impossible to see the external urinary meatus when retraction of the prepuce is attempted, whereas with the normal adhesions the meatus can be exposed, although the rest of the glans remains covered. Forcible retraction of either form may cause radial splits in the skin with subsequent scarring and finally an acquired phimosis.

Phimosis of whatever origin should be treated by early circumcision, it leads to retention of secretion and even of urine within the preputial sac, causing balanitis. It is later responsible for difficult and unsatisfactory sexual intercourse. Carcinoma of the penis is well known to occur almost exclusively in the uncircumcized, but it is primarily a disease of those who cannot retract the foreskin or will not observe simple hygienic rules of cleanliness with regard to the preputial sac.

It is clear that a number of difficulties and some serious disease will be avoided by routine circumcision of infants. Against this must be set the occasional complications of improperly performed operations and the dangers involved in the loss of the protective covering of the glans. Our present mode of living demands that a baby's urine should be confined within its immediate coverings and the vogue for water-tight plastic pants, particularly worn at night, is responsible for a considerable incidence of ammonia dermatitis. This is unpleasant enough on the foreskin, but on the glans and external meatus it causes ulceration with acute symptoms and long-term danger of meatal stenosis. These dangers can, of course, be avoided by proper care and do not constitute a bar to routine circumcision any more than the exceptionally uncommon complications of possessing a normal foreskin demand it.

Hypospadias

Hypospadias is the commonest penile anomaly: it may be only an insignificant variation upon the normal anatomy but in its more severe degrees it is a serious handicap to both urinary and sexual function. Hypospadias implies that the external urinary meatus opens at some point on the ventral surface of the penis, short of the tip. It is due to a failure of complete fusion of the urethral folds, which in embryonic development grow over from either side to form the anterior urethra in the male. These folds are also concerned with the completion of the prepuce; in hypospadias this organ is also un-united ventrally and instead of forming a sheath for the glans it is drawn back as a hood on the dorsal aspect.

In the least severe degree of hypospadias the external meatus is placed on the glans or at the coronal sulcus (Fig. 6.1). The glans distal to the meatus is grooved; on this groove will be found one or two openings leading into short blind ducts, easily mistaken for the normal urethra which is always the most proximal opening. In this situation the meatus is often stenosed and may be responsible for difficult micturition. Indeed, in the newborn period the opening may be plugged by epithelial debris, causing a transient retention of urine. It is then quite difficult to find so that it is often supposed that there is a

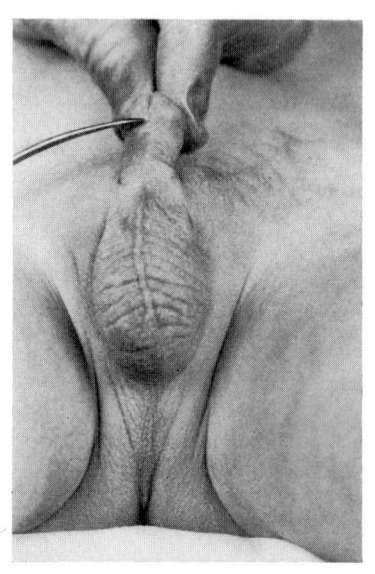

Fig. 6.1. Coronal hypospadias. A very mild anomaly without curvature of the penis or stenosis of the orifice. No treatment is required for this type.

congenital absence of the urethra. However, a search with a fine probe in the region of the coronal sulcus will usually discover the opening and release the urinary stream.

Apart from meatal stenosis, which is easily corrected by meatotomy dividing the bridge of tissue between the urethral opening and the blind ducts lying dorsal to it, there is very little disability involved in coronal hypospadias. The urinary stream may at first seem difficult to direct but children soon adapt themselves to holding the penis at an appropriate angle and very few patients require operation on this account. Parents can be confidently reassured that coronal hypospadias does not hinder normal sexual intercourse, nor impair fertility.

In more severe degrees (Fig. 6.2) the urethral meatus is placed on the undersurface of the penis, or even in the perineum between the two halves of a split scrotum. These last cases, when associated with undescended testicles and a small penis, fall into the intersex category and are discussed in a later section. In all penile and perineal forms normal standing micturition is impossible, though there is no interference with sphincteric control. There is also likely to be some chordee, the penis being subject to a ventral curvature which becomes more acute in

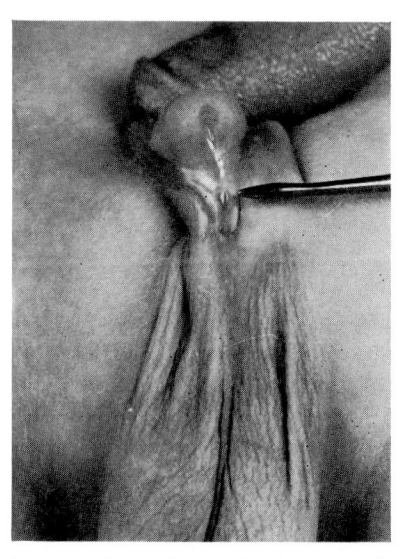

FIG. 6.2. Penile hypospadias. The urethral meatus is near the penoscrotal junction, the penis is short and curved and the orifices of blind sinuses can be seen on the penis distal to the meatus.

erection and which if left untreated renders intercourse unsatisfactory or impossible. This chordee is due to several factors, the most important of which is the presence of a strong fibrous band linking the external meatus to the glans, adherent both to skin and to the underlying corpora cavernosa. In addition the urethra may be shortened and the skin webbed to the scrotum. Correction of hypospadias therefore involves two stages, first the straightening of the penis, second the construction of the terminal urethra and normally placed meatus. The importance of the first stage must be carefully explained to parents, as it usually allows the meatus to drop back further from the tip of the penis and makes micturition even more clumsy. It is desirable that repair should be complete by the time the child goes to school at 5 years of age, but there is little to be gained by an early start and the surgical procedure is easier when the penis is larger. Toddlers do not make the happiest hospital patients and 4 years is perhaps the best time to start surgery. The results of modern operations are on the whole satisfactory and although a perfect meatus is difficult to achieve no lasting disability may be anticipated.

The empirical risk for a younger brother of an index patient with hypospadias is about 1 in 10. The risks for sons of affected individuals is not well established, but almost certainly less than 1 in 10.

Epispadias and Ectopia Vesicae

Although etymologically epispadias appears to be the counterpart of hypospadias, involving a urethral opening on the dorsum instead of the ventrum of the penis, the two conditions have in fact very little in common. Hypospadias is a simple failure of the final stage of urethral formation in the male. Epispadias is an early and fundamental deviation of the normal development of the lower urinary tract and anterior abdominal wall, being only a lesser degree of the ectopia vesicae malformation and affecting both sexes. There is a midline defect in the whole area between the primitive cloaca and the umbilical stalk. In the typical ectopia vesicae (Fig. 6.3), therefore, the bladder lies open on the lower part of the abdominal wall with the umbilical cord, lower than usual in the abdomen, attached to the upper margin. In the male the penis is short and broad with a strip of urethral mucosa continuous with the open bladder along its dorsal surface. In the female the clitoris is split into two elements, each lying lateral to and a little behind a very short urethral strip. The vaginal orifice is small but otherwise normal. In both sexes the anus is placed rather more anteriorly than normal and is frequently complicated by rectal prolapse. Umbilical and inguinal herniae are common. The pubic bones do not meet in a symphysis, they are united by a fibrous band incorporated in the tissue lying behind the bladder.

In the typical ectopia vesicae the urine effluxing from the ureteric orifices is, of course, completely uncontrolled, and causes a good deal of damage to the surrounding skin. In epispadias (Fig. 6.4) the bladder is formed as a saccular organ, but the bladder neck and urethra are deficient in the same way. The penis is therefore the same in appearance as in ectopia, while in the female the urethral meatus is a wide trans-

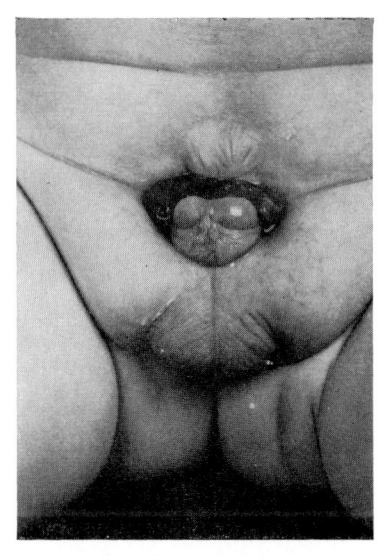

FIG. 6.3. Ectopia vesicae in a boy. The bladder protrudes between the very low umbilical scar and the short, stubby, penis. Bilateral inguinal herniae are present.

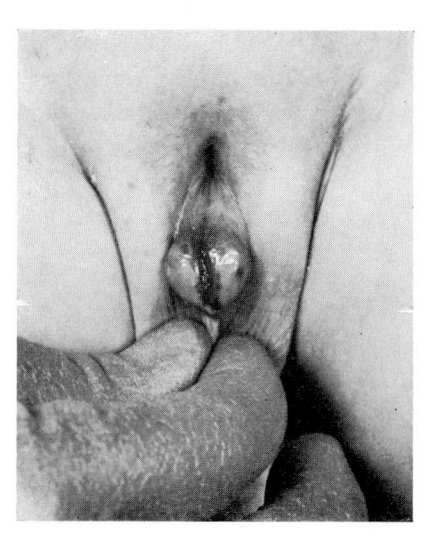

FIG. 6.4. Epispadias in a boy. The urethral strip lies open on the dorsal surface of the penis and the bladder opens through a wide arch under the pubis.

verse slit leading directly into the bladder. The pubic bones again do not meet, but some of the fibrous tissue which unites them lies in front of the bladder. In almost all cases of epispadias there is incontinence, the urine dribbling away continuously. In recumbency, however, the bladder may accumulate some urine which is discharged on sitting up and parents therefore sometimes believe that the small infant with epispadias has a degree of control, an optimism which is usually dispelled in time.

Very rarely an intestinal defect complicates ectopia vesicae, producing a peculiar, and mercifully usually a fatal, anomaly. The anus is imperforate and a portion of the bowel prolapses between a split ectopic bladder. Myelomeningocele often occurs as well.

The ordinary ectopic bladder is an ugly affair and terrifying to parents who are apt to imagine that urgent surgery is required. There is often a feeling that the child will certainly die unless heroic measures are undertaken, yet such is the faith in surgeons that this operation is expected to cure the child completely. This all-or-none approach is easier to grasp than the reality which involves little immediate danger but life-long disability. It is well, therefore, that the general practitioner who first sees the child should have some idea of what the disability is and what methods are available for its relief.

The incomplete symphysis pubis may at first produce a waddling gait with a tendency to external rotation of the lower limbs, but after a few years the stance and walking appear normal. Sexual function in the female is normal; in the male erections are satisfactory although the penis is apt to be pulled against the abdomen and seminal emissions occur from the verumontanum directly unless a urethral repair has been effected. The handicap, and it is a tremendous one, is the urinary incontinence, while the chief dangers to life are the complications of surgical interference. It is true that in the untreated cases metaplasia of the exposed vesical mucosa may in adult years go on to neoplastic change, but in the circumstances of contemporary life hardly any case goes untreated, so that this remote possibility need not be considered here.

A great many forms of treatment have been devised for the ectopic bladder and there is still no consensus of opinion regarding the correct approach, which must indeed vary according to the precise anatomy and to the social circumstances of the child. The exposed mucosa is tender and bleeds easily, but if treated with care, particularly if protected from contact with the napkins with tulle gras, it gives no serious trouble during the first few months of life. The skin around must be protected from the action of ammoniacal urine by creams and by exposure to the air whenever possible. As the infant's activity increases, so the bladder becomes more tender and surgical treatment more urgent.

Surgical reconstruction of the bladder seems the obvious and ideal treatment and it has been attempted at many centres over a great many years. Unfortunately the results have been very disappointing so far, although hope of improvement with new techniques has not been abandoned. Some sort of reconstruction of the abdominal wall and genitalia must of course be performed in all cases and it is therefore reasonable to attempt a bladder reconstruction at the same time in all those in whom there seems a reasonable possibility of useful bladder function. However, reconstruction is not entirely without danger since reflux almost invariably accompanies this condition and reflux from a small-capacity, partially-obstructed bladder can have rapidly deleterious effects upon the kidneys. Functional closure should not therefore be attempted on any very small bladder or one in which there are severe polypoid changes in the mucosa.

In the male the deformity is associated with upward chordee of the penis and this must be corrected by a preliminary operation to lengthen the urethral strip. It is also of value to perform an osteotomy on the iliac bones posteriorly in order to assist approximation of the pubes anteriorly. Reconstruction of the bladder can then be achieved by isolating it, closing it and bringing the abdominal wall structures together. This type of operation can be performed at any stage in early childhood, though it is probably better undertaken before 2 years of age. A careful follow-up by pyelogram and urine examination is essential if upper tract damage resulting from operation is to be recognized early.

Urinary diversion is essential when reconstruction is impossible or has failed. For many years uretero-colic transplantation has been the standard form of treatment for exstrophy of the bladder and it has been responsible for many encouraging results. Long-term surveys, however, reveal dangers and disappointments. As already mentioned, the anus in this disease is abnormal and although it may be adequate for the control of faeces it may allow the leakage of urine, particularly at night. It is therefore essential before advising uretero-sigmoidostomy to be sure that the anal sphincter is functionally adequate. Electrolyte problems in uretero-sigmoidostomy are another cause of complications. Reabsorption of chloride from the urine in the bowel together with loss of potassium can have serious metabolic effects. Ascending infection is also very common and often serious with a chronic pyelonephritis and stone formation. Thus, although uretero-sigmoidostomy, and the variants on it which make use of the anal sphincter for the control of urine, are occasionally very successful and are the only forms of urinary diversion which do not involve the wearing of an appliance, there are serious disadvantages and it is essential that parents should realize if this type of operation is advised that a subsequent revision may be necessary should signs of renal damage appear.

It is possible to avoid some of the infective complications of uretero-sigmoidostomy by performing a proximal defunctioning colostomy, leaving the isolated rectum as a sterile cavity and a substitute bladder. This greatly improves the prognosis in cases where anal sphincter control is adequate, but most parents will reject the idea of a colostomy and would prefer instead a urinary stoma of the abdomen. The urinary ileostomy is, in fact, the most generally applicable form of diversion. In this operation both ureters are transplanted into an isolated loop of ileum, or occasionally to an isolated loop of colon, which can then be brought out on to the surface of the abdomen. The urinary efflux is collected in a stick-on bag which allows no leakage. At first sight this would appear to be a formidable handicap to place upon a young child, yet experience has shown that adaptation is easy and the benefits in terms of urinary control and preservation of the kidneys outweigh its disadvantages.

Rare Penile Anomalies

There are a number of rare conditions affecting the penis which may be briefly listed: micropenis is the only one which most practitioners will have the opportunity to see and even this is diagnosed more often than is justified by the true incidence. Many parents become concerned that the penis remains a small organ until puberty and is apt to be obscured by the suprapubic pad of fat. In the great majority of cases, however, they can be safely reassured that development will occur and there will be no handicap to intercourse. In the true micropenis the organ is very small indeed, though otherwise normally formed. In the months after birth it sometimes becomes lost to sight and the prepuce is invaginated

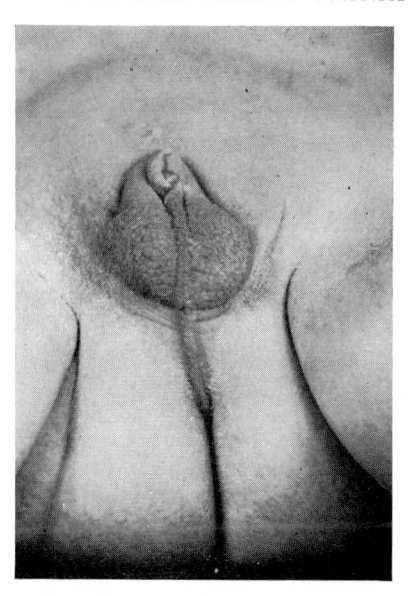

FIG. 6.5. Micropenis. The penis is so small that the suprapubic skin and prepuce are invaginated.

in the midst of the suprapubic fat (Fig. 6.5). There may or may not be an accompanying hypoplasia of the testicles but in any case the prognosis in relation to satisfactory intercourse is poor.

Absence of the penis may occur with normal testicles, the external urinary meatus being in the perineum. Megalopenis is due to an enormous dilatation of the penile urethra with overgrowth of the skin and subcutaneous tissue. Torsion of the penis in which the whole organ, corpora cavernosa included, shows a corkscrew twist through 90°–120°, occasionally accompanies hypospadias. The torsion itself cannot be corrected but it is not a bar to normal sexual function. Diphallus, or double penis, has been recorded in various forms, all of them more or less amenable to surgery.

Testicular Anomalies

At birth there is usually little difficulty in palpating the normal testicle despite its small size. During the first few months the infant puts on subcutaneous fat and the cremasteric reflex becomes more active, so that a much more careful examination is required. The testicle should be sought by stroking gently downwards from the inguinal region with the left hand and receiving it in the scrotum between the fingers and thumb of the right. A rougher or direct approach is apt to stimulate retraction and the normal testicle may, therefore, be mistaken for an undescended one.

Not all normal testicles are fully descended at birth; they may well complete their course within the first year of life. There should always be some hesitation, therefore, in making a diagnosis of absent or undescended testicle in the newborn. Fortunately, in the absence of complications, no treatment is required for this condition until much later. There is, of course, a more urgent diagnostic problem in the intersex cases, which will be discussed later, and occasionally the presence of a large hernia in addition to an undescended testicle demands early treatment.

Hydrocele is common in the newborn period. It is often bilateral and may be reducible if the processus vaginalis is still canalized, although not large enough to allow herniation of the intestine. The reducible hydrocele, like hernia in the newborn, can disappear spontaneously; it may, however, persist and the opening may widen until a hernia is present. Surgical cure is a simple matter of ligation of the processus vaginalis. Irreducible hydroceles which are present at birth are almost always reabsorbed during the first year of life. Aspiration is no assistance in this process and unless the swelling is enormous no treatment should be carried out.

Although it is not a congenital abnormality, torsion of the testis or spontaneous infarction may be mentioned as a rare cause of a hard testicular swelling in the newborn. It is usually explored surgically, although in fact little is gained by operation and the testicle is probably better left *in situ* in the hope that some interstitial cells may survive.

Female Genital Anomalies

Most of the serious abnormalities of the vagina and uterus, agenesis and duplication for instance, produce no symptoms in infancy or childhood and are very rarely diagnosed at this stage.

Labial fusion (Fig. 6.6) is a common and innocuous condition, but often mistaken for something more serious. The labia minora are adherent through the greater part of their length, leaving only a small opening under the clitoris through which urine is passed. This adhesion may be present at birth or may form later during an attack of vulvitis.

Parents and occasionally even doctors are alarmed by this appearance, thinking that the vagina is altogether absent, but once it is seen that the membrane is at the level of the labia minora, and no higher, the diagnosis should not be in doubt. Separation is easily accomplished by the use of a probe. Re-adhesion should be prevented by the regular application of petroleum jelly.

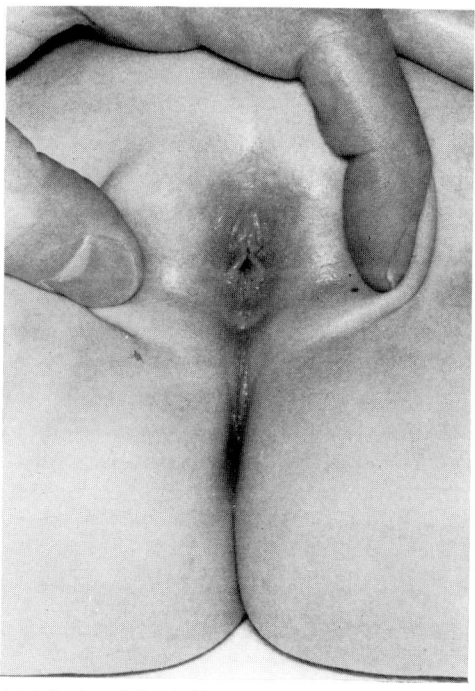

FIG. 6.6. Labial fusion. The labia minora are adherent to one another in the mid-line, but there is no serious anomaly.

Hydrocolpos is due to more serious obstruction to the vagina, causing the accumulation of a large volume of milky secretion in the genital tract. It is often stated to be due to an imperforate hymen, though in fact the obstructive membrane may well originate above the level of the hymen, bulging downwards and even protruding between the labia (Fig. 6.7). The first sign of this anomaly is often the abdominal swelling of the enormously distended vagina, it goes on to cause retention of urine, obstruction of the bowel and oedema of the legs. Most cases are easy and satisfactory to treat: once it is clear that the vagina is completely obstructed but that the urethra is patent there is no diagnostic problem and a simple incision releases the pent-up fluid. The uterus and tubes are rarely affected and the ultimate prognosis in regard to sexual function is good.

Haematocolpos, although due to a similar obstruction, is essentially a disease of puberty and will not be discussed here.

Herniae in the female infant frequently involve the ovary, which slides down the hernial sac. Where a gonad can be felt in the groin of an

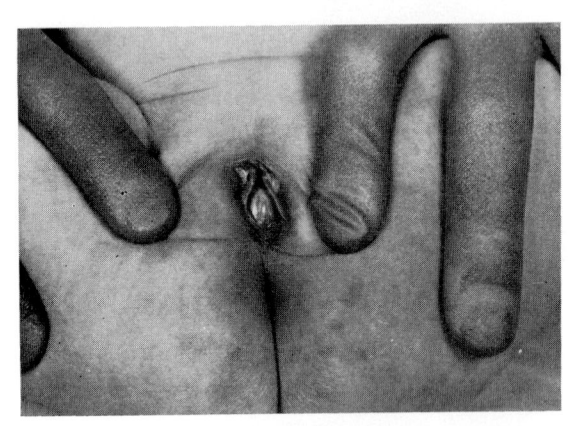

FIG. 6.7. Hydrocolpos.

apparent female, however, the testicular feminization syndrome, described below, must always be considered.

INTERSEX STATES

Of all the abnormalities of the external genitalia none poses so difficult a problem in diagnosis as the child whose external genitalia give no certain clue as to the sex, yet here more than anywhere is an urgent need for final and complete assessment, so that right from the start the child may be brought up in the proper sexual role, untroubled by parental doubts and fears. Many of the psychological disasters spring from early uncertainty and late changes of role, and these it is our duty to avoid. It must be recognized, however, that where there is serious doubt as to the sex, external inspection is not enough for diagnosis. Laboratory tests and occasionally even exploratory surgery are required if mistakes are to be avoided.

Many syndromes are grouped together under the general heading of intersex. These conditions may arise from a primary abnormality of the number of sex chromosomes, as already described in Ch. 1, from mosaicism due to the formation of two or more separate cell lines containing different numbers of sex chromosomes, from abnormalities of the gonads themselves or from subsequent derangements of the normal differentiation of the external genitalia. These last conditions may be due to autosomal genetic factors or to external environmental influences. It will be clear, therefore, that no one simple test will be adequate to decide the sex in which a child should be reared. The chromosome numbers may be estimated from a complete chromosome count, but since this is a complex investigation not readily available a good deal of reliance is usually placed on the observation of the sex chromatin (see Ch. 1, p. 9). Where more than one X-chromosome is present a chromatin granule can be observed in the nucleus of epithelial cells and a 'drumstick' can be seen on the nucleus of polymorph leucocytes. In the ordinary course of events the finding of this sex chromatin granule indicates that the child is female, but several fallacies in this interpretation are encountered and in the first month of life, when diagnosis is most important, the results of the examination are sometimes misleading.

The disorders arising from variations in sex chromosome number may be considered first, though briefly, as in general they do not present problems of diagnosis at birth. These variations in number arise theoretically from a failure of disjunction of the sex chromosome at the reduction division and it may therefore be anticipated that the possible findings in the abnormal cases are XXX, XXY, XO and YO. The last of these is not found clinically and it is presumed that affected foetuses would not be viable. The triple X syndrome is found in female children without specific anatomical abnormality; they may be mentally deficient and are often infertile, but where they have produced daughters these are not necessarily abnormal in chromosome number. The XXY combination is characteristic of Klinefelter's syndrome in which the genitalia are apparently masculine and, indeed, present no abnormality in the infant. The testicles, however, remain small and firm and are mostly incapable of spermatogenesis. The body takes on a eunuchoid appearance after puberty should have occurred and breast development is then a marked feature. In children's clinics these cases are most likely to be found among mentally deficient children. The sex chromatin in them is positive as two X's are present.

The XO pattern where there is only a single sex chromosome present

P

is characteristic of Turner's syndrome, although some of the features of this syndrome may be found in children who have mosaicism, who have normal chromosomes, or occasionally even in the male. The classical example has, however, an outwardly female appearance with a normally developed vagina, uterus and tubes, but the gonads are agenetic, represented by only a thin streak of tissue containing stromal cells alone. These girls present with dwarfism and certain somatic abnormalities such as webbing of the neck or with amenorrhoea during adolescence. In early infancy, however, there is often oedema on the dorsum of the feet and multiple skin folds on the neck which disappear later but which may give an indication of the presence of a chromosome disorder. Slight enlargement of the clitoris also occurs at birth in a few. As only one X chromosome is present these children are chromatin negative and it is important to realize that this does not indicate a male individual.

The next category of intersex conditions which must be considered is that of true hermaphroditism. In these individuals both ovarian and testicular tissue is present. Their chromosome state is variable and a great many patterns have been reported; mosaics are common amongst them, but many cases are apparently simple XX and almost all are chromatin positive on examination of the buccal smear. The anatomy of the genitalia exhibits wide variations, there is usually a penis with some degree of hypospadias, though a complete masculine urethra has been reported. The vagina is almost always present, although its orifice may be hidden within the depths of the urethra. The testicular and ovarian tissue may be fused in an ovo-testis or separate gonads may be present on the same or opposite sides. A testis or ovo-testis is apt to descend into the scrotum, but the ovary remains within the abdomen. The great importance of this abnormality is in the development at puberty, when menstruation and breast development appear at the same time as a deepening of the voice, the growth of facial hair and penile erections. Such a psychologically disastrous situation should never be allowed to occur and its avoidance entails a full diagnosis during the earlier part of childhood, with removal of the inappropriate gonad. Diagnosis, however, requires differentiation from the next class of intersex conditions, the pseudohermaphrodites.

In the pseudohermaphrodites the gonads are normal, being either testicles or ovaries, but the individual has genitalia modified in the direction of the opposite sex. Thus, in the female pseudohermaphrodite ovaries are present but the genitalia are masculinized and in the male pseudohermaphrodite the reverse situation occurs. The sex chromatin in both cases corresponds to the gonad, not to the external appearance.

The great majority of female pseudohermaphrodites are suffering from adrenal cortical hyperplasia, a congenital disorder concerned primarily with a failure in the biosynthesis of cortisol. This process appears to be incomplete and stops short at the stage of hydroxyprogesterone. The absence of circulating cortisol leads to hypersecretion

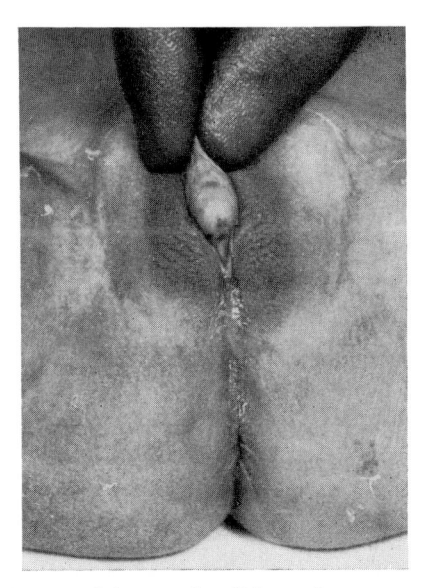

Fig. 6.8. Female pseudohermaphroditism due to adrenal cortical hyperplasia. There is considerable hypertrophy of the phallus, with extreme curvature and a urethral meatus close to the glans. The labial folds are rugose as in the scrotum.

by the pituitary of adrenotropic hormones and therefore to adrenal cortical hyperplasia. As a by-product of this process a large excess of adrenal androgens is produced. The process commences in foetal life so that at birth the child has normal ovaries, Fallopian tubes and uterus, but the phallus is enlarged to the size of an ordinary penis with a degree of hypospadias (Fig. 6.8). The vagina is present but usually opens into the urethra where it is not directly visible. The labial folds take on a rugose appearance reminiscent of a scrotum and may fuse in the midline. The child is therefore not infrequently mistaken for a male. The process of virilization does not cease at birth, however, there is a continuing stimulation both of somatic and sexual development. The child grows more rapidly, develops muscles appropriate to a pubertal male, with enlargement of the phallus, the appearance of pubic hair and deepening of the voice, at perhaps before 4 or 5 years of age. More important in the neonatal stage are the dangers resulting from the electrolyte disturbance. These children suffer from salt loss, leading to Addisonian crises with vomiting, severe dehydration and collapse. There is in fact considerable danger that they will die suddenly before the diagnosis is reached, although biochemical correction is usually possible with the assistance of cortisone and salt administration. Cortisone has in fact remarkable effect in this syndrome and appears to act as substitution therapy. So long as it is continued growth can proceed normally and virilization does not progress. It is therefore of vital importance for the ultimate fate of the child as well as for the immediate avoidance of electrolyte disturbances that this disease is diagnosed as soon as possible after birth, emphasizing the need for full investigations of the child with genitalia of equivocal sex.

Female pseudohermaphrotism due to adrenal cortical hyperplasia is determined by an autosomal recessive gene.

A second and less serious class of female pseudohermaphrodites is provided by those infants who have been virilized during foetal life by hormones in the maternal circulation. Such influences can arise from maternal virilizing tumours, arrhenoblastoma for example, but much more commonly the hormones are administered in the hope of preventing abortion. Testosterone itself has been used for this purpose on a number of occasions, but many of the progesterone preparations more commonly employed also have an androgenic effect, if administered within the first 3 months of pregnancy. The majority of these cases have no more than an enlarged clitoris with otherwise normal openings of urethra and vagina, but in a few the changes are more advanced so that the urethral folds are closed over to form a penis-like organ. This disease is, of course, not progressive and in many cases regression occurs. The clitoris ceases to enlarge and may soon appear relatively normal, but where a canalized anterior urethra has been formed surgical correction will be required. One further form of female pseudohermaphroditism must be mentioned in which there is no evidence at all of endocrine disturbance. It is a purely anatomical abnormality, usually with the formation of a penis-like structure out of fused labia minora, together with stenosis of the urethral and vaginal orifices.

In the male pseudohermaphrodites hormonal changes are not commonly encountered, but two separate conditions must be mentioned. The first is known as the testicular feminization syndrome, although the evidence that the testicles themselves are responsible for the feminization is flimsy in the extreme. This syndrome is familial and all cases present a very similar appearance. The individuals are almost always brought up as girls and on external inspection there is nothing to suggest that an intersex abnormality is present. The clitoris, urethra and vulva are typically feminine. The vagina is short, however, and ends a little above the region of the hymen in a mass of tissue, perhaps representing a uterus, from which two vasa deferentia run to the testicles which are placed either in the inguinal region or intra-abdominally. Most often this type of male pseudohermaphroditism is discovered at puberty when there is complete amenorrhoea with slight breast development only and absent pubic and axillary hair. Some of these children are diagnosed in infancy, however, because of the palpable gonads in the groins, and in all cases where there is an apparent hernia in the female child this condition should be considered. A careful inspection of the vagina will usually give the correct clue. In this syndrome there can be very little hope of changing the sexual role to that appropriate to the gonads, for the tissues which might go to make up a penis are absent. The female role must be accepted and many individuals have married and had sexual intercourse with some satisfaction. It may be necessary at a later time to undertake castration with hormone replacement therapy.

This condition occurs in families with a pattern which suggests determination by a sex-linked recessive gene. Determination by a sex-limited autosomal gene is an alternative possibility, but for practical purposes this gives the same family risks.

In the second type of male pseudohermaphroditism we are dealing with a heterogeneous group; the least severe cases differ only in degree from simple perineal hypospadias in which the penis is small and the testicles undescended. In more severe examples, however, a vaginal canal is present, perhaps opening on the surface, perhaps communicating with the posterior urethra. In these there is often a uterus, usually asymmetrical, with Fallopian tubes. The testicle is retained within the abdomen in most and is sometimes completely absent on one side. Some of these cases are mosaics XY.XO and the absence of the testicle on one side leads to unilateral development of female genital passages. The uterus in these conditions does not exhibit menstrual changes, though infections and bleeding may occur from the genital tract. The general bodily development will be masculine but may be modified by hypogonadism. The psychological orientation depends very largely upon the upbringing, but where the children have been reared as girls they may have severe emotional disturbances in adolescence.

Differential diagnosis in the intersex states, as will be clear now, is a matter of difficulty and it has already been emphasized that clinical examination is seldom adequate. In the child with genitalia of equivocal sex, only where two testicles can be palpated beyond doubt may the examiner be satisfied with external inspection alone. In all other cases the first steps must be the cytological examination of epithelial cells, derived from either buccal smears of skin biopsy, or of polymorph leucocytes for sex chromatin, and the collection of 24-hour specimens of urine for estimation of 17-ketosteroid output. This collection sometimes presents difficulties, but stick-on bags such as are used for colostomies are often satisfactory. The normal level of 17-ketosteroids in a 24-hour specimen of a newborn child is less than 0·5 mg. In adrenal hyperplasia it is usually raised to over 1·0 mg and frequently to higher levels, increasing during the course of the first month of life.

All the intersex females are chromatin positive but chromatin-positive cases are not necessarily female, they may, for instance, be true hermaphrodites or examples of Klinefelter's syndrome. The sex chromatin therefore gives an important lead but not a complete diagnosis. In cases where the sex chromatin is positive and the output of 17-ketosteroids is raised, together with the output of pregnantriol, there can be no doubt that the infant is suffering from adrenal cortical hyperplasia. In chromatin-positive cases where there is a history of testosterone or progesterone treatment during pregnancy, it is reasonable to assume that the latter is the cause of the disorder. In all other chromatin positive cases a careful endoscopic examination must be made to determine the precise anatomy and if necessary a biopsy of the gonads must be performed, for it is only in the latter way that diagnosis of true hermaphroditism can be established.

In the chromatin-negative cases it is likely that the diagnosis is one of male pseudohermaphroditism, but it must be remembered that in Turner's syndrome the clitoris is sometimes a little enlarged and sex chromatin is absent. The latter diagnosis can usually be established from other stigmata. The other chromatin-negative cases spotted at birth are likely to be severe examples of hypospadias with some development of the Müllerian system, which can be verified from endoscopy. In them, however, there is still a chance of true hermaphroditism being present and suspect cases should at least have a laparotomy and biopsy before puberty so that the inappropriate gonadal tissue can be removed.

Pseudohermaphrodite conditions must be suspected in two other circumstances during infancy, where an apparent female has gonads palpable in the groin and where a child with hypospadias has a sudden onset of collapse and dehydration. In the former group testicular feminization syndrome may be responsible; in the latter, adrenocortical hyperplasia in the female.

INTERNAL ABNORMALITIES

Although not immediately obvious in the newborn baby, abnormalities of the kidneys, ureters and bladder are as common as the external deformities and involve a greater danger to life and health. For the most part, exact diagnosis can only be reached from radiological investigations which are beyond the scope of this discussion, but if these anomalies are to be treated before it is too late their presence must be suspected from the early clinical findings so that the practitioner and paediatrician may refer the infants for radiological investigation. The common presenting signs which arouse suspicion are, therefore, of the greatest importance: the first evidence is usually to be found in an abdominal mass, a distended bladder, a raised blood urea or a urinary infection, and the significance of these findings is discussed below. It may be, however, that investigations are started because previous siblings have been affected, as in infantile polycystic disease, adrenocortical hyperplasia or testicular feminization, or because hydramnios or oligo-hydramnios has suggested a disorder of foetal urinary production. Anomalies of other systems sometimes give a clue to urinary tract disorders: the 'Potter' facies is associated with renal agenesis; anomalies of the external ear are said to be (and a single umbilical artery is certainly) accompanied by an increased incidence of urinary anomalies. Agenesis of the abdominal muscles always indicates a urological problem and infants with ano-rectal deformities should have an intravenous pyelogram, as should those with a severe degree of hypospadias.

An abdominal swelling may be found on routine examination of the newborn infant or during the search for a cause of failure to thrive, and urinary tract abnormalities are responsible for most of such swellings. An enlarged kidney at this stage has the same characteristics as in later life, although being lower in the abdomen it is easier to feel. Even the normal kidney is readily palpable in the dehydrated infant, but is much less easily felt as the tissues fill out. A hard renal swelling at birth may well be due to a neoplasm, usually a relatively benign one and perhaps hamartomatous. Adrenal tumours are, however, a more common malignancy in the newborn, A unilateral cystic swelling may be a hydronephrosis with pelvi-ureteric or uretero-vesical obstruction, or if it is very coarsely lobulated, a multi-cystic kidney. Bilateral renal swellings may be due to polycystic disease or hydronephrosis with lower urinary tract obstruction. Sudden renal enlargement after birth may be the result of renal vein thrombosis.

A chronically distended bladder is an important indication of urinary tract anomalies, but it is only in exceptional cases that the distension reaches above the umbilicus. The normal bladder is, of course, palpable when distended but usually the process of examination will stimulate a contraction and after micturition the swelling will disappear. By contrast, bladder distension associated with a slow continuous dribble of urine from the penis indicates obstruction with overflow incontinence. The neuropathic bladder resulting from congenital spinal anomalies is often distended, but expressible: urine is expressed as long as pressure is made on the bladder with the palpating hand. It should never be necessary to catheterize the infant simply for the purpose of determining whether the abdominal swelling is or is not a distended bladder, for catheterization involves grave dangers of infecting an obstructed urinary tract and should not be undertaken unless all preparations are made for the institution of permanent drainage. In the female, bladder distension is uncommon, but hydrocolpos produces a swelling which is not easy to distinguish from the bladder in the abdomen, though it may be recognized from the appearance of the vagina.

Disorders of micturition attract little attention in infancy, for napkins conceal both the frequency and the force of bladder evacuation. Much may, in fact, be learned from the proper observation of micturition, particularly in relation to overflow incontinence, but at least acute retention, with the napkins completely dry over a long period, is unlikely to escape notice. The newborn infant may fail to pass urine for something up to 48 hours without there being necessarily any abnormality of the urinary tract, but in these circumstances the abdomen should be palpated for bladder distension. More serious causes of anuria at birth are complete renal agenesis, which is usually rapidly fatal, or total urinary tract obstruction, in which case the child will not survive more than 2 weeks. The onset of acute retention in later infancy may have a much less serious significance, being due for instance to the pain of meatal ulceration, to impacted calculi, or to a temporary exacerbation of a chronic obstructive process which may still be amenable to surgery.

Incontinence is a term which might be thought inapplicable to the young infant who exercises little voluntary control over micturition, yet there is a sense in which incontinence is an important symptom even in the very young. Normal micturition is frequent but bladder emptying is complete and rapid, the stream of urine powerful. Afterwards the infant will remain completely dry for a definite, although a variable, period: perhaps for half an hour, perhaps for 3 hours. If by contrast the urine is dribbling away continuously and the stream is never forceful, then an abnormality is present. The two most common causes are lower urinary obstruction in the male and neuropathic bladder in both sexes. The diagnosis in the latter case is seldom in doubt because an obvious meningocele is present. Occasionally a congenital spinal deformity producing little external deformity is nevertheless associated with interference with the spinal centre for micturition.

Some other causes of dribbling incontinence, such as epispadias, may be recognized on external inspection, while others, such as the vaginal ectopic ureter in the female, can only be detected by urological investigation. Usually this is postponed until the child is much older, but in fact there is no reason why the diagnosis should not be made in infancy, if the true significance of the continual dribbling incontinence is recognized.

Renal failure is often the first sign of a renal anomaly. It should be recalled that during foetal life the waste products of metabolism are removed via the placental circulation and although urine formation occurs from an early stage, renal function is not essential to normal development, and a newborn infant without functioning kidneys can appear outwardly normal at birth. However, in the extreme case of bilateral renal agenesis already mentioned the infant is usually stillborn or dies within a few hours of birth due to other congenital anomalies. In these cases the complete absence of urine secretion causes oligo-hydramnios which may have some influence in causing deformities of the limbs. A more common circumstance is the presence of grossly inadequate kidneys due to congenital cystic disease, dysplasia or obstruction. The child appears healthy but renal function is inadequate to maintain an independent existence and the blood urea rises rapidly after birth as the child's condition deteriorates. In the case of the obstructions it may be possible to correct the cause but unfortunately some of the infants will have kidneys already too severely damaged for this treatment to have any permanent effect.

In the infant, vomiting, loss of weight and dehydration are usually the first signs of failure. All save clear feeds are rejected, the abdomen becomes distended, the stools loose or constipated. Clearly there is nothing specific about these signs which could be due to many diseases, grave or trivial. It is essential, therefore, to keep in mind the possibility of renal involvement in all infants who fail to thrive and set the appropriate investigations in train. A raised blood urea will of course be found together with an acidosis and low sodium in most cases. A variety of disorders could be responsible for these findings, but if a urinary obstruction is present, it must be urgently relieved at the same time as biochemical resuscitation is carried out.

A urinary infection is a common complication of many abnormalities and it is not infrequently the onset of such an infection in the young infant which draws attention to the defect. At this age urinary infection produces no specific signs or symptoms, the child may have a fever or even a subnormal temperature; feeds are refused, vomiting, diarrhoea, dehydration and sometimes jaundice may occur. Routine examination of the urine is essential; the infant's urine is first collected in a stick-on plastic bag and examined as soon as possible after it has been passed. In most cases the presence of large numbers of pus cells along with organisms will leave little doubt as to the presence of infection, but if the findings are equivocal then a specimen free of contamination must be collected. In the infant this is most easily done by supra-pubic puncture; a fine needle is inserted into the distended bladder immediately above the pubis, the needle being directed backwards and not downwards.

The pyuria may perhaps respond rapidly on antibiotic treatment but all such infantile infections should be thoroughly investigated by pyelography and if necessary cystography. This investigation is the more urgent in boys, particularly if there is any rise of blood urea.

Renal Agenesis and Renal Dysplasia

Absence or gross underdevelopment of one kidney is unlikely to cause any sign at birth, but if both sides are affected the infant is either stillborn or dies within a few hours of birth. Both agenesis and dysplasia are frequently accompanied by other urinary-tract anomalies, such as complete absence of the urinary passages, and by anomalies elsewhere. Potter has noted the association of pulmonary hypoplasia with renal agenesis and has described a facies peculiar to the syndrome; the nose is flat and broad, the ears are large and low-set and there is a marked groove below the orbital space. Clearly no treatment of this condition is possible.

Dysplasia is a term which can apply to many intrinsic renal anomalies: histologically it is recognized by constituents in the renal parenchymal such as cysts, islands of cartilage, immature glomeruli and tubules. Such changes may be present in kidneys which are small, or of normal size, but they are most often associated with some urinary tract abnormality and their existence probably renders the kidney liable to infection and pyelonephritis, going on to renal failure.

Cystic Disease of the Kidneys

Congenital polycystic kidneys may become evident in the newborn period or in early infancy and are usually fatal within a few months. The disease as seen at this age differs from that in later life, it occurs in siblings but not in different generations of the same family. The cysts in infantile form are small and of more or less uniform size, in contrast to the irregular large cysts of the adult form, and there are probably differences in the microscopic connections of the cysts as well. The 'adult' form is autosomal dominant. The 'infantile' form is autosomal recessive and at least two genetic variants exist which appear to breed true within sibships. In the more severe variant death is usually perinatal; in the milder form the condition presents in infancy but the child may survive a few years.

The infant's kidneys may be extremely large and cause enormous distension of the abdomen, but at other times they are only slightly enlarged and have a pelvi-calyceal pattern which is indistinguishable from normal. The appearance with high dose pyelography is characteristic: opaque medium is retained in the tubular cysts throughout the parenchyma for many hours; even, in very severe cases, for days. Renal failure is inevitable and may be accompanied by hypertension. Although some children live on for months or even years, no effective treatment of the disease is possible.

Besides the classical polycystic disease in which the liver, as well as both kidneys, is affected, there are many other forms of renal cyst, though the common solitary cyst of adult life is hardly ever seen in infancy. The unilateral disorder known as multicystic kidney is important, however, in the newborn period as the cause of an abdominal swelling. In this type the kidney is entirely replaced by large irregular cysts, it is functionless and the ureter is often obliterated. It is a harmless condition but unfortunately there is no way of diagnosing it except by exploration, which is necessary to exclude the possibility of a malignant tumour, so that nephrectomy is usually performed.

Fused and Ectopic Kidneys

Horse-shoe kidney, solitary kidney, fused pelvic kidneys and other anomalous formations are commonly found in infants with multiple congenital defects in other systems. They are liable to complications in later childhood, particularly to hydronephrosis, but are of little importance in early infancy. The pelvic ectopic form especially may be palpable as an abdominal mass but the correct diagnosis can be established without difficulty from pyelography.

Hydronephrosis due to Pelvi-ureteric Obstruction

Although due to an anomalous development, hydronephrosis is again chiefly a disorder of later childhood, presenting with severe attacks of loin pain. Occasionally, however, an enormous hydronephrotic sac produces an abdominal tumour in the neonate. It may be obviously cystic and is likely to vary a little in size from day to day, but may be as hard as a neoplastic growth. In the thin infant it may transilluminate. Diagnosis is established by retrograde pyelography or exploration, and treatment is usually a nephrectomy, for renal damage is likely to be severe in this type of hydronephrosis, but if there is a suspicion of bilateral disease, a pyeloplasty must be performed and the kidney preserved even if considerably thinned out.

MEGA-URETER

The ureters are greatly dilated in this condition, although no organic obstructive cause can be found. There are two principal forms: one which may be unilateral, in which there is a sudden and unexplained narrowing of the ureter a few centimetres above the bladder, the other which is bilateral and involves the whole length of the ureter, usually associated with vesico-ureteric reflux. The first may be responsible for attacks of pain, as in the congenital pelvi-ureteric obstruction, but recurrent or persistent urinary infection is the commonest mode of presentation in both forms. The diagnosis, which can be reached only from radiological investigations, is therefore seldom made during infancy, except where renal damage is so advanced that the child becomes uraemic during the first weeks of life. Some cases are amenable to surgical reconstruction of the lower end of the ureters, some mild examples are better left untreated except for chemotherapy to clear the infection, while at the other extreme some are too severe to benefit from treatment at all.

URETERIC DUPLICATION

Double ureter is a common anomaly; it is in fact often a harmless variation of the normal anatomy. However, other abnormalities frequently complicate the duplication and are productive of symptoms. For instance, the ureter from the upper pelvis may end ectopically. When in the female it terminates in the lower urethra or vagina, it is responsible for continual dribbling incontinence. In the male the equivalent ending is in the posterior urethra, the ejaculatory ducts or vas: it is then almost always obstructed and easily becomes infected, so that pyuria and recurrent fevers are the rule. In both sexes many of the ectopic ureters which end in the upper urethra have a cystic dilatation a little above their ending, which bulges into the bladder. This deformity is known as the ectopic ureterocele and can be responsible for many signs and symptoms in infancy. The affected ureter is acutely obstructed and often infected, but the mass in the bladder may also lead to obstruction to the outflow from the bladder and to dilatation of the other ureters. Occasionally, too, the ureterocele itself is pushed out through the urethra and prolapses externally as a pink 'bubble'. Complications may also occur when both ureters enter the bladder, particularly when vesico-ureteric reflux is present, and in these it is more often the lower half of the kidney which is involved. Bifid ureters are liable to another series of disorders, though seldom ones which present in infancy. In almost all cases of duplication, surgical excision of the pathological ureter, together with the corresponding half of the kidney, is the usual method of treatment and is generally very successful.

Urinary Fistula at the Umbilicus

At times there is a wide opening into the bladder at the umbilicus, at others a little urinary discharge from a mass of granulations. The anomaly is often described as a patent urachus, though in fact the urachus is not formed in many cases and the bladder itself reaches the umbilicus. The fistula may be the only abnormality present, in which case surgical closure presents little difficulty, but severe urethral obstruction may be found as well in infants having an entirely different prognosis. A urinary leak appearing for the first time 2 or 3 weeks after birth almost always indicates an obstruction, either congenital or acquired.

Other Vesical Anomalies

Duplications of the bladder of varying degrees or completeness, trigonal cysts and mucosal curtains are reported on occasions, but all are very rare. They present with urinary obstruction or infection and cannot be diagnosed from clinical signs.

Vesical diverticula are more likely to be acquired than congenital: they are essentially herniae of the mucosa through the detrusor layer. Usually these herniae occur only when the bladder is obstructed and the detrusor hypertrophied: they are often multiple and no more than a complication of the primary disorder. Rarely the detrusor covering is deficient over a small area of the bladder and herniation can then occur during a normal bladder contraction, so that a diverticulum is present in an otherwise normal organ. Diverticula are responsible for persistent infection, but seldom give symptoms in the first few months of life.

Bladder-neck Obstruction and Urethral Valves

Severe obstruction to the outflow of urine from the bladder causing chronic retention in infancy is one of the most serious congenital anomalies of the urinary tract. It may be due to a variety of causes but it is much more frequent in boys in whom the common lesion is posterior urethral valves. In girls an ectopic ureterocele is an important cause. It is now recognized that true bladder-neck obstruction due to a disorder of the internal sphincter of the bladder is an exceptionally rare cause in infancy, in most of the previously reported cases it is almost certain that a urethral lesion was overlooked.

Posterior urethral valves are ridges of mucosa running downwards and outwards from the verumontanum. They are an exaggerated form of normal structures but cause ballooning of the posterior urethra above them.

The infants have extremely hypertrophied, sacculated bladders with overflow incontinence, dilated tortuous ureters and advanced hydronephrosis, all resulting from obstruction to urinary flow during foetal life. It is the secondary changes rather than the primary obstruction which are difficult to correct: the bladder saccules and dilated ureters drain poorly and predispose to recurrent infection, while renal damage may be already so severe that there is insufficient functioning tissue to support life for more than a few years.

The first signs of the disorder are usually the effects of renal failure: vomiting and failure to thrive. Examination reveals a full and overflowing bladder; the abdomen is often distended, although the bladder is only partly responsible for this, the intestines too are blown up with flatus. The child rapidly becomes dehydrated and acidotic unless treatment is started. Sometimes urinary infection complicates this picture and demands even more urgent treatment. Simple bladder drainage with the small catheters which can be passed through the urethra will give relief for only a few hours and involves the grave risk of introducing infection. The infant must be transferred to an appropriately equipped surgical unit, where satisfactory urinary drainage can be established (nephrostomies are often required) and electrolyte imbalance restored as soon as possible. The exact anatomical diagnosis can await partial recovery of renal function.

ANTERIOR URETHRAL OBSTRUCTIONS

Abnormalities in this group are rare, and the obstruction produced is seldom so serious as in the posterior urethra. The most common example, meatal stenosis, has already been discussed in relation to hypospadias: stenosis of the normally placed orifice is not usually congenital; it results more often from scarring due to meatal ulceration. Congenital valves, strictures and diverticula occur in the anterior urethra and may produce a visible swelling in the perineum or very uncommonly a congenital fistula.

Absent Abdominal Muscles

In this curious condition there is a defect both of the musculature of the abdominal wall and of the urinary tract. Although great efforts have been made to demonstrate that one of these is due to the other it seems likely that they are associated abnormalities without causal relationship. The lower part of the rectus muscles and the lower and medial parts of the oblique muscles are absent, so that the lower abdominal wall consists of skin, superficial fascia and peritoneum. The skin is usually redundant and this together with its lack of support gives it a wrinkled appearance: 'prune belly' seems the most apt description. Although ugly, there is surprisingly little disability involved in the abdominal defect. The urinary-tract changes, however, endanger the child's life: there is an enormous dilatation of the bladder and the ureters with hydronephrosis and usually a complicating pyelonephritis leading to renal failure. Complete urethral atresia is found in some neonates but in other mild cases the cause of dilatation is not apparent. The bladder muscle does not become trabeculated as it does in most obstructions and perhaps a defect in the musculature of the urinary tract is the explanation. When renal damage is already severe at birth an early demise must be anticipated, but more fortunate cases seem to live for many years, even into adult life. No satisfactory treatment has yet been evolved.

SELECTED REFERENCES

ANTELL L. (1952) Hydrocolpos in infancy and childhood. *Pediatrics* **10**, 306
BLYTHE H.M. (1969) A clinico-pathological and family study of polycystic disease of the kidneys and liver in children. *J. Clin. Path.* **22**, 508
BODIAN M. (1957) Congenital bladder neck obstruction. *Brit. J. Urol.* **29**, 393
BROWNE D. (1949) Hypospadias. *Postgrad. med. J.* **25**, 367
DALGAARD O.Z. (1957) Bilateral polycystic disease of the kidneys. *Op. Dom. Biol. hered. hum. Kbh.* **38**. Copenhagen: Munksgaard
GAIRDNER D. (1949) Fate of the foreskin: a study of circumcision. *Brit. med. J.* **ii**, 1433

GORDON R.R. & O'NEILL E.M. (1969) Turner's infantile phenotype. *Brit. med. J.* **i**, 483
JONES H.W. & SCOTT W. (1958) *Hermaphroditism; Genital Anomalies and Related Endocrine Disorders.* Baltimore: Williams & Wilkins
KJELLBERG S.R., ERICSSON N.O. & RUDHE U. (1957) *The Lower Urinary Tract in Childhood.* Chicago: Year Book Publishers Inc.
LATTIMER J.K., DEAN A.L. jun., DOUGHERTY L.J., JU DAVID, RYDER C. & UNSON A. (1960) Functional closure of the bladder in children with exstrophy. *J. Urol.* **83**, 5, 647.
OVERZIER C. (1963) Ed. *Intersexuality.* London and New York: Academic Press
POTTER E.L. (1952) *The Pathology of the Foetus in the Newborn.* Chicago: Year Book Publishers Inc.
SCORER C.G. (1955) Descent of the testicle in the first year of life. *Brit. J. Urol.* **27**, 347
SORENSEN H.R. (1953) Hypospadias. *Op. Dom. Biol. hered. hum. Kbh.* Copenhagen: Munksgaard
SMITH E.D. (1965) *Spina Bifida and the Total Care of Spinal Myelomeningocele.* Springfield: Thomas
STEPHENS F.D. (1963) *Congenital Malformations of the Rectum, Anus and Genito-urinary Tract.* Edinburgh: Livingstone
WILKINS L. (1965) *The Diagnosis and Treatment of Endocrine Disorders in Childhood and Adolescence.* Springfield: Thomas
WILLIAMS D.I. (1968) Ed. *Paediatric Urology.* London: Butterworths

7

Abnormalities of the Gastro-intestinal System

H. H. NIXON AND A. W. WILKINSON

CLEFT LIP AND CLEFT PALATE

Clefts of the palate may be either median or lateral. A median cleft may involve only the uvula or the soft palate or may extend over the whole of the soft palate and the hard palate as far as the alveolus, but is not associated with a cleft of the alveolus or of the lip. Lateral clefts may involve one or both sides and are associated with a cleft of the lip (Fig. 7.1). A complete lateral cleft involves the lip, nostril, alveolus, hard and soft parts of the palates. Incomplete varieties also occur; the lip alone may be cleft, the extent ranging from a mere notching of the red margin to a cleft running up into the floor of the nostril and dividing the alveolus. The cleft lip may be associated with a cleft of the palate ranging from a cleft of the uvula alone to one extending forward through the alveolus to form a complete cleft.

In the most severe degree of bilateral cleft lip the central part of the lip is represented by a small oval piece of skin on the premaxillary portion of the alveolus which bears the upper incisor teeth. The premaxilla is separated from the maxilla on both sides and projects half an inch or more forwards out of the normal line of the alveolus on a strut formed of the prevomerine bone, the palate also being cleft on both sides of the septum.

Unilateral complete clefts of the lip are associated with an asymmetry of the face so that the nose is deviated away from the affected side and the cleft nostril may be widely splayed out.

The very rare median harelip and cleft palate may be associated with absence of the corpus callosum, a condition associated with mental defect.

In the newborn the soft palate is short and the size of an isolated cleft of the soft palate may be underestimated, and mistaken for a cleft uvula. Even a cleft of the soft palate alone is accompanied by a split

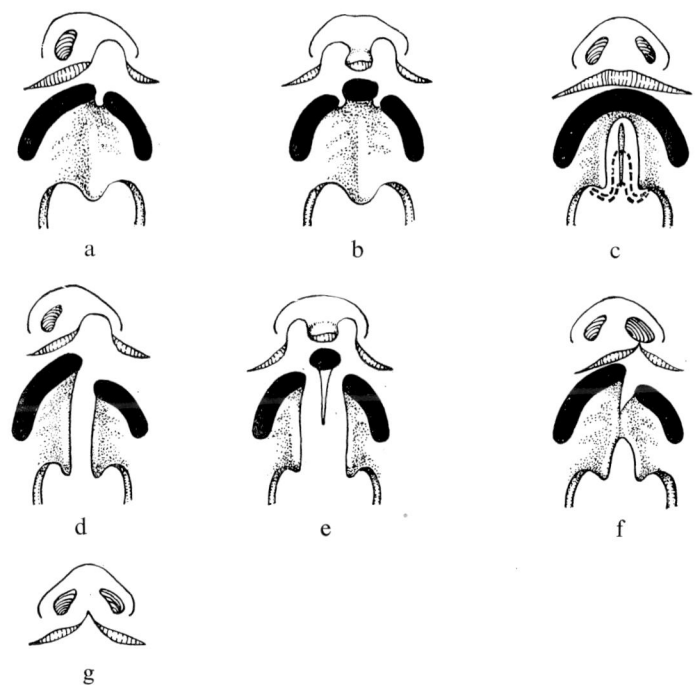

Fig. 7.1
(a) Unilateral harelip (cleft of embryological primary palate)
(b) Bilateral harelip (cleft of embryological primary palate)
(c) Postalveolar cleft palate. The dotted lines indicate incomplete forms of cleft (cleft of embryological secondary palate)
(d) Complete unilateral cleft of lip and palate (cleft of embryological primary and secondary palate)
(e) Complete bilateral cleft of lip and palate (cleft of embryological primary and secondary palates)
(f) Incomplete unilateral cleft of palate and harelip with skin bridge (incomplete cleft of embryological primary and secondary palates)
(g) True median harelip. Rare (often associated with cerebral abnormality)

oronasal sphincter and the inability to close off the nose from the mouth, and such a cleft will produce the cleft palate speech defect just as will a more extensive cleft. The usual wooden spatula is too wide to be convenient to examine the newborn pharynx and the handle of an ordinary teaspoon is a more satisfactory instrument.

The uncommon submucous cleft of the soft palate is easily missed in infancy. The mucosal layers form a complete soft palate although the muscles are separated as in the usual type of cleft. As a result oronasal closure is incomplete and the typical cleft palate voice develops owing to the nasal escape of air. The speech defect is usually the reason for the examination which leads to diagnosis. When the child gags the soft palate is seen to widen without rising and a dimple appears in each side instead of the usual one in the midline. Treatment is by division of the mucous membrane bridge and repair of the cleft in the usual manner.

The immediate problem is that of feeding. Leakage of milk into the nasal cavity through a cleft of the palate prevents the child from producing normal suction at the breast or from the bottle. Sometimes simply enlarging the hole in a large teat is enough to enable the child to feed satisfactorily, but usually the most satisfactory method of management is to teach the mother to feed the baby from a teaspoon, delivering the milk into one cheek and allowing the child to swallow it. A baby with a cleft palate who struggles to feed in an inefficient way takes down more wind than milk and may regurgitate all he has taken, both wind and milk, and become undernourished. A special cleft-palate teat has been designed with a flap to block the cleft in the palate: but this flap rubs against the free borders of the palatal cleft and nasal septum causing ulceration and predisposing to infection such as thrush and leading to scarring which may cause some inconvenience later in the repair of the palate. In addition it is difficult to keep the crevice between the flap and underlying teat clean.

Although isolated cleft of the lip itself does not usually give rise to feeding troubles a severe degree of harelip associated with asymmetry of the cleft alveolar arch may prevent the baby from forming an airtight seal at the breast or on the teat.

An isolated cleft of the palate may occasionally be associated with marked underdevelopment of the lower jaw (micrognathia), the so-called Pierre Robin syndrome. The tongue is relatively large compared with the small lower jaw and tends to fall back through the cleft in the palate, blocking the nasal passage and causing acute difficulty in breathing. Such babies should never be nursed on their backs where they are liable to swallow their tongues, and attempts at feeding may cause choking. The mother should be shown how to push the jaw forward with a finger behind the angle of the jaw while the baby sucks. Sometimes it may be necessary to feed through a plastic nasogastric tube. In severe degrees of this deformity, during a crisis of respiratory distress, it may rarely be necessary to hold the tongue forward with a stitch passed through the tongue. Prone nursing, using a plaster bed if necessary, should almost entirely avert the need for tracheostomy. Provided children with this combination of deformities can be tided over the first 6 to 12 weeks of life, subsequent growth of the lower jaw is sufficiently normal to overcome the initial disability.

The disability from a cleft palate is that of inability to achieve oro-nasal closure and hence normal speech. A secondary result of cleft of the palate is a tendency for the two sides of the arch to fall in together and this is increased by the necessary surgical treatment. The result is that in the more severe cases the middle third of the face tends to grow less than the remainder and produces the 'dish face' appearance as the child grows, with regression of the upper lip and relative prognathism.

Treatment

Clefts of the lip are usually closed at about 3 months of age when the child is thriving and has reached a weight of about 5 kg. Although complete closure of a double harelip with a protruding premaxilla is possible in one operation, some surgeons prefer to close the lip in two stages. At the first operation one side of the lip is attached to the protruding premaxilla and prolabium and at a second operation the other side of the lip is joined to the other side of the prolabium to complete the lip closure. Following this type of operation the premaxilla moves back but the septum may become buckled and the alveolar arches may grow in behind the premaxilla leaving a difficult orthodontic problem. Some surgeons therefore prefer to remove a piece of bone from the prevomerine strut behind the protruding premaxilla to allow replacement of the premaxilla between the lateral alveolar arches. This has the disadvantage that it will lead later to a sinking back of the upper lip, due to regression of the central part of the upper alveolus, again leaving a difficult problem for the orthodontist.

The deformity in harelip combined with cleft palate extends into the nose which also is deformed with a twisted septum and cartilages. In cases of harelip combined with cleft palate the entire middle third of the face may be asymmetric with the nasal spine displaced to the uncleft side and the alveolar arches at different levels. Because of the maxillary deformity correction of the nose is the most difficult part of the harelip repair. Nasal deformity may persist after the primary operation and require later correction for the sake of appearance and to allow an adequate nasal airway. Soft tissue corrections are often made at 4 years of age. The correction of any severe skeletal deformities should be deferred until growth is largely completed at about 12 years of age.

The repair of the cleft palate is usually carried out at about 18 months of age. The object of the operation is not only to close the cleft in the palate but by dissection in the lateral pharyngeal spaces to mobilize the muscles of the oronasal sphincter so as to obtain a functioning muscle sling which can draw the middle of the soft palate up and back against the pharyngeal wall to close off the nasopharynx and allow normal speech. The operation should be carried out before the child has learned to speak. Subsequently most children will learn to speak in the normal way by parental encouragement alone.

Various modifications of these orthodox methods of treatment have been proposed. Repair of a harelip in the neonatal period, originally fashionable more than 50 years ago, is now being tried again in certain clinics. It has been said that interference with maxillary growth results from operation on the palate at the age of 18 months. To avoid this it has been suggested that at this age or earlier, at say 6 months, only the soft palate should be repaired. Closure of the hard palate is postponed till 5 years of age. By this time growth of the palatal ridges will have reduced the residual cleft to a slit. Provided the soft palate is efficient the residual hard palate cleft interferes with speech remarkably little.

Whatever method of treatment is employed a large proportion of children with cleft palate require orthodontic treatment to align displaced teeth and to deal with supernumerary teeth which may grow obliquely in the cleft. Such orthodontic treatment is usually delayed until about 8 years of age when the teeth are sufficiently well developed in the second dentition to allow pressures to be applied. The teeth are moved in the jaws and the improvement in appearance and occlusion make this a very valuable part of the management of a child with cleft palate. In later years the appearance of the child can be improved, if necessary, by a dental prosthesis built on to a dental plate which by providing a smooth roof to the mouth may help to increase the clarity of speech.

Recently interest has been aroused by techniques for aligning the distorted dental arch of children with complete clefts of the palate and lip by the application of corrective sucking plates which can be fitted to the baby from the first days of life. In this way the alignment of the alveoli can be improved before the lip is repaired. Bone grafting may be used to retain the correction. If the maxilla is grossly too small late correction can be obtained by cap splinting, rapid expansion, and bone grafting to retain the improvement. Osteotomies to move the maxillae may be preferred and sometimes osteotomy to reduce the lower jaw in proportion may be wiser.

After repair of cleft palate most children learn to speak satisfactorily from their parents although rather more slowly than the normal child; for those who have difficulty after 6 or 7 years of age speech therapy may be of great value. Speech therapy cannot, however, correct bad speech when the nasal escape is due to the palate being too short or too immobile to close the nasopharynx. Some form of pharyngoplasty may help to reduce the disproportion between the soft palate and the pharynx it has to close, but is not entirely satisfactory.

Children with soft palate clefts are prone to upper respiratory infections and their aural complications, in particular to middle-ear deafness. Because of the gap between nose and mouth the child is unable to develop the air pressure necessary for a sneeze or to clear the nose properly; mucus tends to stagnate and becomes infected and infection may spread to the middle ears.

When a baby with cleft palate or harelip fails to thrive the surgeon is sometimes approached by the physician with a request to repair the cleft in order to help the child in feeding. Such requests should be resisted, for experience shows that children who are unable to thrive before the operation are bad surgical risks even in the absence of other obvious defects such as a cardiac anomaly.

Because treatment of these deformities is so often prolonged through several stages the baby should be seen by a surgeon as soon as possible and a programme drawn up and the situation explained to the parents. Continuity of treatment is probably best maintained by the surgeon.

The parents of a child with harelip and cleft palate may ask for advice on the risks of further children being similarly involved. The chances of further children being involved are as follows:

Harelip with or without Cleft Palate
Both genetic and environmental factors are concerned in the aetiology of this condition, and family studies show that it is aetiologically distinct from median cleft palate. The genetic predisposition appears homogeneous, and is probably multifactorial. Empiric risk figures are given below:

Subsequent sibs, parents normal, no other relative affected   1 in 25
Subsequent sibs, parents normal but another relative affected   1 in 25
Subsequent sibs, one parent affected   1 in 10
Children   1 in 30

Median Cleft Palate
The genetic predisposition for median cleft palate appears not to be homogeneous. In some instances there is little evidence of genetic predisposition, but in others it looks as if a single mutant gene with a variable degree of heterozygote manifestation is concerned. Empiric risk figures are given below:

Subsequent sibs, parents normal, no relative affected   1 in 50
Subsequent sibs, parents normal, but another relative affected
    1 in 10
Subsequent sibs, one parent affected   1 in 6
Children   1 in 50

Clefts of Lip and Palate in Association with Mucous Pits of the Lower Lip
This rare condition is due to a dominant mutant gene, with a 1 in 2 risk to the children of those affected.

Oesophageal Atresia

The various anatomical types of oesophageal atresia and the frequency with which they occur are shown in Fig. 7.2. In all types the upper part of the oesophagus ends blindly about the level of the second to fourth thoracic vertebra; mucus and saliva accumulate in this wide pouch and may overflow and be aspirated into the trachea and bronchi. In the commonest type there is in addition a fistula between the trachea and lower portion of the oesophagus. Through this fistula air may pass down into the stomach and on into the intestines, causing a variable degree of abdominal distension; in addition gastric secretion may be forced up the oesophagus and through the fistula into the trachea, bronchi and the rest of the respiratory tract to cause an irritative broncho-pneumonia. In a small number of children there is atresia without a tracheo-oesophageal fistula; the length of the lower portion of the oesophagus varies from an almost complete segment joined blindly to the trachea or bronchus to a small knob above the diaphragm, the latter being more common. This type of atresia without fistula can be recognized by percussion of the abdomen which remains dull and scaphoid.

A short oblique fistula may exist between the oesophagus and trachea at the root of the neck but without any interruption of the continuity of the gullet.

Although oesophageal atresia occurs only about once in every 1500 live births, it should be suspected in any newborn baby who soon after birth suffers from respiratory distress or cyanosis with an excessive quantity of frothy mucus in the pharynx, especially if frothy mucus

A	B	C	D	E	F	G	H
244 (85%)	4	24 (8%)	2	4	6 (2%)	1	1

Number of Cases

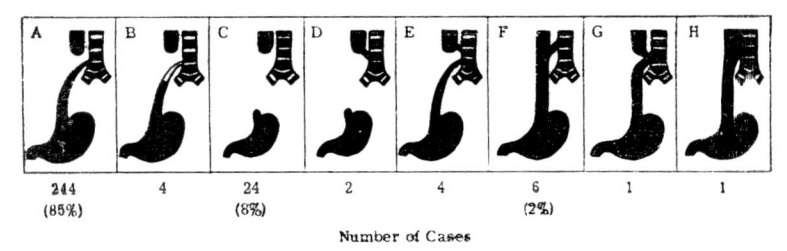

FIG. 7.2. Types and frequencies of oesophageal atresia. After Waterston.

accumulates again soon after it has been cleared by aspiration. A size 10 rubber catheter should be passed through the mouth into the oesophagus; normally such a catheter will pass into the stomach and gastric contents acid to litmus can be aspirated, but if it stops after about 10 cm have been passed this is almost certainly due to oesophageal atresia. In such a circumstance the baby must not be fed but should be transferred without delay to a children's hospital where facilities exist for the immediate operative treatment of the child. At such a hospital the only additional investigation which is necessary is to x-ray the child in the upright position with a radio-opaque catheter in the upper blind segment of the oesophagus. The introduction of opaque oil or other contrast medium into the blind upper pouch is unnecessary and leads almost without exception to the spillage of the medium into the bronchi and lungs causing obstruction to these narrow airways and later a broncho-pneumonia. Provided the x-ray film includes part of the abdomen of the baby the presence of gas in the stomach and intestines will confirm the existence of a tracheo-oesophageal fistula as surely as the arrest of the catheter shows the blind ending of the upper atretic pouch of the oesophagus.

The rare oesophageal fistula without atresia is very difficult to diagnose. Attacks of respiratory distress are accompanied by abdominal distension due to air being sucked through the fistula. It is rarely possible to see the fistula on passing an oesophagoscope or bronchoscope though methylene blue injected down the endotracheal tube may be seen to pass through the fistula. These fistulae are usually higher than those associated with an atresia at the level of the junction of cervical and thoracic oesophagus. Such a fistula may be demonstrated by injecting an opaque medium such as 'Hypaque' through an oesophageal tube which is slowly withdrawn as the behaviour of the medium is watched on the screen of an image intensifier. Cine-radiography is invaluable in recognizing the sudden 'flick' of contrast through a fistula. This type of isolated fistula is probably not as rare as has been supposed and may be missed owing to the difficulty of diagnosis.

All newborn babies with congenital abnormalities of the alimentary tract can be easily and safely taken long distances by road, rail, sea or air to the few suitably equipped hospitals where their anomaly can receive the specialized nursing and surgical care which are essential if the highest possible survival rate is to be obtained. An indwelling gastric tube and regular suction during the journey are mandatory. Babies with oesophageal atresia are no exception to this general rule and the accompanying nurse must have a 10 ml syringe attached to a soft rubber catheter so that she can aspirate mucus from the pharynx and upper blind pouch of the oesophagus when this is necessary.

The results of surgical treatment depend on early diagnosis, the maturity and weight of the baby and the existence of other abnormalities. The most frequent concomitant abnormalities are those of the heart, imperforate anus and duodenal atresia. The longer the diagnosis and ligation of the tracheo-oesophageal fistula are delayed the more likely is the development and the greater is the severity of broncho-pneumonia due to the regurgitation of gastric secretion. Few babies weighing less than 2 kg will survive the primary anastomosis of the oesophageal segments and ligation of the tracheo-oesophageal fistula even in the absence of other anomalies. In such small premature children it is wiser to confine the immediate postnatal treatment to ligation and division of the fistula and the establishment of a gastrostomy or jejunostomy for feeding. The use of a 'Replogle' double lumen tube in the upper pouch averts the hazards of aspiration. When the baby reaches about 3 kg a delayed repair can be performed without hazard. In cases with a gap too wide to bridge (usually those without fistula) a delayed repair by colon transplant is required. The upper pouch is brought out above the left clavicle and repair is postponed about 6 months. In the interval it is important to feed the baby by mouth to accustom him to taste and swallowing. Of course this food discharges from the cervical fistula into a receptacle. The gastrostomy feeds maintain the baby. About 40 per cent of all babies with oesophageal fistula are either premature or have other important and dangerous anomalies. In the remainder who are mature and have no other serious abnormality about 90 per cent should survive a primary operation on the atresia, but up to 45 per cent of these may later need one or more dilatations of the anastomostic stricture. The overall mortality rate remains at about 40 per cent of all the patients treated surgically.

Diaphragmatic Hernia

The presence of a large part of the stomach, small intestine, colon, spleen and liver in the pleural cavity through a diaphragmatic hernia may cause sudden severe respiratory disturbance with cyanosis and the heart may be displaced from left to right. An acute disturbance of this type may come on during feeding. Assisted respiration by face mask may even make matters worse because air forced into the intestinal tract may increase the compression of the lungs. The passage of an endotracheal tube to inflate the lungs directly may be life-saving. It should preferably be undertaken *before* transfer to the surgical unit, an anaesthetist accompanying the baby. Bowel sounds are not always heard in the chest nor are fluid levels invariably seen in an x-ray film of the chest, but unusual gas shadows above the diaphragm, and displacement of the heart, are common. Delay in treatment may be followed by increasing distension of intestine incarcerated in the chest and the mediastinum may be so far shifted that the lung on the opposite side may also be compressed. Sometimes the hernia will partially reduce if the baby is held upright by the shoulders. Urgent operative treatment is advisable using a long transverse incision in the upper abdomen so that any accompanying defects of intestinal fixation or rotation may also be treated.

Oesophageal Hiatus Hernia

Sliding hernia of part of the stomach through the oesophageal hiatus is not uncommon in early infancy. Symptoms occur because the cardia becomes incompetent and reflux occurs from the stomach. Peptic oesophagitis arises with vomiting and there may be haematemesis—'coffee ground' or of frank blood. Older patients complain of pain like heartburn. The symptoms usually date from the first weeks of life and in the first few days there may be haematemesis. The vomiting is usually frequent and occurs after feeds. It may become projectile and then gives rise to suspicion of hypertrophic pyloric stenosis. The hiatus hernia not only mimics pyloric stenosis; there is also an association between the conditions. It should therefore be considered in babies suspected of pyloric stenosis without palpable tumour and also in babies who continue to vomit after operation on pyloric stenosis. A barium swallow may need to be repeated before the herniation is demonstrated. Oesophagoscopy allows assessment of the oesophagitis.

Treatment is primarily postural. The baby is propped up in a 'hiatus hernia chair' to reduce reflux and the feeds are thickened. At first the baby is kept upright continually but later only after meals and at night—the most likely times for reflux. At least three-quarters lose their symptoms on this regime soon after the end of the first year of life. At this time the baby is taking less bulky and more solid food and spends less time lying down. In a proportion the oesophagitis may persist, causing failure to thrive, anaemia or even a fibrous stricture. In these operation may be needed to reduce the hernia. When stricture occurs reflux and vomiting may lessen so that it may be wise to repeat oesophagoscopy in spite of reduction of symptoms. Dysphagia due to stricture may follow. Early strictures can be dilated and the hernia reduced at operation to give a fairly normal anatomy. If fibrosis has progressed to shorten the oesophagus reduction may become impossible. Then surgery can only offer such makeshifts as oesophago-gastrectomy; resection, vagotomy and pyloroplasty; or colonic replacement.

The results of surgery are not entirely satisfactory and operation is considered only when medical treatment has failed. More recent procedures relying more on the maintenance of an intra-abdominal segment of oesophagus than on the formation of an extrinsic 'sphincter' are more successful.

Hypertrophic Pyloric Stenosis

It is arguable whether this condition can be considered as a truly congenital anomaly. Furthermore, the features of it are so well known that detailed discussion is hardly necessary. It may be said, however, that the actual finding of a tumour in the first days of life is an extremely rare occurrence.

It is clear that both genetic and environmental factors are important in the aetiology of pyloric stenosis and the empirical risk figures are:

Brothers of male index patients	1 in 30
Sisters of male index patients	1 in 50
Sons of male index patients	1 in 15
Daughters of male index patients	1 in 50
Brothers of female index patients	1 in 10
Sisters of female index patients	1 in 30
Sons of female index patients	1 in 5
Daughters of female index patients	1 in 10

The relatively high risk to the sons of female index patients is noteworthy.

BILIARY ATRESIA

Obstructive jaundice of infancy persisting beyond the first 2 weeks of life is not common compared with other causes of neonatal jaundice. In about half of the cases the cause is neonatal hepatitis and in most of the others it is atresia of the bile ducts. A few are due to even less common causes such as cholangitis. Unfortunately there is no reliable investigation to distinguish the intrahepatic obstruction by inspissated bile in hepatitis from the mechanical obstruction in atresia. Biochemical tests may be suggestive but are not sufficiently precise to make a definite diagnosis in the individual case. For example, fluctuating blood bilirubin levels and the intermittent presence of bile in the stools may occur, surprisingly, in complete atresia as well as other conditions. Diagnosis therefore depends on biopsy. First one should exclude galactosaemia, cytomegalic inclusion disease, rhesus incompatibility and the extended rubella syndrome. The prothrombin time should also be measured and the albumin level should exceed 3 per cent as evidence of safety of operation. The reliability and safety of percutaneous biopsy have increased greatly with recent experience but we still prefer open biopsy. At this limited operation a cholangiogram is performed if the gall-bladder is present. It may reveal for example an atresia of the lower end of the common bile duct or a choledochus cyst.

Only when the histologist has reported is further treatment considered. This limited procedure is safe and can therefore be advised early so that diagnosis is reached before secondary cirrhosis makes long-term survival unlikely even in the operable cases of atresia. When histological diagnosis is made the surgeon can re-operate and explore the porta hepatis well into the liver in the hope of finding anastomosable proximal ducts with the knowledge that he is not risking damage to collapsed and inconspicuous ducts in hepatitis or cholangitis with inspissated bile, both potentially recoverable.

In the past paediatricians have tended to observe and 'investigate' cases of obstructive jaundice for 3 or more months in the hope that they may turn out to be due to a reversible condition such as hepatitis. But at this stage, even if laparotomy reveals atresia with proximal bile ducts suitable for anastomosis, long-term survival is unlikely for the liver will usually have become irreversibly cirrhotic. They have been discouraged from earlier surgical referral by the realization that extensive laparotomy may jeopardize the life of babies who cannot benefit. The regime suggested above avoids this dilemma.

Atresia may affect the whole of the extrahepatic ducts and extend as far as the interlobular ducts or it may involve the duct system as far down as the junction of common hepatic and cystic ducts with persistence of the (empty) gall-bladder, cystic and common bile ducts. Clearly neither of these obstructions can be relieved by surgery. Less commonly, in about 15 per cent, the duct system may be patent as far distally as the porta hepatis or beyond. In such cases the dilated duct can be anastomosed to the intestinal tract to provide biliary drainage. Unfortunately this last type represents only about one atresia in twelve. So surgery has still little to offer—nevertheless this regime of early biopsy will avoid the situation in which most of the operable cases are doomed owing to secondary cirrhosis even though early cirrhosis may be recoverable. Furthermore it will reveal a few eminently operable cases of cystic dilatation of the common bile duct.

The inoperable case of biliary atresia may retain good health for several months and usually lives for 9 to 12 months, occasionally several years. This can put a great strain on the family. There is an uncommon type of so-called 'intrahepatic atresia' in which the small proximal collecting ducts are atretic but the distal intrahepatic and extrahepatic ducts are normal. In this type the child may surprisingly live for several years, and some cases so diagnosed on biopsy studies have lost their jaundice and reverted to good health. Occasional cases of biliary atresia have short segments of patency within the liver. Small portions of adjacent liver drain into these. They enlarge to form 'bile lakes', aspiration from which may give false hopes that adequate drainage of the liver is possible.

Exomphalos

It is usual to consider two types of exomphalos. In the so-called 'hernia into the cord' there is a narrow neck at the point where the protrusion passes through the skin but the most distal part may be large and may contain much of the small intestine. The intestine can be reduced by twisting the cord and thus squeezing the bowel back into the abdomen, providing that it is not adherent; the cord is then strapped to the abdominal skin to prevent recurrence of the hernia. In the second type of exomphalos the sac appears to be hemispherical with a wide neck. The difficulty of management depends more on the width of the neck than on the total size of the protrusion. When the neck is wide in proportion to the total size, but the protrusion is not large, it is usually possible to mobilize the skin sufficiently to close it over the defect and it may be possible to obtain an independent closure of rectus sheath as well. When the defect is larger it may be possible to close the skin only after widely undercutting the skin and subcutaneous fat from the rectus sheath and external oblique aponeurosis and muscle. The sac should be retained intact to prevent the intestines from adhering to the mobilized skin and fat. Associated intestinal anomalies requiring immediate treatment are too rare to justify the extra problems produced by routine exploration of the sac. Later closure of the muscle layer is feasible in one or more stages.

Some surgeons have returned to the older method of leaving the exomphalos intact, encouraging shrinkage by the local application of antiseptic and sclerosing solutions. It is quite successful but the baby needs to stay in hospital for 3 months or so. Even more recently the development of silastic-covered dacron sheeting has encouraged further trial of prosthetic closure. The sheet is sewn into the defect and tucks may be taken as frequently as every other day obtaining a more rapid enlargement of the abdominal cavity and muscle closure.

Reduction of an exomphalos is made more difficult by distension with gas or fluid of the intestines contained in the sac. The earlier treatment is started the more likely it is to be successful. Until only a few years ago rupture of an exomphalos *in utero* or during delivery was thought to be incompatible with survival. Such children should now be referred at once to a suitable surgical unit, the prolapsed intestine being covered with gauze moistened with warm isotonic (0·9 per cent) saline. The superficially similar condition of gastroschisis may also respond to surgical closure. Here, the bowel protrudes alongside a normal umbilicus and there is no sac. The intestine is shortened and its wall thickened by a chronic fibrous infiltration. Gut motility and absorption will depend on the severity of these changes in the individual case.

Intestinal Obstruction

The four main causes of intestinal obstruction in the newborn period are atresia or stenosis, malrotation, Hirschsprung's disease and meconium ileus due to cystic fibrosis. There are other less common causes but in all kinds of intestinal obstruction in the newborn the most important thing is simply to recognize the presence of intestinal obstruction promptly. In the majority of patients the final recognition of the exact type of obstruction can be made only when the abdomen has been widely opened at operation by a long transverse upper abdominal incision and the entire abdominal contents have been examined. Success in such operations depends directly on early diagnosis. Of the three main signs of acute intestinal obstruction—vomiting, abdominal distension and constipation—vomiting is of most importance in the obstructed newborn baby. It has been shown that the green colour of the vomit is of particular significance and in spite of the general belief that the vomiting of green fluid is common after birth, Nixon found that it occurred in the absence of intestinal obstruction in only two out of a series of nearly 4000 consecutive births which he studied. It may be associated with functional obstruction due to sticky miconium, infection, respiratory distress, or umbilical vein catheters (Howat & Wilkinson, 1970). A similar picture may follow neonatal asphyxia usually in a low birth-weight baby. About one out of every four babies vomits during the first few days of life. The yellow colour which is common in early postnatal vomiting of a transient nature is due to carotene pigments which are derived from colostrum. If doubt exists Fouchet's test should be applied to the vomit or to the stain on the bib or clothing. During the first days after birth repeated vomiting must be adequately explained without delay, since intestinal obstruction is so important a cause of it and if unrelieved is almost always fatal. Only when the obstruction is above the level of the ampulla of Vater will the vomit be unstained with bile. Distension is absent in duodenal obstruction and appears late in lower obstruction of the small intestine. It may become obvious before vomiting in colonic obstruction due to Hirschsprung's disease. Even with atresia there may be a good deal of meconium in the bowel below the point of obstruction, and the passage of this meconium should not be taken as evidence against the presence of an obstruction. Farber's test is of little practical value in the diagnosis of obstruction even when this is due to atresia. It is based on the assumption that atresia arose as a persistence of the solid stage of the intestine and more recent work suggests that atresias are due to intra-uterine infarction at a much later stage of development and swallowed squames may have passed the point of atresia before this was formed.

A baby with duodenal atresia should be carefully examined for signs of Down's syndrome (mongolism) for about one-third have this serious defect. There is no association between jejunal or ileal atresia and mongolism.

Particular types of intestinal obstruction may be indicated by certain clinical features. In complete atresia apparently normal babies usually begin to vomit green fluid within 24 hours of birth and the upright x-ray film shows typical fluid levels. When the atresia affects the lower part of the small intestine and diagnosis is delayed, abdominal distension becomes evident during the second or third day of life. In stenosis the onset of symptoms may be delayed because air may pass the stenosis freely but eventually the narrow place is plugged with meconium to produce complete obstruction. Intermittent disturbances coming on some days after birth should raise the possibility of malrotation of the midgut with secondary extrinsic obstruction of the duodenum. Malrotation presents usually in the first week of life but the onset of obstruction may be delayed for weeks or months and very rarely until adult life. It is particularly important that the intermittent signs of obstruction should be promptly investigated because of the dangers of strangulation of a midgut volvulus.

Hirschsprung's disease commonly first causes disturbance during the newborn period in an apparently healthy child whose abdomen becomes distended before vomiting becomes marked, although the child may not feed properly from the beginning. When rectal examination is carried out as part of the clinical examination of the patient a meconium plug may be passed, followed by a large escape of gas and the deflation of the abdomen. This may be so dramatic that in the past it has been mistaken for the rupture of an anal membrane. After relief of the obstruction the child may remain well for days, weeks or even months before the symptoms of Hirschsprung's disease recur. Repeated relief may be obtained by the passage of flatus tubes and the use of carefully administered rectal washouts. It is usually wiser and safer to make without delay a colostomy proximal to the aganglionic segment in order to avoid the dangers of recurrent obstruction and vomiting in the neonatal period. In the less common type of Hirschsprung's disease with a long segment reaching above the sigmoid colon and perhaps even into the small bowel the clinical features suggest a low small-intestinal obstruction and the diagnosis is usually made only at laparotomy. This disease is in part genetically determined and a history of its occurrence in another member of the family should suggest the diagnosis. Hirschsprung's disease may present in the neonatal period with diarrhoea rather than constipation and obstruction; the frequent passage of fluid stools may be associated with marked distension of the abdomen and vomiting. The distension may be mistakenly attributed to the effects of severe gastroenteritis. The distinction is an important one because Hirschsprung's disease with this so-called putrefactive diarrhoea may lead to death within 24 hours, whereas the repeated passage of a flatus tube to empty the bowel of gas and liquid faeces followed by a colostomy may lead to prompt recovery. Investigation of the family history of a series of Hirschsprung's disease has revealed a number of examples where such a clinical picture in an earlier sibling had been mistakenly attributed to gastroenteritis which caused the death of the child.

Family studies on Hirschsprung's disease indicate that as the length of bowel involved increases from the rectum to the whole of the colon, the sex ratio changes from a marked male preponderance to unity, the risk of recurrence in later sibs increases from a low to a relative high figure, and the length of segment involved in a second affected sib is usually similar to that involved in the index patient.

Empiric risk figures for typical (aganglionic segment extends no higher than pelvic colon) Hirschsprung's disease are, for brothers of index patients, 1 in 20, for sisters less than 1 per cent. For long segment (at least ascending colon involved) index patients, the risks are: for brothers 1 in 6, and for sisters 1 in 8 (Carter, 1963).

Temporary dysfunction of the bowel and anal sphincter can imitate Hirschsprung's disease during the first 2 weeks of life. The baby is usually of low birth-weight and with a history of stressful delivery, whereas aganglionosis is uncommonly associated with low birthweight.

Very rarely intestinal obstruction may also result from the meconium plug syndrome. In this condition mucus immediately within the anus becomes firm and blocks the bowel, the baby is distended and appears to have Hirschsprung's disease but deflates readily on rectal examination assisted perhaps by a rectal washout. This diagnosis should not be too casually accepted because the majority of patients presenting in this way will later have further symptoms and it ultimately becomes evident that they are suffering from Hirschsprung's disease. It is unwise to consider this diagnosis unless rectal biopsy has revealed the presence of normal ganglia in the wall of the bowel.

The faecal plug syndrome is diagnosed during laparotomy for acute intestinal obstruction when concretions in the transverse or sigmoid colon are found as the only explanation of the obstruction. The cause of these hard faecal concretions is not known. Usually even at laparotomy Hirschsprung's disease with impaction of faeces in the narrow segment is suspected and a colostomy is made above the obstruction. In spite of this the bowel may become gangrenous and perforate over the site of the hard faecal masses and they should be removed if they can be felt. Occasionally perforation and peritonitis may be present before laparotomy is done. Unlike the meconium plug syndrome this usually follows a period of passage of normal stools.

When a baby is born with a distended abdomen and soon afterwards begins to vomit, the most likely cause is meconium ileus or meconium peritonitis resulting from prenatal perforation of the bowel. Since respiration is at first almost entirely diaphragmatic, in these patients abdominal distension may so hinder diaphragmatic movement as to cause death from asphyxia within a few hours. It has been suggested that this may be relieved by tapping the abdomen before referring the patient to a surgeon; this kind of tapping is dangerous and should be considered only as a life-saving procedure in extreme respiratory distress. Abdominal distension at birth may be found for reasons other than obstruction, for example in ascites. Distension may also arise from a chylous exudate in association with a mesenteric lymphangioma, or be due to the presence of large mesenteric or enterogenous cysts or giant hydronephrosis. Urinary transudate may fill the peritoneum following gross prenatal urinary tract obstruction. Vomiting is not a feature when the cause is not obstructive.

In addition to the four types of intestinal obstruction which have already been mentioned there are some less common causes which must be remembered. A Meckel's diverticulum which retains an attachment to the umbilicus may cause obstruction due to volvulus.

Certain forms of obstruction which are common later in life may occasionally arise during the neonatal period. Amongst these are pyloric stenosis (in which case, of course, the vomitus will not contain bile), incarceration of an inguinal hernia, or intussusception. Volvulus, incarcerated hernia and intussusception may each lead to strangulation—a matter of extreme urgency.

A mesenteric cyst of lymphatic or enterogenous origin or a duplication of bowel is another very rare cause of neonatal obstruction which may be intermittent or incomplete.

It cannot be stressed too strongly that the baby who is obstructed does not look ill. Investigation must not be delayed because the baby looks so well in spite of vomiting green fluid. By the time the baby begins to look ill the changes in the bowel are far advanced with strangulation due to volvulus or tension gangrene due to over-distension. Without active surgical treatment death is certain.

Oedema and redness of the lower abdominal wall may look like superficial sepsis secondary to umbilical infection, but in the newborn it is also a typical sign of bacterial peritonitis. One must not be discouraged from making this diagnosis because peristaltic movements are heard still to be present; in the newborn peristalsis may persist even in the presence of purulent peritonitis and rigidity does not always develop in the abdominal wall over the peritonitis. Obstructive signs due to infection will not arise until a few days after birth and may be associated with hypothermia and lethargy.

X-ray appearances
Oral contrast radiology is necessary only in the diagnosis of incomplete obstruction after complete obstruction has been ruled out by plain radiography. The function of the oesophagus and the state of the oesophageal hiatus should be examined as well as the pylorus, since many babies with a hiatus hernia vomit in the first days of life. The vomit may not be bile-stained but discoloured by altered blood, and forcible because of pylorospasm, arousing the suspicion of obstruction. A

barium meal may show an incomplete obstruction in the duodenum and only at laparotomy can it be certainly distinguished whether this is due to stenosis of the duodenum or to malrotation of the midgut.

A barium enema will usually diagnose Hirschsprung's disease when carried out by an experienced radiologist. Rectal irrigations should be avoided before the examination because they may deflate the colon and obscure the transition zone. Functional obstruction, usually in a low birth-weight baby, may also imitate the radiological picture. Rectal biopsy will settle the diagnosis but cannot indicate the length of the segment like the barium enema.

The only special investigation which is needed to confirm or refute a provisional diagnosis of acute intestinal obstruction in the newborn child, is a plain X-ray film of the abdomen in the erect position which will show fluid levels in *dilated* loops of bowel above the point of obstruction. Fluid levels are not themselves evidence of obstruction and are seen in normal x-rays of the abdomen of babies under the age of 2 years. When a baby has been crying before examination and has swallowed air there will be many fluid levels but the air will be evenly distributed throughout the bowel and the important point of progressive dilatation of the loops will not be seen. In duodenal obstruction there will be only a gastric fluid level and one in the duodenum. In the rare obstruction of the pylorus only the gastric bubble will be seen and the absence of gas at lower levels is additional evidence of obstruction. In obstruction due to meconium ileus the meconium is so thick that fluid levels may not form. Instead there is very marked gaseous distension of the small intestine and there may be a mottled meconium shadow pattern in the loops of small bowel. *Meconium peritonitis* may be associated with scattered irregular dense shadows suggesting calcification outside the bowel. *Adhesions* resulting from intra-uterine peritonitis may lead to a grouping of the bowel shadows in one corner of the abdomen. Haustration is not always recognizable in the large bowel and it may not be possible to say whether a particular shadow is of large or small bowel. In cases of low ileal atresia the much-dilated blind end of the bowel becomes forced out to a peripheral position in the abdomen and it may imitate the position of the large bowel so closely that it may mistakenly be thought to be evidence of gas reaching the colon.

In *functional intestinal obstruction* due to infection the fluid levels are in dilated loops of bowel but these are of equal calibre throughout the length of the intestine. In *advanced peritonitis* it may be possible to recognize the separation of the loops of bowel by the peritoneal fluid.

Gross diffuse distension of the bowel loops with fluid levels may also be seen in *neurogenic ileus* resulting from intra-partum cerebral damage.

DUPLICATION OF THE ALIMENTARY TRACT

These congenital anomalies usually present after the neonatal period but may cause neonatal intestinal obstruction. They occur at any part of the alimentary tract and vary from tubular duplications so intimately connected to the adjacent bowel that they must be resected together (e.g. 'double-barrelled ileum'), to cystic structures in the mesentery, separate from the bowel (enterogenous mesenteric cysts). They may be classified as

(1) Intraluminal cystic duplications.
(2) Extraluminal cystic duplications.
(3) Mesenteric enterogenous cysts.
(4) Tubular duplications.

Intestinal duplication may be associated with a mediastinal cystic duplication, a sagittaly split vertebra, and allied anomalies (Accessory neurenteric canal, the split notochord syndrome.) Duplication of the hind gut—colon and rectum—may be associated with duplication of the anus.

Presentation may be as intestinal obstruction. This may be due to blockage by an intraluminal cystic dilatation, 'ribboning' of the gut over a mesenteric enterogenous cyst or volvulus of a loop of bowel which is heavy owing to the presence of a duplication. It may be acute, complete and present at birth or it may come on later as recurrent acute attacks or progressive partial obstruction.

Duplications may communicate with the adjacent bowel usually at one end of their extent. In this case symptoms may arise from the collection of material in a 'blind loop' and the end result may be a 'giant diverticulum'.

The lining of the duplication does not always correspond with that of the adjacent bowel. Thus an ileal duplication, for example, may have a gastric mucosal lining. At the site of communication, peptic ulceration can arise just as in a Meckel's diverticulum. This may produce abdominal pain and may be complicated by perforation with peritonitis or by severe haemorrhage causing melaena. The haemorrhage may be so profuse that fluid blood is passed and the child exsanguinated.

Meckel's Diverticulum
This diverticulum of the ileum may present in various ways—not commonly in the neonatal period. Obstruction may result from invagination or from volvulus around a diverticulum retaining its umbilical attachments. Ectopic gastric mucosa may cause ulceration and hence perforation or haemorrhage. The bleeding is usually profuse and passed as dark red fluid blood per rectum. Recurrent minor bleeds are rarely due to Meckel's diverticulum. Finally acute diverticulitis may simulate appendicitis.

ABNORMALITIES OF THE RECTUM AND ANUS

There is still much confusion and controversy about the anatomical classification and therefore the diagnosis and treatment of congenital anomalies of the anus and rectum.[1] Part of the difficulty arises from the difference of opinion which exists about the anatomical details of the abnormalities and their embryological basis. Since broadly speaking there are two different classifications of these abnormalities both will be given and their treatment will be described. Most of these anomalies can be diagnosed at birth by close inspection and their treatment can be decided without special investigation.

These anomalies may first be divided into two different types according to whether there is complete occlusion of the bowel or whether there is an external opening; either indirectly by a fistula into the urethra in males, or by a fistula into the posterior fornix, or by a lower opening into the vagina, vulva or vestibule in the female or directly on to the perineum in either sex. In the absence of any kind of opening (which is uncommon) intestinal obstruction is complete and unless the termination of the bowel approaches the skin surface, which is rare, relief of the obstruction by abdominal operation—definitive or colostomy—is essential for survival. A high fistula (urethral or posterior fornix of vagina) is rarely big enough to alter this situation. In the rare cases in which the blind end of the bowel is nearer the surface a perineal operation may be sufficient. Where a low fistula ('ectopic anus') exists adequate function may be achieved by enlarging the existing opening in some suitable fashion, but it remains a matter of opinion whether such

---

[1] A suggested International Classification has recently been proposed. It is elaborate but should be valuable in assessment and comparison of management and diagnosis.

an enlarged opening is aesthetically as well as functionally satisfactory during adult life. In all cases ultimate function depends on a clear definition of the abnormality being made at the earliest possible stage and on treatment being designed from the onset to suit the individual requirements. The idea that a so-called imperforate anus is a common abnormality and can readily be dealt with by a bold median incision into the perineum is wrong; true imperforate anus, i.e. a septal occlusion of an otherwise normal rectum and anal canal, is found in less than 3 per cent of anomalies of the anus and rectum.

TABLE 7.1

Developed from Browne, D. (1955)	*Ladd & Gross* (1934)	
LOW		
Covered anus	Imperforate anus	type I
	Anal stenosis	type II
Perineal ectopic anus	Imperforate anus with perineal fistula	type III
Vulval ectopic anus	Imperforate anus with vulval fistula	type III
Vaginal ectopic anus	Imperforate anus with low vaginal fistula	type III
HIGH		
Rectal agenesis with recto-urethral fistula	Imperforate anus with urethral fistula	type III
Rectal agenesis with recto-vaginal fistula	Imperforate anus with high vaginal fistula	type III
Rectal atresia	Imperforate anus	type IV
Anorectal stenosis	Anal stenosis	type II
Anorectal membrane	Imperforate anus	type I

These anomalies have also been classified into high and low types according to whether it is believed the termination of the normal part of the bowel lies above the levator ani or extends below it. This classification is compared in Table 7.1 with the other widely used classification based on a different concept of the local anatomical variations. The merit of this classification is its prognostic value. The low anomalies, correctly treated, usually give normal control at the normal time. The high ones rarely do. Delayed or ill-chosen treatment of the low anomalies can destroy the chance of continence.

ABNORMALITIES OF THE GASTRO-INTESTINAL SYSTEM

From this it will be seen that in the anal membrane, which is rare, there is simply a thin membrane closing the anal canal at the level of the anal valves.

In stenosis of the anus there is a small pinhole opening at the muco-cutaneous junction which can usually be treated by repeated dilatation. In the 'covered anus', which is more common in males than in females, there is usually a ridge of skin at the site of the anus which may extend

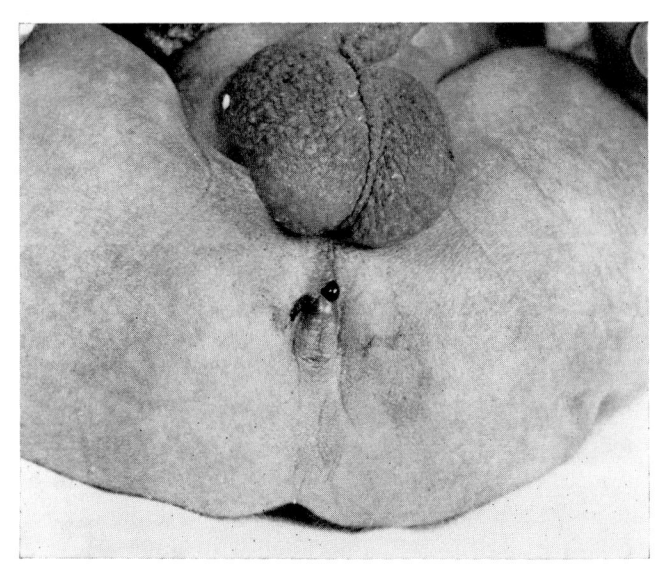

FIG. 7.3. 'Covered anus' or imperforate anus with rectoperineal fistula.

forwards as an abnormal median raphe which can often be seen to be filled with meconium, along the perineum and occasionally even on to the scrotum and penis—(Fig. 7.3). This track may be open, and may then be classed as a rectoperineal fistula. Whichever classification is used, in this kind of anomaly the bowel is complete down to the skin, the anal canal is virtually normal, the relationship of the lumen to the external anal sphincters is normal and prompt treatment is simple and effective. The abnormal skin overlying the anal sphincters should be excised together with any external tract and the skin edges may be loosely sutured to the anal mucosa. The opening thus made is dilated daily, for 3 months at least, to avoid any tendency to contract.

The term 'ectopic anus' assumes that the end of the bowel proper extends below the levator ani and that adequate treatment can be achieved by the enlargement of the natural opening by incision or repeated dilatation. Alternatively these openings may be considered as fistulas from a bowel which ends above levator ani. There is agreement, however, that primary treatment by enlargement may be satisfactory even though opinions differ on what later treatment (if any) is preferable.

The 'ectopic anus' may open at the lower part of the vaginal wall, in the vestibule, the vulva or in the perineum in females. In males it is confined to the perineal type of opening.

When there is a fistula or 'ectopic anus' opening in the vagina or perineum the passage of meconium may mislead the casual observer since the abnormality of the site or size of the opening may be distinguished only by close inspection.

It is important that these 'low' anomalies should be seen early by the surgeon who is going to deal with them. For early simple measures can avert irreversible distension of the rectum which in turn may result in incontinence in just those cases which can be expected to give good results. Indeed, the management of these cases is as important as the operative procedure and no one should begin treatment who is not prepared to continue such supervision for several years if necessary.

In the high type of rectal anomaly the rectum ends blindly above the levator ani but there is usually a fistulous connection with the urethra in the male or the posterior vaginal fornix in females; rectovesical fistula is very rare, and usually associated with other severe anomalies of the urinary system and sacral nerves. These high anomalies produce intestinal obstruction since the fistulas seldom provide an adequate escape for gas and meconium. All high anomalies should therefore be referred to a surgical unit without delay for treatment either by colostomy, the transference of the bowel to the perineum being delayed until the baby has reached a weight of 10 kg, or else less commonly by primary pull-through operation in the first day or two of life.

A recent analysis of more than 300 anorectal anomalies has shown that they are more common in males than in females. About a third of the patients had a 'covered anus' stenosis or an anal membrane. Of the remaining two-thirds, in just over half, the rectum ended above levator ani in an 'atresia' or 'rectal agenesis'. An 'ectopic anus' or low fistula was present in the remainder. Ninety per cent of these cases of rectal agenesis occurred in males and in 75 per cent of these there was a recto-urethral fistula.

SELECTED REFERENCES

BENTLEY J.F.R. & SMITH J.R. (1960) Developmental posterior enteric remnants and spinal malformations. *Arch. Dis. Childh.* **35,** 76

BODIAN M. & CARTER C.O. (1963) A family study of Hirschsprung's disease. *Ann. of Hum. Genet.* **26,** 261

BROWNE D. (1955) Congenital deformities of anus and rectum. *Arch. Dis. Childh.* **30,** 42

CAMERON SIR R. & BUNTON G.L. (1960) Congenital biliary atresia. *Brit. med. J.* **ii,** 1253

CARTER C.O. (1961) Inheritance of congenital pyloric stenosis. *Br. med. Bull,* **17,** 251

CARTER C.O. (1965) 'The inheritance of common congenital malformations', Chapter 3 in *Progress in Medical Genetics,* Vol. IV (ed. Steinberg and Bearn)

CARTER C.O. & EVANS K.A. (1969) Inheritance of pyloric stenosis. *J. med. Genet.* **6,** 233

FRASER F.C. (1963) Hereditary disorders of the nose and mouth. *Proc. 2nd Inter. Conf. Hum. Genet.* 1852–5.

HOWAT J.M. & WILKINSON A.W. (1970) Functional intestinal obstruction in the neonate. *Arch. Dis. Childh.* **45,** 800.

LADD W.E. & GROSS R.E. (1934) Congenital malformations of anus and rectum. *Am. J. Surg.* **23,** 167

NIXON H.H. (1956) Intestinal obstruction in newborn period. *Great Ormond Street Journal,* No. 11, p. i

NIXON H.H. (1961) In Goligher J. *Surgery of the Anus, Rectum and Colon,* 1st edn. London: Cassells

PARTRIDGE J.P. & GOUGH M.H. (1961) Congenital abnormalities of the anus and rectum. *Brit. J. Surg.* **49,** 37

SANTULLI T.V., KIESEWETTER W.B. & BILL A.H. JR (1970) Ano rectal anomalies: a suggested international classification. *J. Ped. Surg.* **5,** 281.

WILKINSON A.W. & COZZI F. (1968) Familial incidence of congenital anorectal anomalies. *Surgery,* **64,** 669.

WILKINSON A.W. (1969) Anorectal abnormality in children. *Proc. Roy. Soc. Med.* **62,** 1234

8

Orthopaedic Abnormalities

G.C. LLOYD-ROBERTS

GENERAL AFFECTIONS OF THE SKELETAL SYSTEM

A catalogue of 'The General Affections of the Skeleton' has been compiled by Fairbank in which he presents in atlas form observations and conclusions based upon an interest in those anomalies which extended throughout his active professional life. It is unnecessary to report the observations made by Fairbank and others upon these conditions because many of the generalized skeletal abnormalities are unlikely to be suspected in very early life. Polyostotic fibrous dysplasia, for example, is so insidious in onset that it is unlikely to be considered until some complication (deformity, fracture or facial asymmetry) or associated sign (skeletal or sexual precocity and pigmentation) arises.

In contrast some generalized skeletal disturbances do declare themselves in infancy and among these are included certain conditions in which early diagnosis is important.

Alkaline Hypophosphatasia
This presents with multiple skeletal deformities and has, when familial, been diagnosed *in utero* by radiography. The appearances in infancy resemble those of florid rickets but it does not respond to antirachitic treatment. The importance of early diagnosis rests upon its association with craniostenosis and the risk of blindness, if irreversible optic nerve damage is not prevented by cranial decompression. It is transmitted by a recessive mutant gene.

Vitamin-resistant rickets does not normally present until after the age when walking begins. There is then usually an exaggeration of the genu varum or of the outwardly curved and inwardly rotated tibiae which are so frequently met at this stage of development. Familial inheritance is common and a short bow-legged parent should indicate the need for radiological examination of the wrists. The serum alkaline phosphatase is high and the blood phosphorus is low. It is transmitted by a sex-linked recessive gene although in some families there may be some clinical abnormality in the heterozygous female 'carriers' of the gene.

Fanconi's syndrome. Signs of rickets may occur in this genetic disorder, which presents after walking begins. It is due to a recessive mutant gene.

Renal rickets. This is seen in infancy only in association with renal agenesis. The radiographic appearances do not resemble those characistic of other forms of infantile rickets, for metaphyseal fractures are more conspicuous than epiphyseal irregularity.

Diaphyseal achlasis (multiple exostosis) can rarely be diagnosed before the metaphyseal osteochondromata become palpable or before there is evident disturbance of growth at the epiphyseal plate, notably at the lower end of the ulna. Other members of the family are frequently affected. The parents should be warned that the child will be short, but not a dwarf. They may be reassured if the question of malignant metaplasia is raised and told that osteochondromata will require removal only if they are causing symptoms. Inheritance is dominant.

Albers–Schonberg's disease (marble bones). This is a rare cause of repeated fractures in young children.

Osteogenesis imperfecta. This is the commonest generalized skeletal disorder requiring and benefiting from treatment in the very young age group. It is fundamental to realize that this disease has a tendency towards spontaneous improvement as the child grows up. This fact dominates the management. Whilst it is, of course, true that some are stillborn, some die in early infancy, and some progress to severe crippling in spite of treatment, yet there is a general trend towards improvement. The diagnosis is seldom in doubt. Multiple fractures or repeated fractures in one bone are usual, the sclerotics are frequently an obvious blue and there is joint laxity. The skull is broad in the bi-parietal plane and is soft so that fractures complicated by subdural haematoma are not infrequent. The face is pinched and small in relation to the skull. The radiograph shows diffuse osteoporosis and a thin cortex with unduly slender bones. Deformity due to the softness of the bones may occur without fracture so that the rib cage may react to the negative pressure within the thorax.

The trend towards spontaneous improvement indicates the need for energetic treatment of the fractures to prevent deformity, which by reducing the mechanical efficiency of the bone may predispose towards refracture in its own right. Prolonged immobilization will increase the osteoporosis so that an attempt should be made to reduce immobilization to the shortest time compatible with satisfactory repair. Healing is sometimes so proliferative that neoplastic change is suspected.

Non-union is uncommon but it is liable to occur when repeated fractures at one site lead to secondary deformity. This is particularly so in the subtrochanteric region of the femur.

Two recent developments re-emphasize the importance of treating these fractures with the intention of obtaining union in an acceptable position. First, intramedullary nailing of long bones prone to repeated fractures has justified itself. The operation is easier if deformity is not excessively severe. Second, recent metabolic studies have demonstrated a disorder of nitrogen metabolism upon which treatment may in the future be shown to have a favourable effect. This will be enhanced if deformity has been prevented.

It is transmitted by a dominant mutant gene.

Infantile cortical hyperostosis. Although probably not a congenital anomaly it may be mentioned at this point for it may present at any time up to 6 months and cause diagnostic difficulty. The onset is sudden, the baby becomes ill and febrile, feeds are resisted, the lower jaws swell and the face becomes increasingly cherubic. The radiograph shows the mandible to be surrounded by a tube of periosteal new bone, and the mistaken diagnosis of osteomyelitis is often made. The prognosis is good, however, and the swellings gradually subside leaving behind a normal mandible. Although the jaw is most commonly if not always involved, other bones can share in this change. The clavicles and scapulae are frequent sities. Affected long bones are indistinguishable from those in scurvy in so far as the periosteum is similarly elevated but the white line of Fraenkel on the diaphyseal side of the epiphyseal plate is absent. Caffey has also drawn attention to the radiographic changes which occur if children's long bones are injured but not broken. These injuries resemble the lesions of scurvy and infantile cortical hyperostosis but in contrast the ensheathing new bone extends beyond the attachment of the periosteum to the epiphyseal plate and small fragments may be seen to be avulsed from the margin of the metaphysis. Lesions are usually multiple and vary in maturity and should be specially sought in babies with inadequately explained subdural haematomas.

Congenital joint laxity. This is now emerging as a clinical entity. It is frequently familial. The laxity presents in a variety of ways from recurrent dislocation of joints to double-jointedness. Recurrent dislocation in infancy is very rare unless joint laxity is present and then the patella–femoral joints are the most frequently affected. Genu recurvatum or markedly valgus ankles may be present at the time the child begins to walk. In general, however, the presentation is that of a floppy baby (see below) in whom the hips may be abducted so that the flexed knees touch the examination couch—an abnormal state of affairs in spite of the often repeated statement that this is the normal excursion of hip joints in infancy. Apart from those cases in which congenital or habitual dislocation occurs the condition is benign. It is not associated with muscular weakness and is perhaps advantageous if the victim becomes a professional contortionist or acrobat.

It is transmitted by a dominant mutant gene.

GENERAL AFFECTIONS OF THE SUPPORTING TISSUES

Diseases of the central nervous system are responsible for many of the conditions which are included under this heading. They come to an orthopaedic surgeon with symptoms which often differ from those for which they are referred to a neurological clinic. The common orthopaedic presentations are emphasized below with an outline of their management.

The *floppy or limp baby* (amyotonia congenita) is a syndrome for which disorder of the nervous system is so often responsible that it may conveniently be mentioned first. These babies have much in common initially. They are 'rag dolls' to a greater or lesser extent so that, as the name implies, they may be folded up into a ball. The muscles are flabby to feel but not paralysed; the tendon reflexes are suppressed or reduced. There is delay in motor development exemplified by a clumsiness in manual tasks and tardiness in sitting, standing and walking. When the child eventually sits up an abnormal thoracolumbar kyphosis may be evident and cause alarm but it is only a postural deformity and a reflection of muscle weakness. On standing, the infantile 'flat foot' and valgus deformity at the subtaloid joint may be grossly exaggerated and knock-knees may be conspicuous. These postural deformities are due to the effect of weight-bearing on mobile joints insufficiently supported by the musculature.

Floppy babies may be regarded as belonging to a group of conditions which includes some in which deterioration is rapid and death from progressive paralysis is early, and some in which there is complete recovery in a variable time. In others the syndrome may indicate the presence of a generalized disease of which the presenting feature is a secondary floppiness.

The neurologist sees relatively more patients with a progressive spinal muscular atrophy (Werdnig–Hoffman's disease) than those with a good prognosis of the benign resolving type. The orthopaedic surgeon on the other hand rarely sees the malignant case but frequently meets the resolving variety.

Amyotonia of good prognosis has the basic features of the syndrome already described but time will distinguish it from progressive atrophy. In the benign there is a history of retarded yet progressive development of motor skills so that finally the child becomes normal. Electromyography may be misleading in that a myopathic pattern may be obtained —but a careful history will establish functional improvement over a period of months and this is of far greater importance. Whilst most recover completely a few cause anxiety by their tardiness in so doing. Others never develop normal muscle power although no muscle is completely paralysed.

Amyotonia of bad prognosis is due either to progressive spinal paralysis or infantile muscular dystrophy. In both the weakness tends to be severe in early infancy and there is demonstrable paralysis. A low intensity radiograph in spinal paralysis may show a decrease of soft tissue shadowing due to muscle and an increase in the fat. The process is progressive and death usually occurs before the age of 4. In spinal paralysis the electromyograph shows denervation patterns and muscle biopsy will confirm this whilst a dystrophy will produce a myopathic electrical discharge and a characteristic histological picture.

The symptomatic amyotonias are well illustrated by the floppiness which may precede the typical signs of cerebral palsy especially if it is of the athetoid or cerebellar ataxia variety. In some, amyotonia persists and atonic diplegia is the final outcome, but in most, development of the central nervous system will allow recognition of pyramidal, basal ganglion or cerebellar dysfunction in the peripheral nervous system. Other examples of symptomatic amyotonia are found in mental deficiency, poliomyelitis, polyneuritis, hypocalcaemia and osteogenesis imperfecta.

Arthrogryposis multiplex congenita or amyoplasia congenita, although rare, can usually be diagnosed soon after birth, for severe deformity is common. The characteristics are (1) rigidity and deformity of joints more evident in the periphery than centrally, and (2) limbs of small circumference which have a featureless tubular appearance. Typical patterns of deformity are a rigid club foot with flexed (sometimes hyperextended) knee and flexed hip or, in the arm, still extended interphalangeal joints, flexed wrist and extended elbow with the shoulder adducted and fully rotated inwards. The trunk is frequently spared. Studies of the morbid anatomy describe scanty muscle fibres with fibrotic and fatty infiltration between these attenuated bundles.

There is a tendency to group patients with this syndrome as a single entity but two clinical types emerge and seem to be quite distinct in aetiology and prognosis. A lower limb type is associated with congenital spinal paralysis (usually spina bifida) and in this type the deformities seem to be determined by peripheral paralysis. It seems probable that *in utero* the paraplegic foetus, being unable to move, grows in the foetal position, so that rigidity and deformity follow, producing the signs of lower limb arthrogryposis. In these children the depth of central paralysis dominates the prognosis but is difficult to assess in the newborn period. The management of these cases will be dominated by the extent of paralysis. In one case correction of a single deformity, such as a rigid club foot, by conservative or operative means, may be all that is required, whereas in others the parents must be warned that their child may grow up to lead a wheelchair life. It is wise to be cautious in manipulating these joints in infancy for the combination of rigidity and paralysis predisposes towards fracture.

The other clinical type of arthrogryposis is not associated with paralysis but with muscular aplasia and dysplasia. In these children the arms are as frequently involved as the legs, unlike those with spinal paralysis. Early care is directed towards non-operative correction of disabling deformities such as club feet, flexed knees and dislocated hips. The deformities of foot and knee often demand operative correction and this need not be unduly delayed although it is prudent to wait until the child is either beginning to walk or making the attempt. If both hips are dislocated, rigidity provides some stability and it is probably best not to attempt reduction. This, however, does not necessarily apply to uni-

S

lateral dislocations. In deciding about operation on the arms, time is the most valuable asset for the function achieved is often surprising. In general, deformities which do not respond to non-operative treatment should be corrected by soft tissue operations rather than osteotomy in the very young.

Gigantism must be distinguished from *hypertrophy*. In gigantism the limb or part of a limb is large and abnormal whereas in hypertrophy there is enlargement in length and girth but the appearance is otherwise normal. Simple hypertrophy is usually of unknown cause and may involve one-half of the body including the trunk and face. It is unlikely to be noted in infancy as the disproportion is seldom great enough to warrant surgical correction even in adolescence. Some difficulty may, in fact, be encountered in deciding whether one limb is too large or the other too small.

Gigantism usually affects one limb or one digit and the enlargement is more commonly in girth than in length when diffuse neurofibromatosis (see below) or a lymph-haemangiomatous malformation is present, but if congenital arteriovenous communications are responsible, overgrowth in length predominates.

Diffuse lymph-haemangioma is usually characterized by blotchy flat angiomatous malformation in the skin which ultimately demands little more than cosmetic surgery or its consideration, but the limb occasionally becomes so massive that it prevents walking and undermines the general health because of deep or superficial bleeding and ulceration. Amputation is occasionally indicated in these cases.

Haemangio-lipomata are sometimes seen in babies' thighs. Spontaneous haemorrhage within them causes pain and further swelling. They are easily removed.

Fibroblastic tumours resemble fibrosarcomas very closely both clinically and at operation. They are however benign and tend to regress if partially excised. Failure to recognise this tumour may result in unnecessary mutilation.

Congenital arteriovenous fistulae are characterized by excessive limb length which is more conspicuous than the increase in girth. Deformities of the hands and feet accompany this not infrequently. The diagnosis is based upon these findings, and the presence, at least in older children, of venous dilatation, warmth and a bruit heard over the main vessel or a large communication. The bradycardia phenomenon is often present and the pulse pressure high. Although the inequality of length may require surgical treatment in the future, the main consideration in infancy is to ensure that the arterio-venous leak is not causing cardiac dilatation with the risk of early failure. This occasionally demands amputation as the multiple communications which exist (some intra-osseous) are not amenable to obliteration by surgical means. In this connection it is important to realize that the excision of what appears to be a single shunt is too often followed by the opening up of others hitherto unsuspected at other levels in the limb. The associated deformities are treated on general lines and the overgrowth in length by epiphyseal arrest at an appropriate age. Ulceration may occur in spite of the hyperaemia if the arrangement of the shunts causes local ischaemia.

Neurofibromatosis is genetically determined. It is of interest to the orthopaedic surgeon because of the variability of its presentation. It has already been mentioned as a cause of gigantism with overgrowth in length associated with diffuse neurofibromatous overgrowth in the subcutaneous tissues. Enlargement of one digit is most commonly due to this disease. The long bones are often infiltrated and radiologically show areas of trabecular density, cyst formation or sclerosis. It is rarely associated with vitamin-resistant rickets but more commonly with one variety of congenital scoliosis and with pseudarthrosis of the tibia (see below). Malignant metaplasia may occur in later life but this is rare compared with the development of spinal-cord compression from intraspinal tumours.

In diagnosis it is important to realize that in infancy and early childhood, the well-known *café-au-lait* patches on the skin are only occasionally present and subcutaneous nodules do not occur. These are later manifestations and consequently the diagnosis is often difficult initially.

Constriction rings. These cause considerable parental alarm—which is not surprising for they sometimes surround the bone so closely that it seems impossible for muscles, vessels and nerves to be contained within the space available. The parents may be reassured, however, that the vital structures are present and that the constriction will not progress and cause a limb to fall off. The rings are amenable to surgical correction by multiple 'Z' plasties which are often best performed in several stages at the age of 3 or 4 years. If the limb distal to the band is relatively swollen it will return to normal after operation. In contrast to the limb constrictions, digital rings may render the finger useless.

Congenital webbing across joint flexor surfaces is most commonly met behind the knees and in front of the elbows, which consequently have fixed flexion deformities. The disability is functional in the legs and cosmetic in the arms. It is important to appreciate that the neurovascular bundle lies displaced within the apex of the web, where it is liable to injury, if the surgeon performing a 'Z' plasty is unaware of the fact. Furthermore, the neurovascular bundle is shortened so that corrections of the skin web alone and stretching of the flexion contracture may cause a traction injury to the nerves. If full correction is desired it is probably wise to shorten the bone.

Haemangiomatous malformations of bone are responsible for the striking progressive absorption and disappearance of long bones or vertebrae which is sometimes associated with angiomatous deposits in regional lymph nodes and erosion of neighbouring structures. In a recent example the thoracic duct was invaded from the vertebrae and the resulting chylothorax and paraplegia was fatal. In long bones the prognosis is more favourable and healing may occur spontaneously or after bone grafting.

THE HEAD, NECK AND SPINE

The Face, Skull and Neck

Asymmetry of the face is most commonly developmental in origin. In this event prominence of one frontal bone is often accompanied by a similar enlargement of the opposite occipital bone (plagiocephaly) in contrast to the asymmetry associated with torticollis or congenital abnormality of the cervical spine which is usually confined to the face, or hemihypertrophy in which the overgrowth involves one side only and is of normal contour.

Wry neck is the commonest deformity of the neck presenting in infancy. Although the majority are due to contracture of the sternomastoid (muscular torticollis) it is necessary in every patient to exclude alternative causes for this deformity. To do this a distinction must first be made between a postural torticollis or an apparent wry neck and a fixed or structural one. In the postural category are those in whom the neck can be moved passively through a full range of movement when traction is applied to the head against counter-traction to the extended arms. Such cases include those who simply hold their heads to one side and those with a degree of moulding (frontal and occipital on the opposite sides) sufficient to simulate fixed deformity. This is sometimes associated with infantile idiopathic scoliosis of good prognosis (see below).

Structural torticollis is characterized by limitation of passive movement and frequently asymmetry of the face which is enlarged on the side which is tilted 'to face the sun'. Unlike the similar moulding deformity the occiput is not flattened on the opposite side. This is sometimes secondary to other deformities including Sprengel's shoulder, congenital or idiopathic thoracic scoliosis and Klippel–Feil syndrome. Less commonly tumours or inflammatory disease of the cervical spine may be responsible. The latter include forward or rotary subluxation of the atlas on the axis which is more likely to be secondary to upper respiratory infection than injury at this age.

Muscular torticollis implies that the sternomastoid muscle is shortened so that the ear approaches the shoulder on the affected side and the chin is rotated towards the opposite side. Facial asymmetry may be present from an early age and is progressive if the contracture is not corrected. The cause is unknown but one possibility is that intra-uterine malposition causes ischaemic changes in the muscle which may make it vulnerable to injury during delivery, which is frequently abnormal. Sometimes the contracture is associated with a hard globular tumour within the substance of the muscle or a history of its presence in infancy and subsequent disappearance. The sternomastoid tumour contains fibrous tissue which appears to be replacing degenerate muscle.

Hulbert reviewing 100 patients with idiopathic torticollis emphasizes the natural history of this tumour and its relationship to prognosis. Typically it is noted within the first months and begins to disappear after 3 months, being seldom palpable after 6 months. Only those babies with a tumour appear to be liable to persistence of muscle contracture and of these only about 20 per cent in fact develop deformity if stretching exercises are instituted when the diagnosis is made. The management of muscular torticollis therefore should include stretching exercises for all patients regardless of the presence or absence of a tumour for, if transitory, it may have been overlooked. If the contracture persists, operation should be performed at about the age of 3 years by which time non-operative correction will have manifestly failed or be unlikely to succeed. Furthermore, at this age the neck will be growing rapidly so that deformity of the neck and face will have become both conspicuous and progressive and the structures, which must be exposed in the root of the neck, are of a size that makes their recognition simpler and less hazardous.

Klippel–Feil syndrome is characterized by a short, stiff and often wry neck, low hair-line and often skin webbing as seen in Turner's syndrome, but it is not confined to girls. The vertebral abnormalities vary from aplasia or congenital fusion to gross maldevelopment of the bodies with neural arches which may be normal or bifid and possibly associated with a cervical meningocele, dermoid or diastematomyelia.

Sprengel's deformity, or congenital elevation of the scapula, may be part of the Klippel–Feil syndrome accentuating the deformity and adding limitation of shoulder abduction to the disability.

Treatment of the Klippel–Feil deformity (if indicated) should be delayed for some years, is largely cosmetic and not usually very rewarding. Correction of the skin web, division of sternomastoid and upper thoracoplasty, all have their place. The scapula, if elevated, must also be included in the operation and that part which lies above and including the spine is removed together with the omo-vertebral bone if this is present. Brachial neuritis may be caused by nerve-root compression but the onset of spastic paralysis should focus attention on the possibility of a dermoid cyst in the cerebral posterior fossa rather than cord compression within the cervical spine. Sprengel's deformity alone, in children under 6, may be satisfactorily treated by displacing the whole scapula caudally.

Cervical rib rarely presents in the very young but if so venous congestion and a blue hand is the usual symptom.

The Spine

Scoliosis in infancy is always structural. It is either congenital, in which case the vertebrae are manifestly abnormal in development, or idiopathic, when curvature occurs in spite of vertebrae which are initially complete in all respects but which later undergo secondary changes due to the unequal stresses imposed upon their growth centres by the curvature. Neurologically determined scoliosis is very rare in infancy though intra-uterine poliomyelitis may be a cause. It is perhaps surprising that spastic hemiplegia does not initiate structural scoliosis. Scoliosis is an almost constant late complication of the myopathies and contributes towards the eventual death which is usually due to respiratory insufficiency. A curve showing acute angulation over a short distance with apparently complete vertebrae should suggest that neurofibromatosis is the underlying disorder and that neurofibromata may be the cause of cord compression later if the sharpness of the curve is not responsible.

Congenital scoliosis infers that one or more vertebrae have developed abnormally and it is important to realize that structures in the same developmental segment may also be involved. A not uncommon example is aplasia or fusion of ribs attached to the abnormal vertebrae together with either a diminished respiratory efficiency and pulmonary agenesis and congenital disorders of the cardiovascular system, or a defective diaphragm with an associated hernia. In general, however, the clinical problem is either cosmetic or neurological. The latter will be mentioned only in outline as it seldom demands treatment in infancy. Cosmetically even the most florid and extensive lesions may have a relatively good prognosis in contrast to some types of idiopathic scoliosis which may at first appear as a trivial variation on the radiograph. This is because localized anomalies such as a single hemivertebra cause a localized sharply angled scoliosis which allows ample room for development of secondary compensating curves above and below. Exceptions are at the thoraco-cervical and lumbar levels above and below which the spine is too short. Secondly these deformities often neutralize each other if, for example, there is a left hemivertebra at one level and a right at a lower level. The prognosis for this type of curve is therefore somewhat unpredictable but is, in general, better than an early radiograph suggests.

The neurological associations are important, if relatively rare. They include myelodysplasia at the level of skeletal abnormality and spina bifida enclosing a congenital tumour or diastomyelia, which should be especially looked for if there are changes in the overlying skin such as a hairy mole, haemangioma or lipoma. Congenital angular kyphosis alone is due to failure of development of the anterior part of the vertebral body and places the cord in jeopardy as the deformity increases and if kyphosis is associated with congenital scoliosis, the risk of local cord compression is greatly increased.

Idiopathic scoliosis may appear at any level of the spine and at any age up to skeletal maturity and is a subject of some complexity. (Although there may well be some hereditary predisposition the subject cannot be dealt with in full here and only the type seen within the first year will be considered.) One prognostic generalization, however, is of value and deserves mention. This proposes that the earlier the onset, and the higher in the spine the apex of the curve, the worse the prognosis.

Diagnosis must be critical or some babies may be included who are simply wriggling or flopping to one side. The diagnosis demands that there be both a fixed lateral curvature and rotation. The former is confirmed by an antero-posterior X-ray with the baby suspended by the arms—the latter either by asymmetry of the pedicles on this picture or more readily by observing the unilateral hump of the backwardly rotated ribs. The mother will have noticed either the scoliosis, the hump, creases on the concave side of the back or a disinclination to turn the head towards the convex side, so that wry neck is suspected. The angle of deformity should be measured on this radiograph so that subsequent progress becomes a matter of certainty rather than nebulous 'feelings'.

The prognosis varies from complete and permanent resolution to relentless progression which, if not halted, leads to the most hideous and crippling of all types of scoliosis. Fortunately, however, most are of the resolving type. James has reviewed the prognosis in 212 babies with infantile idiopathic scoliosis, of which only seventy-seven resolved. This is probably a low figure because the material was selected in so far as most were babies referred to a scoliosis clinic because of unsatisfactory progress. In unselected patients the incidence of spontaneous resolution is more likely to be between 70 and 80 per cent and this estimate is supported by Pilcher who has continued to study the natural history of this curve pattern. Correction, if it is to occur, is usually complete in 2 years, the lateral curve disappearing before the rib hump. The radiological measurement of angle of curvature is less of a guide to prognosis than age of onset, associated moulding and the presence or absence of compensatory curves. If the curve is noticed at less than 3 months, associated with head moulding and without compensatory curves (i.e. it is one long curve), spontaneous resolution is likely to follow in as many as 90 per cent. It should be emphasized that no treatment is given. Physiotherapy is of no value in any type of structural scoliosis nor are cradle splints in scoliosis of infancy.

Progressive infantile curves usually appear nearer to the first birthday, have no moulding and are associated from the onset with compensatory curves. Their treatment is difficult and the prognosis remains dismal in 80 per cent.

Lumbo-sacral Spina Bifida
There are three ways in which paralysis due to spina bifida may engage the orthopaedic surgeon in infancy and it must be realized that in each

category the laminal defect is often invisible in the radiograph of the very young and may be overlooked, especially if there is no indication of its presence on the overlying skin. First there are the isolated deformities which prove unusually resistant to treatment. Examples are club foot, pes cavus or calcaneus and paralytic rigid flat foot. Secondly, intrauterine paralysis may cause a type of arthrogryposis confined to the lower limbs and characterized by foot deformities, flexed knees and often dislocated hips all of which are rigid. Thirdly there is flaccid paralysis resembling poliomyelitis which frequently involves the calf, and the extensors of the knee and hip. Treatment begins immediately the diagnosis is made. In order of priority it aims to correct primary deformity, to prevent the development of secondary deformity and lastly to restore muscle balance when this is possible. The nature of the disease, however, imposes its own limitations on treatment. Loss of sensibility, especially position sense, may prejudice the result of successful correction of deformity and muscle imbalance. Operative correction of spinal deformity may be indicated to improve balance, allow the fitting of calipers or correct pelvic obliquity. Furthermore, dislocation of the hips in spite of efforts at prevention may result from the paralysis. A dislocation present at birth may be either so rigid that reduction, if this is not supported by osteotomy and ileopsoas transplantation, simply results in a stable stiff hip in a different position, or so flaccid that reduction is unstable.

THE UPPER LIMB

The Hand

It would be inappropriate to enumerate in catalogue fashion the many congenital derangements which affect the hand, which are more varied than those of the foot. They indicate generalized abnormalities more frequently than those of the foot and it is necessary in this context to remember some of the commoner associations of this nature. The trident hand of achondroplasia, the curved fifth finger and abnormal palm creases of mongolism, the short fingers in dysplasia multiplex congenita and long fingers in arachnodactyly, are but a few to illustrate the many generalized disorders reflected in deformity of the hand.

In considering the management of those deformities confined to the hand, an important fact must always be in the surgeon's mind—the normal hand, unlike the foot, is a precision instrument absolved from the cruder demands of weight bearing. Consequently mobility and dexterity take precedence over stability. It follows from this that shape is of less importance than the properties of pinch and grip, which are accomplished in the normal hand by opposing the thumb to a digit and by flexion of the fingers of the ulna side of the hand against the palm. Furthermore, the hand is a paired structure and if one is normal it will become the dominant partner. If its handicapped fellow can grasp and is controlled by an arm which can give the hand the properties of a motivated paper weight, near full function will develop. In this connection it will be recalled that even congenital absence of the hand constitutes but a minor disability to those who do not attempt skilled manual work in striking contrast to the serious consequences of loss of the hand in later life. Nor, indeed, is this the end of the story for structure in a growing child adapts itself to the demands of function in a remarkable way and apparently insuperable handicaps may be overcome by the passing of time and structural adaptation.

Absence of the thumb illustrates this principle well, for mobility may develop at the metacarpo-carpal joint of the index finger to such an extent that this digit replaces functionally its absent neighbour so that pinch is restored.

The implications of this proposition are that in most patients no decision should be taken to alter the structure of the congenitally abnormal hand until some years have passed and the functional disability has become apparent beyond peradventure. Two further observations of a precautionary nature should be made at this stage: first, if it is thought possible that surgical treatment may be needed in the future, no part of the hand should be removed early for cosmetic reasons; it is vital to preserve working stock and the sacrifice of a supernumerary digit, for example, may deprive the surgeon of skin or bone which might be of value to him later; secondly, congenital deformity of the hand often simulates closely an abnormality in the hand of one or other parent. Be cautious, therefore, lest you be tempted to offer a prognosis whilst the father's hands remain in his pockets.

In considering the individual deformities, only those which require treatment in infancy will be mentioned.

Congenital amputation demands reassurance which is both authoritative and confident, based on the premise that in life, one does not miss that which one has never had, and an appointment at a limb-fitting centre at about the age of 1 year.

Radial club hand. In this anomaly, the radius is absent or, more rarely, represented by a rudiment. The hand lies opposed to the radial border of the forearm, the thumb is frequently absent and the forearm is short. Surgery should in general be confined to unilateral deformity if at skeletal maturity or thereabouts it is demanded by cosmetic or very rarely functional considerations. Ulna–carpal fusion is the operation of choice. About 1 in 5 are associated with congenital disorders of the heart (Holt–Oram syndrome).

Congenital adduction of the thumb. Most babies clutch their thumbs within their palms but occasionally this is accompanied by a contracture of the first web space. Having excluded cerebral palsy, early stretching and fixation in plaster in gradually increasing abduction is indicated and correction is the rule—but relapse may occur if the extensor tendon is absent, in which case early transplantation is necessary.

Trigger thumb, a misnomer, for stenosis of the tendon sheath causes flexion at the interphalangeal joint rather than the intermittent locking that the name implies. Common though this is, it is frequently misdiagnosed, though the clinical picture is characteristic. In addition to the flexion deformity, there is a palpable thickening of the tendon sheath which encloses a nodule on the tendon just proximal to the transverse crease at the base of the thumb. Spontaneous correction may occur but persistence is the rule. Division of the tendon sheath at about 1 year resolves the problem.

Syndactyly usually demands operation, but this is best postponed for 4 or 5 years.

Polydactyly and supernumerary digits may be amputated early provided that no further operations are contemplated on the hand and that the activated digit of a pair is not removed in error, leaving a thumb or finger of more normal appearance, less well endowed for movement.

Congenital contracture of the fifth finger is best left alone, for stiffness in flexion allows it to be used in grasping, whereas treatment will probably cause stiffness in extension, which is usually an indication for amputation in any finger.

Genetic implications. Certain of these malformations behave in individual families as if determined by a dominant mutant gene. This is true of polydactyly, ectrodactyly (lobster-claw hand or foot) and

The Arm

Aplasia of one or other forearm bones has already been mentioned. Absence of both bones, in whole or in part and with or without a corresponding loss of the humerus is, as would be expected, associated with deformity and loss of function, so serious that surgery has little place compared with the baby's natural adaptability. Partial absence of the ulna may occur in neurofibromatosis and in children with this condition and some others surgical radio-ulna synostosis is worth considering. Congenital amputation is most common in the upper third of the forearm; consequently flexion of the elbow is preserved and a useful hook will result. Reference to a limb-fitting centre should be considered at the age of about a year.

Congenital dislocations at the wrist or elbow are less disabling abnormalities. The former is a dorsal dislocation of the ulna at the inferior radio-ulna joint (Madelung's deformity) which is associated with bowing of the radius. The disability is cosmetic only and so may be ignored in childhood and although resection or shortening of the prominent terminal ulna may be requested, it should not be done until after skeletal maturity is reached. Similar considerations apply to congenital anterior dislocation of the head of the radius. It is characterized by prominence of the radial head in front of the elbow and occasionally limitation of flexion. Failure to resist an appeal or temptation to excise the radial head may result in a dislocation of the inferior radio-ulna joint, owing to the loss of radial growth which operation causes.

In common with the lower ulna dislocation and in contrast to acquired dislocation, disability is negligible. These congenital types may be distinguished from the traumatic upon this issue and the associated changes which involve neighbouring bones—i.e. curved ulna and small capitellum. In addition the head of the radius may dislocate following paralysis, notably Erb's.

Synostosis of the radius and ulna causes loss of forearm rotation—but happily the position is usually that of full pronation, which in relationship to the function of the hand is ideal. Consequently this is seldom noted in infancy and even later it may be disguised by increased mobility of the shoulder. Good function precludes correction even if it were possible to restore active rotation, which is improbable. The diagnosis may need to be clinical if cross-union is not seen on the radiograph, but then there is likely to be bowing of the ulna and an abnormal relationship at the superior radio-ulna joint. Clinical diagnosis must, however, distinguish between pronation congenitally determined and that due to flaccid or spastic paralysis of long standing.

Recurrent dislocation of the elbow is due to failure of development of the ulna coronoid process and is very rare. Because of the technical difficulty of repair, this should be left until the child is older.

Bony ankylosis of the elbow. The need or otherwise for correction will depend upon the position of the forearm which should be such that the hand readily reaches the mouth.

Arthrogryposis may be the cause of extended elbows. Restoration of function is complex and should be deferred until a decision as to the relative indications for osteotomy and tendon transplantation become clarified.

The upper arm is an area of relative tranquility so far as local congenital deformity is concerned, though it is not immune from the effects of generalized disorders of the skeleton and soft tissues. The humerus for example is one of the more frequently fractured bones in osteogenesis imperfecta and may require nailing. The shoulder joint is, however, sometimes affected by congenital abnormality.

Humerus varus resembles coxa vara in that there is often shortening and limitation of abduction—in this case due to the great tuberosity impinging upon the acromium at about 90°. Excision of the acromium will increase the range of movement but the disability barely warrants even so trivial an operation. On occasions the head of the humerus becomes the socket for a globular glenoid, but again disability is mild.

Congenital pseudarthrosis of the clavicle is a curious condition found almost exclusively on the right side and unrelated to any general disorder. An attempt to obtain union should be made.

Disorders of the soft tissues include:

Recurrent subluxation of the shoulder in congenital joint laxity;

Absence of part or all of trapezius, deltoid or pectoralis major—the last is sometimes associated with absence of the breast or congenital abnormality of the cardiovascular system.

Lesions of the brachial plexus. It seems appropriate to mention briefly traction lesions of the brachial plexus, for although not congenital in the literal sense, they are present from birth. Diagnosis follows the observation that one arm is used less than its fellow and if hemiplegia or birth fracture are absent, the cause is likely to be found in the brachial plexus, especially if birth has resulted in arrest of the head with traction on the arm or body. In the very young, swelling and bruising in the supraclavicular region or even axillary vein thrombosis may be seen. Fractures of the clavicle or proximal end of the humerus are sometimes associated.

Although it is customary to divide these nerve lesions into upper root (Erb) and lower root (Klumpke) types, there is frequently overlap between them and sometimes the whole plexus is involved. The upper-arm type involving C5 and C6 roots is by far the commonest and fortunately carries the best prognosis, though recovery may be delayed for up to 2 years before it is complete. As abduction and external rotation movement of the shoulder are the most commonly involved, there is a danger of an adduction and internal rotation deformity developing during this time which will prevent the benefits of recovery from becoming apparent. It is therefore important that the mother be taught to put all the joints of the arm through their full passive range of movement at least once a day and that the surgeon satisfy himself periodically that contracture is not developing. Late reconstruction for residual paralysis by either tendon transplantation or arthrodesis is occasionally indicated but osteotomies to correct secondary deformities, especially internal rotation of the shoulder, are more often necessary and more frequently rewarding.

The lower arm (C8 T1) and the whole plexus types have a poor prognosis and little can be done to improve the function in either, for loss of sensibility is added to the motor paralysis and secondary contracture, a situation seen characteristically in the severely clawed and insensitive hand of Klumpke's paralysis.

THE LOWER LIMB

THE LEG ABOVE THE KNEE

The anomalies of the upper femur and the hip joint are relatively constant in presentation. Detection of abnormality as opposed to differential diagnosis is our primary responsibility in infancy. Fortunately this can be achieved by a simple method of clinical examination which will confirm or deny shortening between the iliac crest and the knee and limitation of abduction of the hip. There is no condition demanding urgent attention in infancy which is not accompanied by one or other or both of these signs.

These essential signs must be sought by a method which, because it must be so often used in a newborn baby or a restless and resentful infant, needs to be rapid and simple.

The fundamental clinical examination requires that we carry out two manoeuvres with the child lying down on a flat hard surface.

(1) Both knees are flexed to beyond the right-angle with the feet in contact and the tips of the big toes in the same horizontal plane. At this point the observer, who faces the feet, looks at the levels of the highest point of both knees. A difference means that the legs are of different length.

(2) Both legs are now widely abducted with the knees and the hips still flexed; any difference between the range of movement of either hip is noted.

These signs of shortening and limited abduction are enough to alert the examiner to the fact that there is an abnormality in one femur or hip joint. If a bilateral abnormality is present, detection is more difficult. Restriction of abduction (now symmetrical) is the basic observation, but it requires the examiner to be experienced in examination of the normal, if he is to appreciate that an abnormality exists. Fortunately, however, only in bilateral congenital dislocation is a moderate delay in diagnosis harmful and in this condition there are other signs to help—notably approximation of the trochanters to the iliac crests, broadening of the perineum and pelvis and restriction of internal rotation when this is tested with the hips in flexion.

Clinical examination followed by a radiograph will confirm or exclude the presence of frank dislocation. Sometimes an early diagnosis of acetabular insufficiency may be made. Dislocation or early degenerative arthritis of such sub-standard (dysplastic, subluxated) joints gradually develops. This is the cause in perhaps 20–25 per cent of all patients suffering from 'idiopathic' osteo-arthritis sufficiently disabling to demand operative treatment—especially and significantly in those who are relatively young in relation to the disease incidence as a whole. It may be prevented by early treatment.

The abduction sign in bilateral disorders, although important, is open to misinterpretation. It can be responsible for unnecessary exposure to radiation if it is believed that abduction in infancy normally allows the knees to touch the examination couch. This is quite untrue.

Other signs, including unequal creases, absence of femoral heads from beneath the mid-inguinal points, and telescoping, belong only to the examination hall. In practice, being often unreliable and difficult to elicit, they are misleading in comparison with the abduction and leg-shortening tests.

Screening of hips in the newborn is of great contemporary interest for in most treatment of dislocation or subluxation in infancy will be entirely successful. Certain points require emphasis if consistently good results are to be obtained.

(I) The examiner should use two tests—the abduction in flexion as already described and Barlow's test. This involves pressure with the thumb backwards over the head of the femur with the hip and knee flexed to 90°. A 'clunk' which is audible, palpable and frequently visible denotes instability of the hip which allows backward dislocation of the femoral head. Pressure in the reverse direction by the fingers behind the great trochanter produces a similar clunk of reduction. It should be emphasized that only a clunk is significant—clicks are common and of no importance.

(II) It is vital that the examiner realize that a positive Barlow's test diagnoses hip instability and therefore potential dislocation rather than frank dislocation.

(III) In frank dislocation with adduction contracture a 'clunk' will not be obtained for the femoral head is habitually out and cannot be reduced. The abduction in flexion test will be positive and so will the radiograph.

(IV) The early management of these babies depends upon the clinical findings.

(a) The hip is habitually in position but can be dislocated. In these Barlow's first manoeuvre will be positive, i.e. a 'clunk' on backward pressure with the thumb. The hip is unstable but is likely to become stable very soon. The baby should be re-examined at regular intervals to confirm this and an X-ray taken at 4 months when the femoral ossific nucleus is visible. A normal hip is to be expected but mild dysplasia requiring a short period of abduction splinting may be found.

(b) The hip is habitually dislocated but will reduce easily with restoration of full abduction. Barlow's first manoeuvre will be negative, his second and Ortolani's test will be positive. These require splinting in full abduction.

(c) The hip is habitually dislocated and will not reduce. Barlow's and

Ortolani's tests are negative and abduction in flexion is limited (adduction contracture). It is necessary to restore full abduction and reduce the hip by traction before a splint is applied.

The differential diagnosis of limitation of abduction requires distinction between unilateral signs (asymmetrical abduction and leg length) and bilateral (symmetrical though reduced abduction and equality of leg length). These are considered separately.

Unilateral signs
(a) *Unilateral congenital dislocation* in contrast to subluxation will be manifest on the radiograph. Because of the good results which follow simple splinting in abduction in cases of subluxation and pelvic obliquity (see below), a somewhat cavalier attitude has arisen in the minds of some towards the management of a dislocation diagnosed before 6 months of age. Whilst simple abduction in a Frejka pillow splint or preferably a Denis Browne abduction splint (which maintains abduction, without interfering with nappy changes or washing and forbids the mother any discretion which may be exercised in the wrong direction) may certainly correct dislocation at this age, it will not always succeed. The decision to use this simple out-patient method demands that full passive abduction be obtainable when the splint is applied. Full abduction may follow gentle pressure applied to the leg held high on the thigh so that a short lever is employed. This may be accompanied by a palpable and often audible click (Ortolani) which is merely manipulative reduction without anaesthesia. If full abduction is not readily obtained it is wiser to admit the child and obtain full abduction by traction or, if this is, for some reason, not possible, by reduction under anaesthesia. In either event, abduction should be maintained until the radiograph indicates that the femoral head is congruous with the acetabulum which in depth resembles that on the other side. Even in favourable cases this may take up to a year. Failure of primary reduction may declare itself either immediately or later but its management is beyond the scope of this book.

(b) *Unilateral acetabular insufficiency* or primary subluxation depends for diagnosis upon unilateral clinical signs and careful and critical scrutiny of the radiograph.

Inspection must be critical for any tilting of the pelvis will tend to reduce the depth of the acetabulum as seen in profile. If, however, the pelvis is correctly positioned and a deficiency of the acetabulum is apparent on the side which is clinically suspect, treatment should be instituted as for a frank dislocation. If this is carried out promptly and efficiently, the outcome is usually excellent. If the radiograph is doubtful but the clinical signs unequivocal it is wiser to treat the child.

(c) *Fixed pelvic obliquity* may be secondary to some other condition or primary. Among the secondary variety are those due to intra-uterine paralysis and subsequent contracture, causing fixed abduction in spina bifida and abduction in cerebral palsy or skeletal deformity such as thoracolumbar congenital scoliosis. Treatment is related to the cause.

Primary obliquity, however, is unexplained. It is important because the signs may be exactly those of dislocation, since fixed adduction both limits abduction and causes apparent shortening. The radiograph does not confirm the suspected dislocation but the tilted pelvis may again lead the unwary to diagnose acetabular insufficiency, when it is not present. Pelvic obliquity is often associated with head moulding and structural scoliosis of infancy as a feature of the 'moulded baby syndrome'.

Unnecessary treatment may not be harmful to the child, for it is likely to be discarded as no longer necessary before walking begins, but it may result in a too favourable conclusion about the results of conservative treatment in hip-joint dysplasia. Forced manipulation under anaesthesia (a most undesirable procedure in all circumstances) on a mistaken diagnosis of dislocation may, because of sudden capsular tension, destroy the blood supply to the capital epiphysis of a normal hip joint. Abduction stretching exercises by the mother will correct the contracture rapidly.

(d) *Congenital coxa vara and short femur* present with the same signs whether they exist together or separately. Ring has recently reviewed such patients. Coxa vara is difficult to diagnose radiographically before the capital epiphysis is ossified but the short femur characteristically shows abnormal bowing and sclerosis in the sub-trochanteric area. This is often mistakenly regarded as due to a birth fracture. A prognosis may be offered with some confidence and accuracy and a rough estimate of final shortening is less than $2\frac{1}{2}$ in. if there is no associated coxa vara and more than 4 in. if there is. Treatment is not necessary in infancy but sub-trochanteric osteotomy and equalization of leg length will need to be considered later.

(e) *Osteomyelitis, pyogenic, arthritic and obstetrical injuries* are mentioned for completeness.

Bilateral Signs
With the exception of fixed pelvic obliquity, all of the conditions mentioned may be present on both sides to tax the diagnostic abilities of the most experienced. To these must be added some general afflictions including gargoylism, achondroplasia, osteochondrodystrophy and protrusio acetabulae. It is easy to overlook these conditions, especially in bilateral dislocation with joint laxity. Pleas for early diagnosis (which amount so often to but thinly disguised criticism) are best made by those of limited experience, abounding self-confidence and short memories. Careful examination will of course often bring its own reward but there is little substitute for experience, intuition and luck in the early diagnosis of bilateral, symmetrical, congenital disorders of the hip joint. Treatment will follow diagnosis along the lines of that indicated for unilateral disorders but in general prognosis is less favourable.

Genetic Implications (of Congenital Dislocation of the hip)
Empirical risk figures for the younger sibs of female index patients are about 1 in 30 (probably higher for sisters than brothers), but about 1 in 10 for the young sibs of male index patients (both brothers and sisters). The higher risks are associated with the presence of familial joint laxity and perhaps the presence of familial acetabular dysplasia.

The Leg below the Knee

Congenital deformities of the lower leg may be divided into abnormalities of length or shape, or both of these.

Abnormalities of Length
The tibia and fibula may be too long in idiopathic hemi-hypertrophy, congenital deep arterior-venous communication, superficial haemangiomatous malformation and neurofibromatosis. The limb is large but of normal contour in hemi-hypertrophy but in the others, the signs of the underlying condition are apparent. The tibia and fibula may be too short in association with a congenital short femur or as a result of cerebral palsy, spina bifida, arthrogryposis or poliomyelitis acquired *in utero* or in infancy. Neonatal osteomyelitis is more likely to cause lengthening than shortening if treatment has been prompt and effective.

Abnormalities of Shape

Internal rotation of the leg. This is normal in the newborn. If it persists apparent bow legs and a pigeon-toe gait develop, but the ultimate prognosis is excellent. Internal rotation is sometimes associated with persistent foetal alignment (anteversion) of the femoral neck and is demonstrable by increased internal rotation of the hip in extension at the expense of external rotation. Rarely the reverse occurs.

Bowing without significant shortening may be lateral, medial, posterior or anterior. Except for the last, these are benign conditions which usually correct spontaneously, or if not, may be readily cured by osteotomy. Lateral bowing may, however, point to a diagnosis of congenital or acquired rickets. Anterior bowing with an intact fibula is a serious sign, especially if the tibial shaft is radiologically abnormal at the apex of the bow. Such a tibia being likely to be affected by neuro-fibromatosis or fibrous dysplasia is prone to fracture and non-union (congenital pseudarthrosis of tibia) and should on no account be operated upon to correct deformity. If the diagnosis is made before the fracture occurs, an attempt should be made to by-pass the abnormal area by an autogenous cortical graft applied across the concavity posteriorly. If fracture has occurred, we are presented with one of the most difficult reparative problems in orthopaedic surgery and amputation is the not infrequent outcome.

Abnormalities of Length and Shape

Congenital amputations are rare in the lower leg but can usually be satisfactorily fitted with an artificial limb.

Absence of the fibula and tibia are characterized by anterior bowing and shortening. If the fibula is absent there is frequently valgus deformity and loss of the fifth toe and associated metatarsal. Repair is difficult. Amputation is frequently the ultimate outcome and a Symes amputation will produce a good functional result. The alternative is tibial lengthening with or without shortening of the opposite leg to compensate for a discrepancy at maturity. If the tibia is absent, a short leg is associated with a dislocated and unstable knee so that there is seldom an alternative to disarticulation at the knee.

THE KNEE

Osteochondromata are the commonest bony tumours found in this area.

They arise by displacement of growing epiphyseal cartilage cells. Among intra-osseus bone cysts in this region we should remember that *non-osteogenic fibroma, metaphyseal fibrous defect* and *angiomatous bone cysts* have their greatest incidence in this region and are developmental in origin. The epiphyseal cartilages of the knee contribute more to growth than any other, so that disorders of growth are often manifest in a radiograph of this area.

Fixed flexion of the knees at birth may be associated with congenital skin webbing across the concavity of the popliteal space. This deformity resists gradual correction by plaster or traction which is perhaps fortunate, for the neurovascular bundle lies in the superficial margin of the web and is thus liable to traction injury unless the femur is shortened to an extent that will allow extension without tension. True arthrogryposis or intra-uterine paralysis, usually with a myelo-meningocele, may result in flexed knees which, however, may be safely stretched though the hamstrings and posterior capsule may need to be divided.

Genu-recurvatum may be a manifestation of arthrogryposis but may also exist as a single abnormality which will usually respond readily to gradual correction by adhesive strapping or plaster applied as early as possible. Obstinate contractures require quadriceps-plasty to restore flexion. Sometimes a minor variation of this deformity is found in older children in which either hyper-extension or full extension is accompanied by a loss of flexion. Most are due to quadriceps fibrosis secondary to injections or infusions in the neonatal period and operative relaxation is needed.

Congenital dislocation of the patella may be inherited from a near relative and demands operation which, however, should avoid transplantation of the tibial tubercle lest growth at the upper tibial epiphysis be inhibited.

Bow legs (*genu varum*) in infancy often generates parental concern which is usually unwarranted. Most represent persistence of the outward curve and inward rotation, seen so often in normal babies. Nutritional or inherited rickets may be excluded by a radiograph but care must be taken not to diagnose the rare osteochondritis of the medial tibial epiphysis (*Blount's disease*) too freely for the beak of the medial epiphysis is frequently prolonged medially during infancy in idiopathic varum.

Lastly, two very rare conditions are worth mentioning.

Ulceration over the front of the knee joint may be found at birth, due possibly to intra-uterine compression upon the flexed knees of the foetus; healing is rapid and in spite of its position the scar causes no permanent ill-effect.

Sciatic nerve palsy may be the cause of the baby being unable to bend the knee actively in the presence of full passive movement. The prognosis may be good if this is due to obstetrical traction during delivery but it is less likely to improve if an injection of Niketamide or kindred substance has caused ischaemic neuritis.

The Foot and Ankle

The foot and ankle are the site of several important congenital deformities which tend to follow uniform patterns, and which, with the exception of club feet, do not require operative treatment in the first year.

Congenital amputations. These occur typically at the meta-tarso-phalangeal joints, tarso-metatarsal joint and immediately distal to the calcaneus and talus. All of these have a relatively good functional prognosis and require only special shoes or minor operations of a 'tidying up' nature, to make shoe-fitting easier.

The lobster-claw foot is the counterpart of a similar deformity seen more commonly in the hand. The management of these is the same as for congenital amputations.

Toes may be abnormal in number, size or shape. The treatment of polydactyly or hypertrophy will be dictated by the needs of the shoe-maker. Syndactyly is common and of no importance.

Congenital curly toes in which the third or fourth toe is rotated laterally and flexed at the proximal interphalangeal joint, frequently worries parents. Sweetnam found that about one-third straightened spontaneously as the children grew, and straightening was not influenced by the traditional treatment of strapping the toe. Furthermore, curly toes do not tend to cause symptoms in adult life.

In contrast, however, there are four varieties of congenital angular deformity of toes, which may give rise to symptoms later.

(1) *Interphalangeal valgus of the big toe.* This may cause a painful callosity to form on the convexity overlying the joint, thus indicating the need for arthrodesis or phalangeal osteotomy later. It is not the same as valgus at the metatarso-phalangeal joint—hallux valgus, which is seldom if ever seen in infancy.

(2) *Hallux varus* is a deformity similar but in the opposite direction to hallux valgus and seen in infancy. It may be associated with a fused double big toe or an abnormally short first metatarsal. Correction is by operation.

(3) *Congenital hammer toe* is characterized by flexion at the proximal interphalangeal joint at the second toe which is too long.

(4) *Congenital contracture of the fifth toe* is a deformity of medial rotation and elevation so that it overlies the fourth toe on its dorsal aspect.

Both (3) and (4) are potentially troublesome and frequently require surgical correction or ablation in later life. Considerable improvement and sometimes correction may be obtained if seen in infancy and manipulated assiduously by the mother in directions opposite to the deformity.

An absent fifth toe and complete or *partial duplication of the forefoot* suggest the possibility of an anomaly of the tibia or fibula.

Metatarsus atavicus implies that the first metatarsal is short and mobile, simulating a thumb. This sometimes causes a pronation deformity (valgus) to occur in the hindfoot, for only by this means can the head of the metatarsal be brought in contact with the ground and share in the task of weight-bearing.

Primus metatarsus varus is due to the first metatarsal lying more medially than it should, either as an isolated deformity or as part of a deformity involving all the metatarsals. Primus varus is of interest as a potential cause of hallux valgus later on.

Metatarsus varus consists in a medial position of the metatarsals with which supination and adduction is often associated. This, however, is important because it is frequently treated unnecessarily and sometimes not treated when it should be; most cases are of no significance, for the deformity is postural and can be readily over-corrected passively and often actively by the baby, in response to judicious tickling of the lateral side of the foot. The anxious mother may with benefit be taught to correct the deformity passively and told that when walking starts, the inner border of the shoe will ensure that correction is maintained.

In a small number of patients the deformity is not amenable to immediate passive correction and treatment is indicated. There seem to be two distinct varieties; the first is associated with other stigmata of a club foot which may be mild and easily overlooked and the second, a deformity in its own right accompanying a lateral dislocation of the navicular on the talus. In either event, treatment should initially be as for a club foot and the parents warned that operation may be necessary later.

Pes cavus is very rarely seen in infancy but should it present, the probability of an underlying neurological deficit should always be suspected.

Congenital talipes equino-varus (club foot) has a prognosis which in any one patient is almost unpredictable. The results of treatment are still far from satisfactory.

The attitude is one of equinus at the ankle, and varus at the subtaloid joint. There is adduction of the forefoot. Our first duty must be to establish whether this is a structural or postural deformity. If postural, the little toe of the newborn infant may be made to touch the outer side of the leg without undue force; such cases need concern us no further, for the foot is normal. If the deformity cannot be so overcorrected, a club foot exists and demands not only treatment but also further attention, lest it be associated with arthrogryposis or spina bifida. Most, however, exist as isolated deformities (unilateral or bilateral). In the more severe examples, additional signs are present such as wasting of the calf, forefoot cavus and inversion and dimpling below and in front of the lateral malleolus.

Before beginning treatment the mother should be warned that, although an uncomplicated course and wholly satisfactory outcome cannot be promised, her child will not become a cripple and may be expected to walk at a time which is either normal or at least not unduly delayed. This is important because the mother of such a baby frequently has preconceived and erroneous notions of the probable outcome. She must also be warned that the management of the child demands her assiduous and regular attendance at hospital which, because of a tendency to relapse after initial correction, may extend over 5 years. It is advisable to avoid the term 'club foot' in this discussion.

Early treatment is important and ordinarily a start should be made on the first day of life. Whilst there are unquestioned advantages to be gained by an immediate and energetic approach to correction, it is unfortunately not axiomatic that early treatment will produce a good result in all cases. It seems, however, to offer the best prospect of success.

There are several methods of treating club feet in infancy which may be summarized in general terms as repeated manipulation (common to all) and either maintenance by repeated plasters of the correction obtained or maintenance and continuing correction in splints such as Denis Browne's or by strapping in the manner attributed to Robert Jones. The various methods are all capable of producing good results in a comparable proportion of feet in the hands of exponents who are familiar with and skilled in the application of the particular technique which they choose to practice.

My own preference is for Robert Jones' strapping because it requires the least special equipment. Being easily applied, it can be readily changed or adjusted at frequent intervals, by a suitably instructed nurse or physiotherapist, between visits to the surgeon. It is, furthermore, the safest, being the least likely to cause pressure sores or embarrass the circulation.

The following routine is suggested. The surgeon manipulates the foot into abduction and valgus, being careful not to force dorsiflexion until the heel is at least corrected to the mid position, for there is otherwise a danger of spurious correction of equinus at the mid tarsal joint, rather than at the ankle. Adhesive felt about $\frac{1}{2}$ in. wide is now put around the forefoot to encircle it and another $\frac{1}{2}$ in. square placed above the lateral malleolus. Adhesive strapping $\frac{3}{4}$–1 in. broad is applied from just below the medial malleolus, around the heel, up the lateral side of the leg (under tension), over the top of the flexed knee, ending on the medial side of the upper third of the leg. Another strip begins on the dorsal surface of the adhesive felt at the level of the fifth metatarsal—this encircles the forefoot and from its starting place is carried, with tension, over the top of the flexed knee to the medial side of the upper leg.

It is our practice to change the strapping once a week when the opportunity is taken to manipulate the foot gently. On two other occasions during the week, the physiotherapist 'takes up the slack' by placing new strips of strapping over the existing ones, with slightly more tension. The mother is taught to stretch the foot several times each day.

This routine is followed until over-correction is obtained with particular emphasis on the heel. This may take from 3 weeks to 6 months and then Denis Browne removable bootee splints may be used to maintain rather than obtain correction.

Unfortunately there are a substantial number of feet (about 30 per cent) which do not respond rapidly and wholly satisfactorily to early treatment. The management of these resistant or relapsed deformities is beyond the scope of this book but one point requires emphasis. Failure to correct equinus early and completely bodes ill for the final outcome, particularly if the os calcis is small and inverted, for in these, any pressure applied to the forefoot is likely to be expended on the midtarsal joint producing a false correction of equinus here rather than at the ankle. A lateral radiograph with the foot as near as possible to a right angle to the leg will demonstrate the danger. Posterior displacement of the fibula is an added danger signal. We have been encouraged recently by the results of elongation of the tendo-achilles, posterior capsulotomy of the ankle and division of tibialis posterior as early as the third month. The operation will often allow the heel to be brought under control and false correction is then eliminated. We regard this operation as an incident in treatment which does not interfere with continuation of the strapping method which is re-applied in the operating theatre and continues as though an operation had not been performed. In this connection a significant observation recently made suggests that the os calcis of the infant moves into valgus more readily when the talus is in calcaneous than in equinus. This would account for the fact that uncorrected equinus is too often associated with both a failure to over-correct heel varus and with a gradual relapse into varus again of such correction as is obtained.

Genetic Implications
Empirical risk figures for the younger sibs of index patients are about 1 in 30, but are about 1 in 10 if a parent is also affected. Risks to the children of patients are not yet established.

The *calcaneo-valgus* foot is as common and as striking as the equino-varus (club foot). Here the resemblance ends, for in most cases it is readily corrected and the prognosis is good. Diagnosis is simple, for the foot lies against the outer border of the leg in such a way that the fifth toe often lies in contact with it. Passive equinus is prevented by structural deformity. Commonly associated conditions, such as congenital dislocation of the hip, arthrogryposis and spina bifida should be excluded. The mother may then be given an encouraging prognosis and the assurance that this is not a club foot. She should be taught to stretch the foot into equinus and varus whenever she feeds the baby or changes the nappy. By this means, correction is usually readily obtained, though in a few a flat foot with some fixed valgus of the heel and plantar flexed talus may persist as a mild cosmetic blemish, but with good function.

Congenital vertical talus is sometimes confused with calcaneo-valgus deformity because dorsiflexion of the forefoot is common to both.

Congenital vertical talus, however, is comparatively rare and is characterized by equinus of the heel as distinct from calcaneous, by rigidity as opposed to relative mobility at the sub-taloid joint, and by a prominence on the medial border of the sole. Associated conditions are common, the prognosis for correction is poor and the usefulness of early operative treatment, as opposed to late correction by triple arthrodesis when symptoms arise, is not yet established with certainty.

The alternative name given to this deformity is congenital flat foot, so that it seems appropriate at this point to digress briefly upon the subject of infantile *flat feet*—a condition often suspected and even diagnosed but very seldom present as a definite abnormality. If the joints of the foot are fully mobile and all the muscle groups acting upon them are working, the foot is normal. By applying these criteria we can be certain that the feet are normal, however much the medial side of the sole bulges or the heel tilts into valgus—common postural deformities adopted by the child when he first stands and accentuated if standing is delayed for any reason or if benign hypotonia or ligamentous laxity are present. Restriction of movement, passive or active, may indicate a vertical talus, cerebral palsy, arthrogryposis, paralysis due to spina bifida, poliomyelitis or muscular atrophy. Fixed valgus is sometimes caused by a synostosis between the os calcis and either the talus or the navicular, as yet in pre-osseous cartilage, and so invisible on the radiograph. Restricted dorsiflexion may point to either cerebral palsy or a congenitally short tendo-achilles with compensatory hypermobility of the joints distal to the ankle and frequently an accessory navicular bone. All of these are potentially the cause of pain or disability.

SELECTED REFERENCES

BLOUNT W.P. (1937) Tibia var. *J. Bone Jt. Surg.* **19,** 1
BROWNE D. (1956) Splinting for controlled movement. *Clin. Orthop.* **8,** 91
CAFFEY J. (1946) Infantile cortical hyperostosis. *J. Paediatrics* **29,** 541
CHANDLER F.A. (1948) Muscular torticollis. *J. Bone Jt. Surg.* **30A,** 556
FAIRBANK SIR THOMAS. *An Atlas of General Affections of the Skeleton.* Edinburgh: Livingstone
HARRIS R.J. & BEATTY T. (1948) Hypermobile flat feet with short tendo Achilles. *J. Bone Jt. Surg.* **30A,** 116
HULBERT K.F. (1950) Congenital torticollis. *J. Bone Jt. Surg.* **32B,** 50
JAMES J.I.P. (1955) Kyphoscoliosis. *J. Bone Jt. Surg.* **37B,** 414
JAMES J.I.P., LLOYD-ROBERTS G.C. & PILCHER M.F. (1959) Infantile idiopathic scoliosis. *J. Bone Jt. Surg.* **41B,** 719

Key J.A. (1927) Congenital joint laxity. *J. Amer. Med. Assoc.* **88,** 1710
Kite J.H. (1950) Congenital metatarsus varus. *J. Bone Jt. Surg.* **32A,** 500
Lloyd-Roberts G.C. (1953) Humerus varus. *J. Bone Jt. Surg.* **35B,** 268
Lloyd-Roberts G.C. (1955) Osteoarthritis of the hip. *J. Bone Jt. Surg.* **37B,** 8
Lloyd-Roberts G.C. & Spence A.J. (1958) Congenital vertical talus. *J. Bone Jt. Surg.* **40B,** 33
Lloyd-Roberts G.C. (1960) Suppurative arthritis of infancy. *J. Bone Jt. Surg.* **42B,** 706
Lloyd-Roberts G.C. & Pilcher M.F. (1965) Structural idiopathic scoliosis in infancy. *J. Bone Jt. Surg.* **47B,** 3
Lloyd-Roberts G.C. & Swann M. (1966) Pitfalls in the Management of Congenita. Dislocation of the Hip. *J. Bone Jt. Surg.* **48B,** 4
Lloyd-Roberts G.C. & Lettin A.W.F. (1970) Arthrogryposis Multiplex Congenita. *J. Bone Jt. Surg.* **52B.** 3
Logue V. & Till K. (1952) Posterior fossa dermoid cysts with special reference to intracranial infection. *J. Neuro. Neurosurg. and Psychiat.* **15,** 1
McCarroll H.R. (1950) Clinical manifestations of congenital neurofibromatosis. *J. Bone Jt. Surg.* **32A,** 601
McKenzie D.Y. (1958) Arthrogryphosis. *Proc. Roy. Soc. Med.* **52,** 1101
Osmond-Clarke H. (1956) Congenital vertical talus. *J. Bone Jt. Surg.* **38B,** 334
Ring P.A. (1959) Congenital short femur. *J. Bone Jt. Surg.* **41B,** 13
Schlesinger B., Luder J. & Bodian M. (1955) Rickets with alkaline phosphatase deficiency; an osteoblastic dysplasia. *Arch. Dis. Childh.* **30,** 265
Shaw N.E. (1960) Neonatal sciatic palsy. *J. Bone Jt. Surg.* **42B,** 736
Smellie J.S. (1951) *Injuries of the Knee Joint.* Edinburgh: Livingstone
Sofield H.A. & Miller E.A. (1959) Intramedullary rod fixation of deformities of long bones in children. *J. Bone Jt. Surg.* **41A,** 1371
Swann M., Lloyd-Roberts G.C. & Catterall A. (1969) The Anatomy of Uncorrected Club Feet–a Study of rotation deformity. *J. Bone Jt. Surg.* **51B,** 2
Sweetman R. (1958) Congenital curly toes. *Lancet* **2,** 398
Walton J.N. (1956) Amyotonia congenita. *Lancet* **1,** 1023
Wechesser E.C. (1955) Congenital flexion adduction deformity of the thumb. *J. Bone Jt. Surg.* **37A,** 977
Wiberg G. (1939) Studies in dysplastic acetabulae. *Acta Chir. Scand.* **83,** Supp. 58

9

Abnormalities of the Skin

E. J. MOYNAHAN

Skin anomalies are easy to see and after birth a careful note should be made of any abnormality which may be present. Its site, size, shape, colour, consistency and any other physical sign should be accurately recorded. A diagram or sketch should be made whenever possible in domiciliary practice, and a photograph in all investigative studies. Details of the family history, mother's previous obstetric and health record, illnesses and events during the pregnancy, age of mother and father, birth order, season of conception, consanguinity, as well as the usual obstetric events during the labour, should all be noted.

The lesion should be followed up throughout its natural history. We need much more information than we possess of the natural history of many congenital skin anomalies, e.g. congenital urticaria pigmentosa, naevoxanthoma, incontinentia pigmenti, the ichthyoses. The family doctor is particularly well placed to gather such information, since he is the only trained observer likely to follow the infant until he reaches maturity.

There is a great deal to be learned about the incidence, pathogenesis, developmental biochemistry and the precise inheritance of most skin blemishes before we can usefully attempt to prevent them.

EMBRYOLOGY OF THE SKIN

The skin is derived from two of the primary germinal layers of the embryo: the ectoderm, which gives rise to the epidermis and its appendages and the mesoderm from which the dermis or corium is derived.

Epidermis
The early embryo is covered by a layer of flat or cuboidal cells derived

from the general surface ectoderm, but by the end of the first month, when the embryo has attained a length of 5 mm, two layers are present. The superficial layer, called the periderm or epitrichium, becomes keratinized and is eventually shed during the fifth and sixth months to form, with the sebum from the skin, the vernix caseosa. It is sometimes retained until after birth and may then give rise to one of the forms of congenital ichthyosis. The deeper layer becomes the basal layer of the epidermis from which a stratified squamous epithelium develops. Keratinization does not begin until the fourth month of intra-uterine life and is delayed until the sixth month in the palms and soles. On the other hand, the melanocytes have reached their definitive sites by the end of the third month. The melanocytes are derived from the neural crest, the cells composing it migrate to the epidermis and other sites where they are found. They do not produce pigment until they have completed their migration, but melanocytes do not do so at all of their definitive sites. A similar 'eclipse' or 'de-differentiation' of the melanin-producing cells occurs during the resting phase of the hair cycle, when it is difficult to detect their presence by present histochemical techniques, and it is tempting to assume that the melanocytes associated with the hair follicle also lose their 'identification marks' when they migrate with the resting hair follicle. Loss of the capacity to produce pigment is one of the manifestations of ageing of the hair follicles. Premature greying is met with in several syndromes, each controlled by a different gene.

Vigorous pigmentary activity can be seen before birth in the epidermis of Negroes and dark-skinned races, but there is usually little evidence of such activity in the epidermis of the white foetus, apart from the melanocytes associated with the growing hairs. There are no racial differences in the numbers of melanocytes per unit area, although there are marked regional differences, common to all races.

Hairs and the Hair Follicle

Emergence of the first hairs begins at the end of the second month, in the eyebrows, upper lids and chin; development elsewhere on the body does not begin until a month later. Hair follicles are formed singly but tend to be grouped in threes. Each follicle arises as the result of the downward growth of a column of cells from the basal layer of the epidermis. A bulge makes its appearance on one side of the column close to the epidermis and from this the sebaceous gland eventually differentiates. Meanwhile, the base of the column swells to give rise to the bulb of the hair follicle. This in turn hollows out so that it becomes cup-shaped and embraces the condensed mass of connective tissue cells, which was pushed in front of the column and now constitutes the dermal papilla. The subsequent production of hair by the follicle depends upon the close association between the dermal papilla and the epithelial cells forming the base of the hair follicle; should the papilla be destroyed or seriously damaged through disease or any other cause, no further hairs will develop in that follicle. The hair itself is produced as a result of cell division in the lowermost epithelial layer of the follicle. The hair follicle shows great variations in mitotic activity which correspond with the phase of growth of the hair concerned, and its mitotic rhythm is quite independent of that of the surface epidermal cells, though both rhythms may come into phase in conditions such as exfoliative erythroderma, when the mitotic rate of the surface epidermis is greatly increased; under such conditions follicles may be unable to produce hair. Congenital universal hypertrichosis of the lanugo hair is a rare anomaly in which there is great overgrowth of the silky lanugo hairs all over the body.

Sweat Glands

Sweat glands may be either eccrine or apocrine; the former open freely on to the surface of the skin and are not associated with hair follicles, whereas the latter usually discharge their secretion into the hair follicle through a straight duct which runs parallel with the follicle from which it develops as an outgrowth in early embryonic life.

Sweat glands first appear in the scalp, forehead, palms and soles, as small epidermal buds, which extend downwards into the dermis as solid cords during the fourth and fifth months. Later the cords become tortuous to give rise to the characteristically coiled secretory portion of the sweat glands (both apocrine and eccrine) with a spirally coiled duct traversing the dermis and epidermis to discharge the sweat directly on to the skin surface in the eccrine glands, in contrast with the straight duct already mentioned, of the apocrine glands.

Eccrine sweat glands begin to show presumptive evidence of secretory activity by the eighth month and may be functional in the ninth month of intra-uterine life. Apocrine glands are still incompletely formed at birth and do not attain full development until sexual maturity.

The Dermis

The dermis arises from mesenchyme which lies just beneath the surface ectoderm. In the earliest month this consists of a dense network of fusiform, stellate cells with little evidence of gross fibre formation, but delicate fibrils begin to appear during the second and later months. The reticular layer can be distinguished from the overlying papillary layer during the fourth month, by the presence of fine and coarse collagenous bundles in contrast to the delicate fibrils to be seen in the papillary layer. Elastic fibres do not appear until near term; most of them appear after birth and they continue to increase in number as the skin continues to grow.

The earliest blood vessels begin as simple endothelial lined structures which differentiate out of the mesenchyme, but with growth of the skin, new capillaries bud out from these. Some of these vessels acquire muscle coats through differentiation of the surrounding mesenchyme to become arterioles and arteries; others, through which a return flow of blood is established, also acquire muscular coats and become venules and veins. Throughout intra-uterine life and later, new plexuses are continually formed in the skin, as in all growing tissues, to give rise to new vessels (neo-angiogenesis), whilst the unwanted transitory vessels normally disappear. The simplest explanation of the pathogenesis of the commoner vascular anomalies seen in the skin and other tissues, such as the commoner strawberry marks, is that it represents a developmental flaw in which certain transitory and possibly surplus endothelial lined vessels or cords persist, which should normally disappear. However, there are differences between the vascular elements composing the lesion reflected in the enzymatic activity of the endothelial lining of the lesion, which may be important functionally.

Lymphatics may develop in two ways; most arise as outgrowths from venous endothelium, others arise from mesenchymal spaces which, early in development, join together to form continuous lymphatic channels and ultimately discharge their contents into the venous system; certain lymphangiomata show their venous origin by containing blood from time to time.

Whatever their primary origin, further development of lymph vessels takes place by budding from the walls of pre-existing lymphatics. It is probable that lymphangiomas arise in a similar fashion to haemangiomas by a process of neo-angiogenesis, although some may represent embryonic rests.

ANOMALIES PRINCIPALLY AFFECTING THE EPIDERMIS

I. Disorders of Keratinization

A. THE ICHTHYOTIC GROUP

Ichthyosis is the general term applied to a group of disorders characterized by dryness and scaliness, sometimes associated with a variable degree of warty overgrowth of the horny layer of the epidermis. A decrease in sebaceous and sweat-gland secretion may occur, and in the severest forms there may be complete absence of sweat glands and hair follicles. Amentia may be associated with ichthyosis as in the Sjögren–Larssen syndrome.

A rich nomenclature has grown up since Avicenna described the fish-scale disease as albarras nigra, and current synonyms include alligator skin disease, sauriasis, xerosis, xeroderma, congenital hyperkeratosis, collodion-skin and harlequin foetus.

Our knowledge of this group of disorders has been greatly advanced by the clinical and histological studies of Dr R. S. Wells, whose work on the population genetics of these maladies is a model of its kind. Stemming from this work, it is clear that there are at least four distinct clinico-genetic forms; five if that associated with atopy be regarded as a separate genetic entity, and it may reasonably be predicted that other distinct morbid entities will be brought to light, since it is already known that keratinization is controlled by several genes.

Ichthyosis Simplex

This is the commonest form and its severity may vary from mild dryness to considerable thickening of the epidermis often with diminished sweating. The scales in this form tend to be quadilateral or polygonal in shape, with free and up-turned edges, which give the skin a rough shagreen-like texture. The extensor surfaces of the limbs are more severely affected than the flexor surfaces with complete sparing of the major joints and the skin of the back is more severely involved than the ventral surface of the trunk. The palms and soles may be dry and wrinkled, while the skin of the hands and other exposed surfaces tends to chap and fissure in the winter months, but the face is only mildly affected as a rule. The condition is rarely evident before the sixth month after which the scaliness and dryness usually increase reaching a maximum between the second and sixth birthday.

Aetiology. The disorder is clearly gene-determined but until the precise molecular disturbance has been identified in each of the forms of ichthyosis, the mechanism whereby this is achieved will remain obscure; it is clear that a number of genes control normal keratinization and several of these display pleitropy.

Genetics. It has now been established by Wells that ichthyosis simplex is transmitted by a single autosomal gene, which behaves as a dominant, but the phenotypic expression of the gene may vary considerably not only in different families but also in the same sibship.

Prognosis. Ichthyosis simplex tends to be lifelong, with increasing severity of symptoms from birth to the second year, and even until the sixth in some families. There is little change until adolescence when the condition usually improves thanks to the increased sweating and greasiness of the skin consequent on the attainment of sexual maturity.

Differential Diagnosis. The characteristic diamond-shaped scales, forming a reticulate pattern over the extensor surfaces of the limbs and the back with sparing of the skin of the flexural surfaces of the major joints, serve to distinguish it from both the X-linked form and from that of the congenital ichthyosiform erythrodermas. The absence of the blistering rules out the bullous form of the latter.

Treatment. There is no specific remedy for ichthyosis in any of its clinico-genetic forms, but frequent bathing using the emollient unguentum emulsificans or ung. emulsificans aquosum as a substitute or supplement to soap is of the greatest value. Bathing helps to hydrate the desiccated skin of the ichthyotic, and the emollient preparation, by permeating the horny layer itself as well as forming a lipid film on the skin surface, helps to prevent or slow up desiccation of the horny layer by restricting evaporation of water molecules from the skin surface. The addition of common salt to the bath water or the overnight application of an ointment containing 5 per cent sodium chloride in emulsifying ointment also helps to rehydrate the over-dried horny layer by increasing the water binding capacity of the polar groups in the keratin molecules. Higher concentrations of the salt (10–25 per cent) may be used in order to assist in the removal of thickened hyperkeratotic horn in the severest cases. There is no place for thyroid treatment in any of the forms of ichthyosis, although it may be specific in dealing with the xeroderma (dry skin) which occurs with hypothyroidism, including cretinism.

Vitamin A in high dosage has only a limited place in the management of ichthyosis simplex, in contrast with other forms, where good results may be obtained in some patients.

X-linked Ichthyosis (sex-linked ichthyosis)
This form is restricted to males, and differs in several important clinical features from ichthyosis simplex. It manifests itself at birth and tends to increase in severity throughout childhood and adolescence. The flexural surfaces of the major joints are involved while the thickened scaly skin is often pigmented at certain sites, thus the schoolboy is often wrongly accused of not washing his neck because of this pigmentary change.

Aetiology. The disorder is also gene-determined, but the precise step in the biosynthesis of keratin which is at fault remains to be identified.

Genetics. Wells has shown that the gene is not only borne on the X chromosome but through linkage studies with Race and Sanger, he has shown that this is close to the X(g) blood group locus.

Differential Diagnosis. Involvement of the joint flexures and progressive severity throughout childhood distinguishes the X-linked form from simplex; absence of erythroderma and blistering serves to distinguish it from the ichthyosiform erythrodermas.

Treatment. Routine measures as for simplex are always helpful and may suffice in mild or moderately severe cases. Intensive high dosage of vitamin A (250,000 international units to 1,000,000 units daily for 10–14 days depending upon the age of the patient) given in one or more courses with intervals of 4 weeks between courses are sometimes very effective in dealing with the ichthyosis. However, it should be borne in mind that in these dosages the vitamin is toxic and may cause acute internal hydrocephalus, skin irritation, erythema and exfoliation (probably resulting from acute lysosomal damage), limb pains and cessation of growth. Hepatomegaly, *per se*, is not necessarily a sign of vitamin A intoxication, because large quantities of the vitamin may be stored, harmlessly in liver cells—not unlike that of the polar bear.

B. THE LOCALIZED OR REGIONAL KERATODERMAS

The Keratoses Palmo-Plantares
These are a group of disorders, with a regular mode of inheritance for each type in the group, in which the hyperkeratotic changes affect the palms and soles and occasionally other regions as well. In rarer in-

stances, other structures including the teeth may be involved in the dysplastic process.

Keratoderma plantaris et palmaris or Tylosis
This is by far the commonest form met with in clinical practice and may become manifest soon after birth. There is characteristic thickening of the plantar and volar skin, which may be reddened to begin with, but later assumes a yellow colour as the skin thickens and fissures begin to appear. All degrees of severity, from mild parchment-like thickening to extensive hyperkeratosis, are met with and familial cases closely resemble each other.

Aetiology. Most cases result from the action of a single gene which clearly affects keratinization of skin devoid of sebaceous glands and hair follicles.

Genetics. Keratoderma palmo-plantaris is inherited as a simple autosomal dominant.

Prognosis. The disorder tends to get progressively worse and may incapacitate the patient or severely restrict his choice of occupation.

Treatment. Vitamin A in appropriate dosage, combined with saline ointment and emollients for washing, all have their place in treatment.

Keratoderma Palmo-plantaris striata
Differs from the foregoing in the tendency for the hyperkeratotic lesions to form strands or islands on the palms and soles. There may also be patches of ichthyosis on the extensor surface of the limbs, with leukoplakia-like changes in the buccal mucosa. The nails are sometimes grossly thickened. The disorder is fully developed during the first decade.

Genetics. The disorder shows a simple dominant inheritance, but sporadic cases have been recorded.

Differential Diagnosis. The disorder resembles pachyonychia congenita in many respects, but differs in its evolution, absence of keratosis pilaris and blistering.

Keratoderma Palmo-plantaris Papulosa
Rarely met with before puberty.

Keratoderma Palmo-plantaris (Transgrediens) Greither).
This is an inherited disorder, transmitted by a dominant gene which is characterized by symmetrical yellow to black thickening of the palms

and soles. Separated from the normal skin by a narrow livid zone. Later the forearm and dorsum of the feet begin to become irritated and slight hyperkeratosis appears on the affected areas. Hyperhidrosis is frequent, involvement of the palms may be sufficient to interfere with manual work.

Keratoderma Palmo-plantaris Hereditaria Transgrediens (Mal de Meleda)
Similar to the foregoing, but rarely manifests at birth. Typically appears between the sixth month and second year. The internal malleoli and extensor surfaces of the knees and elbows and occasionally the dorsum of the hands may be affected. The disorder is inherited as an autosomal recessive. It gets its name from an island in Dalmatia, where inbreeding has led to a relatively high incidence of the malady.

Treatment of both consists in warm baths using ung. emulsificans and the use of 15–25 per cent sodium chloride in vaseline applied every night before washing.

Keratoderma Palmo-plantaris with Periodontosis (Papillon–Lefevre Syndrome)
This is a very rare variety which appears to be due to a single autosomal recessive gene. The hyperkeratosis appears on the soles during the first year of life and may be associated with hyperhidrosis; later, as is often the case in this group of disorders, the palms assume the characteristic parchment-like thickening. The milk teeth are lost through periodontal disease, and the same fate is shared by the permanent teeth as a rule, so that they are nearly all lost before adult life. The gingival anomaly may be due to increased collagenase activity. No effective treatment is known for this dental condition but treatment along the lines suggested above will help the keratoderma.

Keratosis Pilaris
This is an extremely common minor abnormality in which cornified material forms at the pilo-sebaceous orifices, giving a peculiar nutmeg-grater-like appearance and feel to the affected skin. The extensor and lateral aspects of the thighs and upper arms are the sites of election for the eruption, but any part of the body may be involved. The horny plug, composed of keratin and sebum, may occasionally prevent the lanugo hair from reaching the surface and as a result the hair coils up inside the affected follicle. It is often present at birth in a mild form and is usually most prominent during adolescence. Keratosis pilaris is met with in

several conditions in which keratinization is disturbed and is a prominent feature of vitamin A deficiency.

Aetiology. The frequent familial occurrence points to an autosomal dominant gene in a large number of cases, but environmental factors play an important part.

Pathology. There is a hyperkeratosis of the mouth of the hair follicles and coiled-up lanugo hairs are present in some, as in scurvy.

Genetics. The condition appears to be inherited as a simple dominant in most cases.

Prognosis. The condition is benign and is often most marked during adolescence, improving with the attainment of sexual maturity, as with many of the milder ichthyotic conditions.

Treatment. Frequent warm baths, using an emollient preparation such as ung. emulsificans as a soap substitute is usually effective in milder cases. Keratolytics sometimes help.

Pityriasis Rubra Pilaris
Pityriasis rubra pilaris is a rare hereditary disorder of the skin which shows a familial incidence in a majority of cases. It is characterized by the appearance of nutmeg-grater-like follicular hyperkeratosis especially on the dorsa of the hands and fingers, the extensor surfaces of the forearms and wrists, the anterior fold of the axillae and the elbows and knees, often with horny plugs. The skin of the face becomes thickened, reddened and scaly. The disease first appears in childhood and may be present at birth, when it is often confused with other erythrodermic or ichthyotic disorders. It is transmitted by an autosomal dominant gene, but penetrance and expressivity is very variable. Vitamin A in high dosage is sometimes very effective in controlling the disorder.

Porokeratosis of Mibelli
The disorder, which may appear in early infancy and principally affects males, begins with one or more small raised papules which slowly enlarge peripherally and undergo atrophy at the centre, so as to produce a circinate or ovoid lesion with a sharply raised border, resembling a stitched seam, and a smooth atrophic centre. Neighbouring lesions, which also arise from single papules, may join together to produce polycyclic lesions. Lesions are usually found on both surfaces of the hands and feet, the face, scalp and sides of the neck. The mucosae may be involved.

Pathology. There is a well-marked hyperkeratosis especially round sweat ducts and hair follicles. Horny plugs block the sweat ducts.

Genetics. The disorder seems to be inherited as a simple dominant with partial limitation to males.

Prognosis. The disorder tends to be progressive and lifelong, epitheliomatous changes have been recorded.

Treatment. None is of any avail, local excision does not stop the process.

Epidermodysplasia Verruciformis

Epidermodysplasia verruciformis is a very rare dermatosis in which the lesions may be present at birth and which is of some importance because squamous cell epithelioma may eventually develop in some of them. It begins with the appearance of small oval or polygonal papules with grey or greasy scales anywhere on the skin surface; ultimately the whole body may be covered by the lesions. The aetiology has been much disputed, and treatment is unsatisfactory.

Keratosis Follicularis (Darier's Disease)

Darier's disease is a fairly rare inherited congenital disorder which manifests itself by the appearance of pinhead papules covered by a dry horny crust, with more or less extensive involvement of the skin surface. The gene rarely manifests itself in infancy.

Genetics. The disorder is inherited as a simple dominant with irregular transmission in both sexes.

Treatment. Vitamin A sometimes helps, but many patients are not benefited by any form of treatment.

Congenital Ectodermal Dysplasia

Congenital ectodermal dysplasia is the name given to certain rare hereditary disorders, in which there is partial failure of the epidermis and its appendages to develop. Two main types are recognized: one, the so-called anhidrotic type, is associated with complete absence of the sweat glands and often of the sebaceous glands as well; in the second type, some sweat glands, as well as sebaceous glands, are present, so that it is referred to as the hidrotic type.

The most severe cases of the dominant form occur only in males, and such patients present with the following signs: small stature, poor physique, dental anomalies ranging from deficiency to total absence of teeth. The teeth when present are hypoplastic and conical in shape resembling those of a shark, the sweat, sebaceous and mammary glands are absent, the nails show dystrophic changes, the hair is deficient and there may be alopecia of the scalp, eyebrows and eyelashes. Secondary bony changes lead to depression of the nose, hypoplasia of the jaws and the lips tend to be protruding and everted. All except the dental defects, and those associated with them, may be present at birth. The mucosae may exhibit atrophic changes and tear secretion may be impaired. Patients with this condition who lack sweat glands tolerate heat badly.

In the milder form several of the signs may be lacking or minimal, and females as well as males may be affected.

Aetiology. This is a genetic disorder in which the gene exerts its effect during the third month of intra-uterine life when the development of the epidermal appendages—hair, follicles, sweat glands and nails—is in active progress; other tissues and organs may be affected at the same time.

Genetics. The genetics of the malady is of considerable interest. Two types of inheritance are known. A sex-linked recessive type and another with milder defects due to a dominant mutant gene.

Prognosis. Life is not shortened by the disease, but precautions may have to be taken to prevent heatstroke in warmer weather. Occupational choice by the patients is limited to the less strenuous jobs.

Treatment. None is available. Dentures will be necessary, wigs may have to be worn. Dry skin can be managed along the lines mentioned for ichthyosis.

II. Epidermal Anomalies associated with Blistering

There are several congenital disorders which are characterized by the production of blisters in the skin and sometimes in the mucous membranes as well; of these the most important is epidermolysis bullosa, but bullous forms of Darier's disease, Brocq's congenital ichthyosiform erythroderma, ichthyosis foetalis and keratoderma palmo-plantaris and urticaria pigmentosa also occur.

The Epidermolysis Bullosa Group

These disorders form a group in which blisters appear at or soon after birth and then involve the mucous membrane as well. The advent of the electron microscope has greatly increased our knowledge and understanding of these distressing maladies. Studies with it have not only clearly demonstrated the site and mode of production of the primary defect in each form, but at the same time these findings lend powerful support to the concept that each variant results from the mutation of a single gene and that more than one locus must be concerned.

Epidermolysis Bullosa Simplex

The lesions in this form of epidermolysis are strictly limited to the skin, never arise spontaneously, but always follow mild mechanical injury, unlikely to produce blistering in normal skin, and the blisters heal without scarring. The mucosae never blister, and there is no deformity or loss of nails or hair, and the dentition is completely normal. Blistering is more likely to be provoked during the warmer months of the year, indeed chilling the skin will inhibit experimental blistering.

Aetiology. All cases are gene-determined and despite reports to the contrary 'acquired' cases must be looked upon as misdiagnosed.

Genetics. The disorder is transmitted as a simple Mendelian autosomal dominant, the gene is fully penetrant and this is usually completely expressed.

Pathology. Ultrastructural studies show that the lesion is produced as the result of an exaggeration of the response of the epidermal cells in the normal individual to minor mechanical injury. This is revealed by the electron microscope as perinuclear oedema, which is completely reversible in the normal skin, whereas the oedema spreads throughout the cytoplasm of the injured epidermal cell in this form of epidermolysis, leading to the disintegration of the tonofibrils, mitochondria and other organelles until the cell is completely disorganized. The basement membrane at the dermoepidermal junction appears to be normal and remains intact.

Prognosis. Excellent with respect to life; sufferers learn to live with their disability from an early age. All of the disorders in this group tend to improve during adult life, and those with the Herlitz variant are often blister-free by the second or third year, should they survive.

Epidermolysis Bullosa Localized to the Soles

(Cockayne's recurrent bullous eruption of the feet, 'genetic hot-foot'.)

This variant, which is a distinct clinico-genetic entity, is transmitted as a simple autosomal dominant and is characterized by the strict limitation of blistering to the soles of the feet and the warmer months of the year.

Prednisone in small doses may tide the patient over bad spells due to weather or working conditions.

Epidermolysis Bullosa Dystrophica (Dominant)
This form may be clinically indistinguishable from the recessively transmitted mild dystrophic form. Blistering in these patients occurs on the mucous membranes as well as the skin, the nails may be shed or become dystrophic, scarring and milia formation are also features of this and indeed all the dystrophic variants. Blisters lie deep in the skin and contain blood, indicating that the dermis is involved.

Genetics. The disorder is transmitted as an autosomal dominant. The gene appears to be fully penetrant.

Pathology. The lesion has been shown by electron microscopy to lie in the collagenous tissue of the dermis in each of the dystrophic variants, tending to extend deeper in the more severe forms and to be restricted to the uppermost part of the papillary layer in the milder forms, whether dominant or recessive. The basement membrane and epidermis remain intact and appear to be normal, but become detached as a result of the accumulation of blister fluid. Involvement of the dermis often leads to permanent scarring, as well as loss of hair and nails. Dental defects are also due to the involvement of collagenous tissue.

Prognosis. Good as to life; scarring is mild, as a rule and the disorder often 'burns out'.

Treatment. Prevention of sepsis and treatment with steroids in the more severe cases.

Epidermolysis Bullosa Dystrophica Mitis
(Milder variant of dystrophic epidermolysis transmitted as an autosomal recessive.)

Almost identical with the dominantly inherited variant, but tending to be more severe, with deeper involvement of the dermis.

Epidermolysis Bullosa Dystrophica Gravis
In this variant the pathological defect extends deeper into the dermis; dysphagia may interfere with nutrition; hyperkeratosis on palms and soles may replace bullae in the older child and adolescent. The trait is transmitted as an autosomal recessive.

Treatment. Steroids help to ameliorate the disease and by alleviating the dysphagia encourage normal growth and development.

Epidermolysis Bullosa Dystrophic Gravior
This is the severest variant of the dystrophic form of the disease, life is threatened throughout the greater part of infancy, growth is stunted because of severe dysphagia and in some children the fusion of detached bands of pharyngeal or oesophageal epithelium have demanded the use of an oesophageal bougie. Colonic transplant and gastrostomy have been required. However, prednisone or similar steroids given in *adequate* dosage, i.e. sufficient to control blistering, will not only prevent or relieve dysphagia, but prevent the crippling syndactyly which may proceed to total loss of the prehensile function of the hands.

Epidermolysis Bullosa Letalis (Herlitz)
This variant was so named by Herlitz because few survived beyond the neonatal period. The defect is located in the basement membrane itself, and results in failure of the epidermis and dermis to adhere to each other, though both appear to be normal in all respects. Scarring, nail dystrophy and the like are rarely met with in this form, as is to be expected in a disorder limited to the basement membrane. Prednisone is life-saving, when given early, and in sufficient dose to control fresh blistering (upwards of 120 mg daily may be needed to achieve this initially). Furthermore, treatment is rarely required after the first year in those who survive, because the blistering soon becomes trivial. There is still a relatively high mortality because of sepsis and it may be necessary to treat the infant in a germ-free insulator.

OTHER CAUSES OF BLISTERING

Bullous Congenital Ichthyosiform Erythroderma
This disorder was first recognized by Brocq, who clearly distinguished the two varieties of congenital ichthyosiform erythroderma—the dry form (already described above) and the bullous form which is much rarer, and can be recognized by four chief features.

(1) The skin lesions are always evident at birth.

(2) The first symptoms are blisters which sometimes appear on normal skin, but more often on areas of erythroderma. The blisters are flat, superficial and heal rapidly without scarring.

(3) The whole skin may become involved in the erythrodermic process after several weeks and months, hyperkeratosis may begin to appear,

especially at certain sites such as the wrists, the anterior axillary folds, the lower abdomen and the leg.

(4) The verrucous hyperkeratoses are more friable and greasy than those seen in non-bullous ichthyosiform erythroderma. Fatal cases are met with in early infancy.

Aetiology. The disorder is gene-determined.

Genetics. The gene concerned is transmitted as a simple Mendelian autosomal dominant, penetrance appears to be complete and the expressivity is not very variable.

Pathology. The epidermis shows degenerative changes with acanthosis and dyskeratosis and vacuolation of the prickle cells, whose nuclei are often swollen. Clefts appear in the granular layer and blisters tend to form in the superficial portion of the epidermis.

Differential Diagnosis. From epidermolysis bullosa dystrophica, porphyria.

Prognosis. Some cases are fatal, death occurring within a few days or weeks of birth. The blistering becomes less severe as the child gets older, though the ichthyosis generally becomes more pronounced.

Treatment. As for the dry form, but corticosteroids should be tried in the severe cases.

Keratosis Follicularis Bullosa (Bullous Form of Darier's Disease)
The bullous form of Darier's disease is extremely rare, but is of some importance because it is likely to lead to early death of the affected infant and has been likened, in this respect, to harlequin foetus. It is characterized by the presence of a large number of blisters at birth, which is followed by the appearance progressively at the classical sites (forehead, flexures, scalp, palms and soles) of the typical greasy scaling lesions of Darier's disease. The disorder is inherited as an autosomal dominant but the expressivity of the gene is very varied.

Treatment. Unsatisfactory, but some patients respond well to high-dosage vitamin A therapy.

III. Neuroectodermal Anomalies

Pigmented Naevi and Allied Conditions

There has been some confusion in the dermatological literature about the use of the word naevus. Some American authors would restrict it to the common pigmented mole or melanocytic naevus and its congeners, whereas with most British authors the word is used for many benign tumours of the skin, both of ectodermal and mesodermal origin.

The English word mole, derived from Anglo-Saxon mal, meaning a skin blemish, is usually limited to pigmented (melanocytic) naevi, with or without hair, and has no temporal implications. Darier offers a more satisfactory definition of naevi as 'difformites circonscrites de la peau, d'origine embryonnaire ou évolutive, survenant à un age quel-conque et évoluant avec une grande lenteur', and it is in this sense that the word will be used here. The word 'hamartoma' introduced by Albrecht in 1906 to designate tumour-like, non-neoplastic malformations of tissues with abnormal 'Gerwerbsmischung', has not come into general use, although histopathologists find it valuable.

Naevi are extraordinarily common. All races appear to be equally liable, although for obvious reasons the pigmented, which is by far the commonest lesion, will be recognized most often in light-skinned subjects. They occur in all regions of the skin, but are more frequent at certain sites than others.

Classification of Naevi

It will be seen from the foregoing that a satisfactory logical classification is a difficult task, particularly if an attempt is made to group together the histopathological and clinical findings and reconcile them with the pathogenesis and the observed mode of inheritance. However, naevi may be classified.

A. Group of pigmented naevi originating from the pigment-producing cells derived from the neural crest.

(1) Simple pigmented naevus or mole; (2) cellular naevus or naevus molle; (3) naevus pilosus or hairy mole; (4) blue naevus; (5) amelanotic naevus; (6) naevus of Ota; and (7) Sutton's naevus.

B. Group of naevi arising from cells derived from the surface ectoderm of the embryo.

(1) Naevus verrucosus, or warty naevus, including naevus unis lateralis, ichthyosis hystrix, linear naevus and the like; (2) comedo naevus; (3) sebaceous naevus; (4) naevus syringocystadenomatosus papilliferous (syringocystadenoma); (5) woolly hair naevus (naevus

ulotrichus capilliti); (6) sweat gland naevus; (7) familial sebocystomatosis.

C. Naevi originating from or associated with hamartomatous derivatives of the neural crest.

(1) von Recklinghausen's disease (neurofibromatosis); (2) tuberose sclerosis (Bourneville's disease).

Preliminary Embryological and Epigenetic Considerations of Naevi and Pigmentary Anomalies

It will be recalled that the ectoderm produces three main organs or organ systems. The surface ectoderm gives rise to the epidermis and its derivatives, whilst the mid-dorsal ectoderm produces the central nervous system by forming a long thick-walled tube, from which the anterior motor nerve roots sprout in series. The posterior sensory roots and their ganglia arise from the neural crest, a mass of ectodermal tissue which just misses incorporation into the neural tube as it closes. The neural crest also gives rise to the sympathetic ganglia, the melanocytes wherever they are found in the body except the eye (but see below), the Schwann cells of the peripheral nerves and several mesenchymal structures including the leptomeninges and odontoblasts. It is this neural crest material which is important histogenetically in any discussion of the naevus cell; many, if not all, of the elements found in von Recklinghausen's disease (neurofibromatosis) derive their origin from the neural crest and it is known that cells from this source play a very important role in the pigmentary metabolism of the body—both of melanin and carotenoids (vitamin A). It is likely that a special phenylalanine or tyrosine metabolism is peculiar to the neural crest and there is evidence that phenylalanine itself, at least in urodeles, can induce pigment production not only in neural crest derivatives but in ventral ectoderm. It is of interest, too, in view of the occurrence of hypopigmentation and achromotrichia in phenylketonuria, that phenyl-lactic acid, when substituted for phenylalanine in the tissue culture experiments, although permitting the differentiation of other derivatives, effectively prevented pigment production.

The embryonic origin of the pigment cells in the eye has not yet been established with certainty but it seems likely that some at least arise from homologues of the pia mater, itself a derivative of the neural crest. The differences in embryonic origin of the intra-ocular melanocytes and those elsewhere in the body may well be reflected in such phenomena as the marked radiosensitivity of melanocarcinomas of the iris and ocular conjunctiva, the rarity of intra-ocular vitiligo and the earlier (pre-adolescent) occurrence of melanoma inside the eye. The association of naevi with neoplastic melanosis of the meninges demonstrates the link between cutaneous and meningeal melanocytes. The pigmented epithelium of the retina never gives rise to melanocancers, neither do the melanocytes of the hair follicle.

The neural tube is of importance in the development of skeletal elements (vertebrae and cranium) which surround the central nervous system and any failure in neurulation will have important consequences. It is not without interest that most of the common major malformations are due to failures of closure, separation or skeletal investment of the neural tube. Those which are associated with cutaneous anomalies include spina bifida occulta and the centro-facial neuro-dysraphic lentiginosis of Touraine.

Pigmented Naevi

Pigmented naevi or moles are present at birth in about 3 per cent of white infants but in 15 per cent of Negroes, and increase in number fairly rapidly during infancy and childhood. The lesions at birth should present no diagnostic difficulty, but when they are particularly plentiful other conditions should be looked for. The distribution of moles varies somewhat, but they tend to be least numerous on the extremities and commonest on the head and neck. Malignant change is extremely rare before adolescence but infants have been born with metastases from a maternal melanocarcinoma.

Aetiology. It is now virtually beyond dispute that the benign melanoma or mole is a hamartomatous derivative of the neural crest; it is developmental rather than a genetic defect as a rule, but their universal occurrence in all races is perplexing, especially as such lesions are extremely rare in lower forms, the grey mare being a notable exception.

Genetics. Little is known about the genetics of these lesions, except Turner's syndrome, the recently recognized cardiomyopathic lentiginosis and certain patients with neurofibromatosis.

Histopathology. The typical naevus cell is oval with a homogeneous cytoplasm and a large, pale vesicular nucleus. The cells tend to be arranged in cords or columns, in intradermal lesions, and are surrounded by bundles of collagen. Melanin is often present as fine granules in the cytoplasm. The naevus cell tends to become more spindle-shaped the deeper it lies in the corium. The majority of naevi in children are of the so-called junctional type in which the naevus cells appear to be dropping off the epidermis into the dermis; during adolescence most naevi become separated from the epidermis. Junctional activity after childhood denotes potential malignancy, and tends to be retained at certain sites including the hands, feet and external genitalia.

Diagnosis. In early life the characteristic brownish macule is unmistakable and cannot be confused with any other lesions. Freckles (ephelides) appear only after exposure to the sun.

Prognosis. The overwhelming majority of pigmented naevi remain quite innocent, but junctional naevi, and those situated at sites liable to repeated injury, may undergo malignant transformation during adolescence or later in life.

Treatment. No treatment is required as a rule, but careful excision is necessary when considered to be appropriate.

Naevus Molle or Cellular Naevus

The soft or cellular naevus is a fairly common lesion which is palpable as well as visible, and represents a stage in the life-history of the pigmented naevus. The pathology differs in no way, neither does its management.

The Hairy Mole

Hairy moles, with or without pigment, are also fairly common lesions in older children and adults and should present no diagnostic difficulties. They are characterized histologically by the presence of hair follicles in association with the naevus cells and rarely undergo carcinomatous change. Occasionally they may be very large and occupy the so-called bathing-drawers area where extensive pigmentation may be seen: such lesions are often associated with overgrowth of lanugo hair. Malignant change is fortunately rare *but should be borne in mind.* The treatment of these cases presents considerable difficulties and extensive plastic surgery will often be necessary. It is important to distinguish such lesions from the hypertrichosis seen in association with occult spina bifida in the lumbosacral region—so-called faun's tail or satyr's tail, but the strictly central siting over the vertebral column should prevent confusion.

The Blue Naevus

The blue naevus is a collection of naevus cells situated deep in the dermis, and because of its colour it may be mistaken for an angioma. Histologically the naevus cells are spindle-shaped and tend to form

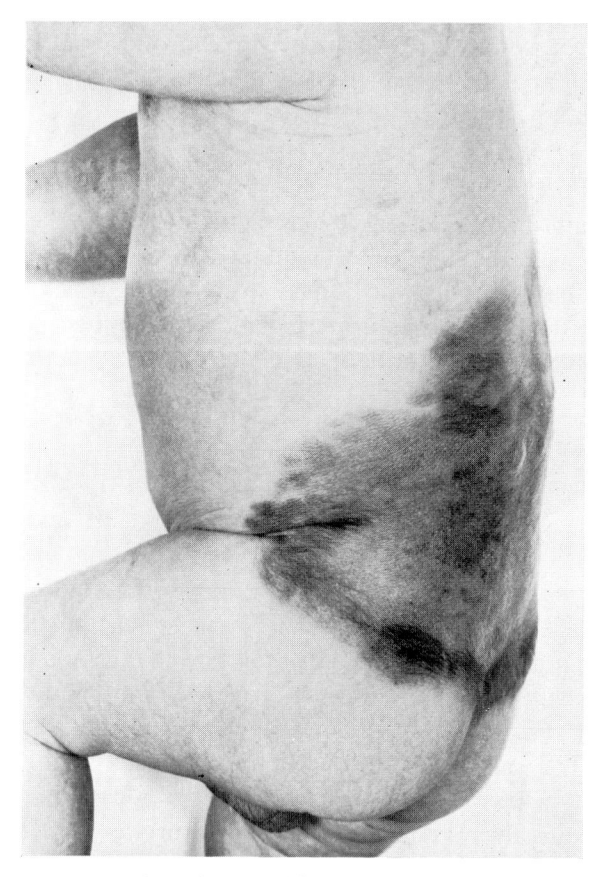

FIG. 9.1. Pigmented hairy naevus of back.

irregular bundles in the lower half of the corium. It is usually quite benign but may require excision for cosmetic reasons.

Amelanotic Naevus

These naevi differ in no way from the pigmented lesions except that they lack pigment; occasionally they may be larger and cerebriform, in which case plastic surgery is indicated. Lack of pigment is no guarantee against malignant change, albinos have succumbed from amelanotic melanocarcinoma. Discrete, widely distributed amelanotic naevi may be present at birth in tuberose sclerosis.

The Naevus of Ota
The naevus of Ota is an extensive blue naevus usually situated on the face and often involving the conjunctiva and other ocular structures. Histology is that of a blue naevus or Mongolian spot. Melanocarcinoma may develop later in life.

Sutton's Naevus
This is an unmistakable lesion, less rare than is supposed, characterized by a central pigmented naevus surrounded by a depigmented halo. It is possible that these lesions secrete a substance which inhibits the tyrosinase system of neighbouring melanocytes; vitiligo may make its first appearance round a mole.

Epithelial and Allied Naevi

Epithelial naevi are derived from surface ectoderm and receive no contribution from the neural crest. They therefore contain no melanocytes and *ipso facto* cannot undergo transformation into melanocarcinoma. They are nearly always congenital or appear soon after birth and may occur at any site. They show a very wide variation in size, shape and colour, with multiple lesions as a rule. They often present a linear or ribbon-like configuration running longitudinally along a limb or in a zosteriform fashion around the trunk, nearly always ending abruptly at the midline. The lesions are usually warty or become so, but may remain smooth and are always devoid of hair. The warty excrescences may be considerable and the affected skin as a result may resemble that of a porcupine or hedgehog. The celebrated Lambert family exhibited this bizarre appearance. Mucosal lesions have been recorded. Nails and hair may show changes as well.

Aetiology. Unknown.

Genetics. Further studies are urgently needed of this group of disorders.

Pathology. There is an enormous overgrowth of the papillae with thinning of the prickle cell layer and gross hyperkeratosis.

Differential Diagnosis. Linear naevi are usually unmistakable but extensive ichthyosis hystrix may be difficult to distinguish at birth. Acanthosis nigricans may closely resemble linear naevi.

Prognosis. The lesions are usually harmless.

Treatment. Small lesions may be locally destroyed; extensive lesions will need careful plastic surgery, many are best left alone.

Naevus Syringocystadenomatous Papilliferus (Syringocystadenoma)
Syringocystadenoma is another rare naevoid anomaly in which there are isolated or confluent small papular lesions of a pinkish hue. Some of the papules may be umbilicated and translucent so that they resemble molluscum contagiosum. Histologically there is dilatation and cyst formation of the sweat ducts; naevus cells abound in the corium and may encroach into the dilated sweat ducts. Excision is the only treatment.

Naevus Ulotrichus Capilliti (Woolly hair naevus)
This is a rare naevoid lesion in which an area of the scalp produces woolly hair amongst otherwise straight hair. No treatment is required.

Familial Sebocystomatosis (Hereditary sebaceous cysts)
This is an unusual familial disorder in which sebaceous cysts may be found anywhere on the skin, in one or more members of the same family. The lesions contain an odourless, greasy material which has a composition different from sebum and body fat; they rarely give rise to any symptoms but are unsightly. Smaller lesions can be destroyed with diathermy and larger ones should be excised for cosmetic reasons. The condition may be localized to the scrotum.

Neurofibromatosis (von Recklinghausen's Disease)
Neurofibromatosis is a slowly progressive, familial disorder, the manifestations of which tend to increase as the patient grows older. It is characterized by pigmentary changes in the skin, in which sessile or mobile nodular tumours may occur, and tumours of the nerves. Lesions may occur elsewhere, especially in the skeleton, eyes and the viscera. The lesions may be slight and trivial or so extensive as to produce gross deformity with gigantism or elephantiasis of the limb or part affected. Lesions may be present at birth, and are sometimes quite extensive then, but the manifestations of the disorder in infancy and childhood are usually mild and inconspicuous. Epilepsy is sometimes a feature of the

disorder, when lesions are present in the brain. Small, pea-sized tumours in the skin or nerve trunks may appear and increase slowly in size and number during childhood, but adolescence is the epoch in which the disease becomes conspicuously manifest. Extensive plexiform neuromas which may be present at birth are rare, but disfiguring, leading to a grotesque appearance, especially when the face or a limb is involved. Tumours of the cranial nerves, especially the auditory nerve, are very common, leading to deafness in older patients, but lesions of the optic, trigeminal and vagus nerves are more common in childhood. Retinal lesions, consisting of whitish plaques (phakomata) may occur and the skeletal lesions sometimes lead to spontaneous fractures, through erosion of the bone, or gross hypertrophy leading to local gigantism. *Formes frustes* are frequent, especially in other members of a family known to have the disease, and an undue tendency towards 'freckling', often zosteriform in various regions of the body, is seen in some patients. A diffuse bronzing of the skin has also been reported. It is not a rare malady and many of the milder cases are never recognized as such.

Aetiology. The heredo-familial nature of the disorder points to a gene-controlled dysplastic process as the cause. The pleiotropic effect of the gene must be exerted fairly early in embryonic life in view of the associated defects in tissues of mesodermal origin and the widespread lesions in the skin and nervous system. However, the genotype as a whole must play a very big role in influencing the clinical manifestations of the disorder, and thus account for the relatively high incidence of *formes frustes*.

Pathology. The disorder, a classical hamartomatous one, is characterized primarily by overgrowth of nerve-sheath structures, but other tissues often participate in the dysplasia. Histologically the affected nerves show diffuse enlargements here and there; occasionally the whole nerve trunk may be involved. The enlargement is due to overgrowth of endoneural and perineural tissues, without involvement of the nerve fibres themselves. The tumours are rarely well-demarcated but intermingle closely with the surrounding tissues. Whorls and bundles of collagenous tissue abound in the lesion. Malignant neoplastic changes may occur in the lesions at any age and the histological picture may be very varied. Some resemble fibrosarcomas, others exhibit myxomatous change and a few are highly pleomorphic.

Genetics. The disorder is almost certainly inherited as a dominant, but its very rare occurrence among siblings born to normal parents points towards the possibility that there may be a recessive form of the disease. A single autosomal gene with incomplete penetrance will account for nearly all cases and discrepancies between the expected and reported incidence of the disease in affected families can be explained by the inconspicuous nature of the lesions in some members of the sibship or the death of the bearer at or before birth. More severe forms of the disease produce disfigurement which militates against marriage and reduces fertility, yet the disease is relatively common in the population suggesting a high mutation rate for the gene.

Differential Diagnosis. The diagnosis is simple when the classical triad of signs is present—*café-au-lait* patches, sessile or pedunculated tumours of the skin and tumours of the nerves. Some difficulty in diagnosis may arise in certain disorders characterized by abnormal pigmentation in early infancy. Urticaria pigmentosa should not be confused with neurofibromatosis, as the lesions in the latter never urticate.

Complications and Associated Disorders. Malignant change in one of the lesions which is fortunately almost unknown in early life, is the most serious complication to be feared. Gigantism of the limb or gross overgrowth of a part, which may necessitate extensive and sometimes mutilatory surgery, is a rare manifestation of the disorder. Imbecility and epilepsy are met with in a small number of cases.

Prognosis. The condition is lifelong and lesions rarely regress once they have appeared. There is a tendency for puberty and pregnancy to lead to an increase in the number and size of the lesions.

Treatment. The majority of lesions should be left alone; surgical intervention may be necessary, even in early life, when extensive plexiform neuromas are present, or in cases with gigantism.

Tuberose Sclerosis and its Cutaneous Manifestations (*Leucodermic Macules, Adenoma Sebaceum, Angiofibromatosis*)

Tuberose sclerosis is the name given to an inheritable neurocutaneous disorder, because of the resemblance of the lesions in the brain to plant tubers, especially the potato. White (non-pigmented) macules are present on the skin, usually widely dispersed, and varying in size from that of a millet seed or lentil to large band-like patches of leucoderma often with a zosteriform distribution. As these leucodermic macules or patches may indeed be the only expression of the gene in an individual from a family with another grossly affected member, it is important that they should be looked for, especially when genetic counsel is sought. They are easy to see, with the aid of Wood's light, even in the lightest of untanned skin, but *the whole of the skin surface should be carefully inspected* if their presence is to be detected.

The first neurological manifestation of the disease may also appear as early as the first day of life, but more usually during early infancy, with seizures, often of the so-called salaam or infantile spasms type, with characteristic changes in the E.E.G. There may be a severe degree of mental handicap.

The lesions of so-called adenoma sebaceum may first appear round the mouth and nose of the infant towards the end of the first year as pin-head pink macules. These may be evanescent to begin with but soon become raised and feel hard to touch. The term adenoma sebaceum should be abandoned because few lesions, in fact, include sebaceous gland, the essential changes being confined to the vessels and connective tissue. *Café-au-lait* patches are present in nearly half of these patients. Late skin changes include sub- and periungual fibromas, and the so-called shagreen patches which usually elect the lumbosacral region or forehead as their favoured site. Phakomata may be present in one or both eyes and congenital anomalies such as polycystic kidneys, cardiovascular anomalies and skeletal disorders may form part of the clinical picture.

Histology. Histology of the white macule reveals that melanocytes are present but little or no pigment is produced; adenoma sebaceum shows variable angiofibromatosis; shagreen patch and fibromata show increased collagen tissue.

Genetics. The disorder is transmitted by an autosomal gene, with a very high spontaneous mutation rate, so that new genes are continuously replacing those lost through early death or reproductive failure, in the population concerned. The gene is found in all races and the bearer of the gene may be identified at birth in upwards of 60 per cent of cases.

IV. Anomalies of Pigmentation

The colour of the newborn baby's skin is largely a racial character and as such depends upon the genetic contribution received from each parent, particularly the genes which control the production of melanin. Four other pigments—haemoglobin, oxyhaemoglobin, carotene and melanoid—also contribute to skin colour, but this is masked by melanin in the darker-skinned races. The white colour of lighter-hued races results from the scattering and reflection of incident light by the colloidally dispersed protein and other aggregates in epidermal cells, after the light has traversed the translucent horny layers. The characteristic

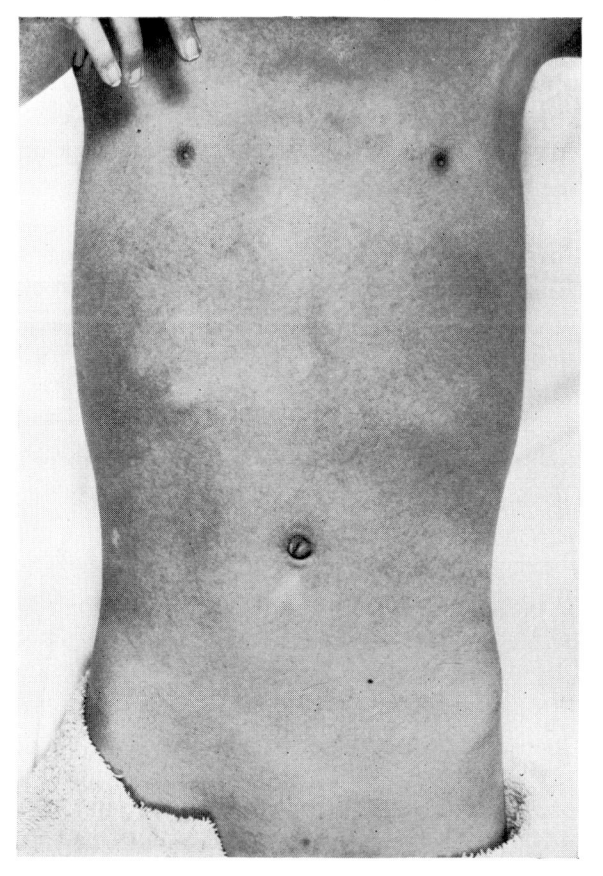

FIG. 9.2. Albinotic macules—when present at birth are pathognomonic of tuberose sclerosis ('epiloia').

pinkish hue of the newborn white infant is a consequence of the thinness of the epidermis at this age, which permits the colour of the blood in the venules of the upper cutis to be seen. Melanin is formed from tyrosine (and possibly tryptophane) by enzyme oxidation to 5·6 indole quinone which is then polymerized to yield the pigment. However, the final stages are not well understood. Melanin is normally only produced by melanocytes or the pigmented epithelium of the retina, but the photoreceptive cells of the latter may begin to synthesize melanin as in retinitis pigmentosa. The production of melanin is influenced by many factors both within the melanocyte itself and in the adjacent tissues, and by more remote factors such as the melanocyte-stimulating hormone of the pituitary, by oestrogens and androgens and possibly by the melatonin secreted by the pineal body. The colour of melanin varies from yellow to black, and may depend upon the degree of polymerization. Tyndall scattering of the shorter waves of the incident light gives a blue colour to melanin granules when they are situated deep in the skin, well demonstrated by the Mongolian blue spots, and in certain pigmented naevi situated in the lower scrotum. It is of some phylogenetic interest that certain of the lower Primates, such as the baboons and drills, display brilliant Tyndall blues on their cheeks and buttocks, produced by melanin deposits in the dermis of the regions affected. Multiple Mongolian spots in coloured babies may be mistaken for bruises, and I have seen more than one such child who was thought to be a 'battered baby' because of this.

Differences in the colour of the skin of different races of mankind are a purely physiological and not a morphological character, depending upon the rate at which melanin is synthesized rather than the number, size or gross structure of the melanocytes themselves. The number of melanocytes varies from region to region in the same individual, being most plentiful on the face, but there are no racial differences in this respect. Red-heads tend to produce different melanin granules from those found in dark or blond-haired people.

Albinism
Albinism is the most striking of the congenital anomalies affecting the pigmentation of the skin, especially when it occurs in members of a dark-skinned race. For this reason it has long been recognized and we find good descriptions in the works of classical writers such as Pliny. Albinism is known to be an inheritable defect involving the melanocytes which results in a failure to produce melanin. It is a disorder which is met with in all of the vertebrate phyla and has been described in many different species. It should be emphasized, however, that complete or total failure to produce any melanin at every site in the body has yet to be met with in man, or for that matter among carnivores although it is common among rodents. Complete or perfect albinism will be familiar

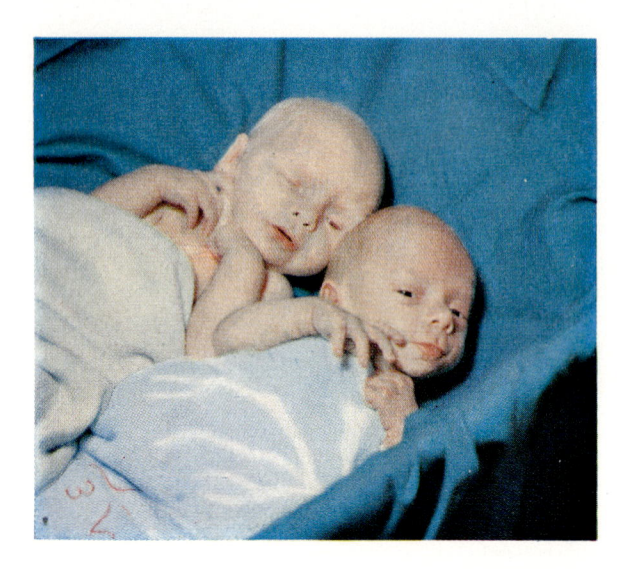

FIG. 9.3. Albinism — 2 children showing an albino baby with a normal fair-haired child of the same age.

to those who have any experience of the common laboratory animals.

Albinism may be classified on a clinico-genetic basis, according to the extent to which the melanocyte system is involved and the mode of inheritance of the anomaly.

The anomaly is easy to recognize and is conspicuous from birth, the skin being milky white in affected areas in all races whilst hair colour may range from faint yellowish-white in a European to a yellowish-brown in a Negro infant. There is usually some pigment present in the irides of albinos of all races, though the amount may be insufficient in some cases to screen off the colour of the blood in the vessels. Eye colour is usually a light grey at birth and the pupil may appear red. Hair and eyes often darken as the child grows older and there is also a tendency for the skin to produce a little pigment with increasing age. The fundus oculi of the albino has usually a bright orange-red hue with a characteristically uniform pink macula.

Histopathology. The skin of the albino is normal in every respect except for absence of evidence of tyrosinase activity. Melanocytes are normal in number and distribution: they fail to produce melanin or produce only minute amounts of the pigment.

Prognosis. There is a tendency for pigmentation to increase with age, especially in the eyes, so that visual handicap may decrease as the patient grows older. The anomaly does not shorten life, but there is an increased risk of skin cancer in the unpigmented exposed skin, especially in those living in the tropics.

Treatment. None is known. Piebalds may stain skin with dihydroxyacetone and obtain an acceptable cosmetic result on exposed surfaces of the body.

Acanthosis Nigricans
Acanthosis nigricans is an anomaly which may be present at birth or appear later in life and is characterized by hyperpigmentation, papillomatosis and warty hyperplasia of the affected skin or mucous membrane. Two varieties of the disorder are recognized: (a) benign, which is usually met with in early life; and (b) malignant, which is much more frequent in adults, although it may be seen in very young patients, and is associated with a cancer. The disease presents with very marked hyperpigmentation of the skin of the axillae, neck, genitalia and limb flexures, with occasional involvement of the soles and palms as well as the buccal and other mucous membranes. The skin in the affected areas is thickened,

convoluted and is usually hyperkeratotic. The hyperpigmentation may be present at birth or appear later in the juvenile or benign form of the disorder.

Aetiology. The aetiology remains unknown. Familial cases have been described.

Histopathology. The microscopic appearances are virtually diagnostic since the marked hyperkeratosis, acanthosis and hyperpigmentation with pronounced papillomatosis can hardly be confused with any other condition.

Differential Diagnosis. Certain pigmented naevoid conditions may be difficult to distinguish, especially naevus unius lateralis. It is probable that abortive forms of the disease are frequently overlooked or misdiagnosed, particularly if naevi are present, as they often are, to complicate the picture of a rare disease.

Prognosis. The benign or juvenile form of the disorder nearly always disappears. The associated neoplasm determines the prognosis in the other forms.

Treatment. Overnight application of an ointment containing 10–20% sodium chloride in appropriate base and washing with ung. emulsificans as soap gives good cosmetic results.

Incontinentia Pigmenti (Bloch–Sylberger Anomaly)
Incontinentia pigmenti is a rare disorder, often familial, which principally affects girls and is characterized by the appearance of vesicles and small bullae at or soon after birth. Papules soon replace the vesicles and may persist for a variable period; pigmentation becomes evident as the papular elements fade and this may persist for many months or years. Several episodes of vesiculation and blistering may occur in the early months of life; in some babies the greater part of the skin surface may be involved. The distribution of the lesions is such that very striking and bizarre patterns may be displayed by the residual pigment, producing an extraordinary array of brownish or bluish streaks, whorls and curlicues. The initial lesions are nearly always blisters or vesicles, and these are almost always followed by lichenoid or warty papules which leave the characteristic brown staining as they fade. Other congenital malformations may be present affecting the eye and the central nervous system, where polymicrogyria and hypoplasia of the pyramid have been reported.

Aetiology. The disorder is almost certainly the result of gene mutation.

Genetics. The very marked preponderance of girls with the disorder, and the frequency with which the trait is transmitted from mother to daughter, points to a dominant sex-linked mode of transmission. I have seen it in three generations of a kindred—grandmother, mother and two girls, while Cockayne reports its occurrence in a father and both of his children. The rarity of males with the disorder has led to the speculation that the gene is lethal for male conceptuses, death occurring early in

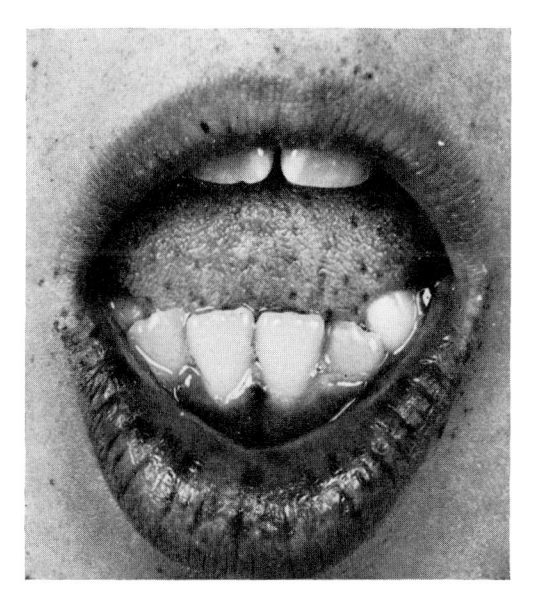

FIG. 9.4. Polyposis—buccal mucosa.

embryonic life. The suggestion that males with the disorder may have Kleinfelter's syndrome with XXY karyotype is not borne out by cytogenetic studies in the three male cases known to me.

Treatment. Blistering in the newborn can be controlled by systemic steroids.

Pigmentation of the Skin and Mucosae with Intestinal Polyposis
(*Peutz–Jeghers Syndrome*)
Pigmentation of the skin and mucosae associated with multiple polyps in the intestine is a very rare anomaly which may be present at birth. There are small patches of pigmentation and black spots to be seen on the buccal mucosa, particularly on the lips, cheeks, palate and gums. The skin round the mouth and nose may bear black spots resembling

freckles, and pigmentation may be seen on the tips of the fingers and toes. Polyps are usually found in the small intestine, but the whole intestinal tract may be involved.

Aetiology and Genetics. An autosomal dominant gene is thought to be responsible.

Histopathology. The skin lesions show proliferation of the rete pegs with acanthosis and spongiosis with increased amounts of pigment in the basal layer. The pigment is melanin.

Prognosis. The skin and mucosal pigmentation gives rise to no symptoms, but the intestinal polyps may produce intussusception at any time.

Xeroderma Pigmentosum

Xeroderma pigmentosum is a rare congenital disorder characterized by hyperpigmentation, atrophy and telangiectasia, sooner or later followed by malignant change and ulceration in the affected skin. Excessive freckling and extreme susceptibility to sunburn on exposed surfaces is an early feature of the disorder, which usually reveals itself during the infant's first spring or summer, when he is badly burned by the sun. Telangiectases and freckling begin to appear on the ears, nose and around the mouth with areas of atrophy in the pigmented patches. Later, warty and scaly lesions begin to appear in the affected regions of the exposed skin; eventually malignant changes supervene in the skin, lips and conjunctivae. Photophobia is a feature in older children. Dark-skinned races are not immune from the disease, which has been reported in Africans, a surprising occurrence until the true pathogenesis was demonstrated.

Aetiology. It is now known that the disorder results from an inherited defect in the mechanism for the repair of damage to the D.N.A. of the cells. It is clear, too, from studies of this repair mechanism in cultured fibroblasts from the skin of patients and their parents, that there are at least two genetically and biologically distinct conditions, in the milder of which the defect appears to be restricted to the skin, whereas other tissues may be involved in the more serious variant leading to oligophrenia, short stature and other anomalies.

Genetics. The disorder is transmitted by an autosomal recessive gene; consanguinity is common, but not invariable; the genes concerned are quite independent in each variant. Heterozygotes may exhibit a tendency to profuse freckling without the other changes.

Differential Diagnosis. Confusion with any other malady is unlikely in the typical case. Symmetrical freckling of the axillae or zosteriform freckling may be met with in neurofibromatosis, but there is never telangiectasia or squamous cell metaplasia.

Prognosis. Untreated cases will develop multiple cancers on the exposed skin and death will follow at an early age from metastases.

Treatment. Uvistat light screen and Uvistat lipstick should be applied before going out of doors at all times. Flurouracil is of some value.

V. Metabolic Disorders

Congenital Porphyria
Congenital porphyria is the rarest of the porphyrias, and is a heredofamilial disorder transmitted as an autosomal recessive trait, though there appears to be an excess of boys in reported cases. It is characterized by striking photosensitivity, due to presence of abnormal porphyrins in the lysosomal membranes of cells in the upper dermis. Blistering is produced after exposure to sunlight, through release of acid hydrolases and other enzymes following damage to the lysosome. Hypertrichosis is another feature. Teeth may be discoloured when they appear.

Treatment. Consists in avoidance of direct sunlight and protection through use of a light screen such as Uvistat.

Hypercholesterolemic Xanthomatosis
This condition is one of the more striking of the lipoidoses in its cutaneous manifestations. The lesions are present at birth and tend to increase in size and number as the patient grows older. In the majority of cases, however, the disorder does not manifest itself until well on in adult life. The essential features of the condition are the presence of numerous yellowish nodules at certain characteristic sites—over the bony prominences, the eyelids and buttocks, but lesions may be found anywhere—and a very great increase in the level of the blood cholesterol. Pigmentation of the skin around the eyelids is a feature in a number of cases. The error in cholesterol metabolism is inheritable and appears to be transmitted as a dominant, but relatively few patients develop xanthomata.

Histopathology. The presence of the characteristic Touton foam cells, containing cholesterol, xanthophylls and carotenoids, with more or less fibrosis in the tumours, is pathognomonic.

Genetics. The metabolic error is inherited as an autosomal dominant, but the inheritance of the tendency to produce tumours is irregular.

Aetiology and Pathogenesis. The exact nature of the metabolic defect has not yet been determined.

Differential Diagnosis. Juvenile xanthoma can be differentiated by normal blood cholesterol level and negative family history.

Prognosis. There is a high incidence of vascular disease, especially coronary and cerebral thrombosis, in this disorder and the expectation of life is appreciably reduced. Gall stones and biliary obstruction producing jaundice may occur but diabetes appears to be rare.

Treatment. Restriction of intake of animal fats sometimes helps to lower the blood cholesterol level and may retard the growth and appearance of tumours.

Juvenile Xanthoma (Naevo-xantho-endothelioma)
This condition is characterized by the appearance at birth, or in the first weeks of life, of one or more yellowish papules or nodules on the skin, commonly on the head and neck, but the lesions may occur elsewhere. Plaques are sometimes formed, and when they occur on the scalp the resulting alopecia may be permanent. The condition is not a true lipidosis and bears no relationship to Hand–Schuller–Christian disease, to hypercholesterolaemic xanthomatosis or any similar metabolic disorder.

Aetiology. Unknown.

Genetics. In contrast with the lipidosis there is no evidence of familial incidence of this disease.

Histopathology. The microscopic appearances are characteristic with numerous endothelial cells arranged in whorls, a number of round cells in groups and a few plasma cells. A few of the endothelial cells, however, may resemble foam cells and fat is present in the majority.

Differential Diagnosis. Urticaria pigmentosa is distinguished by characteristic histology and by the fact that the lesions tend to urticate when rubbed. Other forms of xanthomatosis can be distinguished by the family history, blood chemistry and the histology, in which foam cells are usually plentiful.

Progress. Invariably good. The lesions often disappear in early infancy and rarely persist beyond puberty. Scarring may occur in some of the lesions.

Treatment. None required in most cases, but for cosmetic reasons

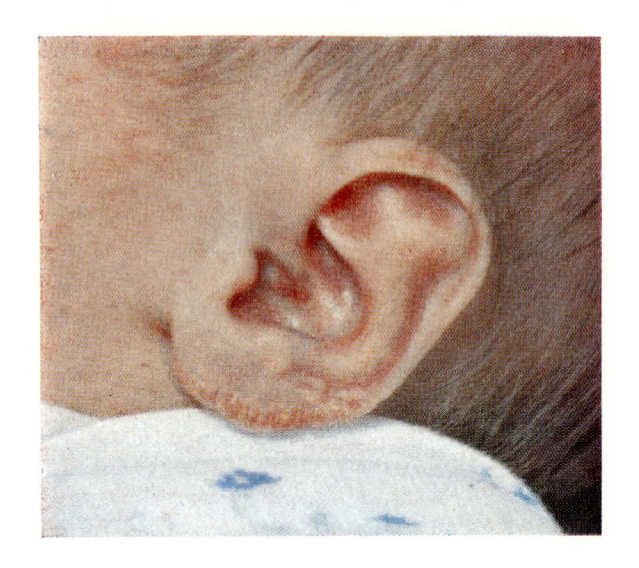

FIG. 9.5. Juvenile xanthoma.

scarred plaques, especially in scalp, may require excision and very occasionally grafting.

VI. URTICARIA PIGMENTOSA (MAST CELL DISEASE)

Urticaria pigmentosa is a relatively rare, sometimes congenital, anomaly in which collections of mast cells accumulate, usually in the skin but other tissues may also be involved. The condition is almost always benign but there exists a malignant form of the disorder, in which there is progressive systemic involvement of tissues as well as the skin, especially the lymph nodes, bones, liver, spleen and blood-forming tissues.

The juvenile type, which accounts for over 50 per cent of all cases, appears during the first 6 months of life but as many as 10 per cent of cases display lesions at birth. Both sexes are equally affected, despite earlier reports that it was commoner in males. Most reports concern patients of European origin or descent but the disorder also affects Negroes and often other racial groups. The cutaneous lesions usually include macules, papules and nodules but vesicles and bullae occur in about 10 per cent of infants affected. Telangiectases may occasionally be present. Typically, the disease presents as pigmented macules which urticate (weal) when rubbed. The macules increase in number during the first 6–18 months or so and tend to become nodular with a somewhat yellowish hue, although the colour is very variable. The mouth may be involved. Solitary lesions occur or there may be dozens, with the trunk as the site of election for the early lesions. The face, scalp, palms and soles are not involved until late and the eruption is usually sparse at these sites.

The recognition, in recent years, of the possibility of systemic involvement has yielded an increasing number of cases with infiltration of the lymph nodes, bones, liver and spleen as well as changes in the blood picture associated with the disease. Various types of anaemia and abnormalities in bleeding and coagulation of the blood have been recognized and mast cell leukaemia has been reported.

Aetiology. The cause is unknown; it has been regarded as a naevoid disorder by some, others consider it to be genetic, but familial cases are relatively few. It has been attributed to a defect in one of the enzymes concerned with mucopolysaccharide metabolism, but the tendency of the juvenile form to clear spontaneously, often before puberty, in contrast with the life-long duration of the adult form of the disease is perplexing. It is likely that the two types have different origins.

Genetics. A familial incidence of the disease has been observed on several occasions but there is insufficient evidence, as yet, to establish the probable mode of inheritance. 'Sporadic' cases far outnumber those in which more than one member of a family is affected though the

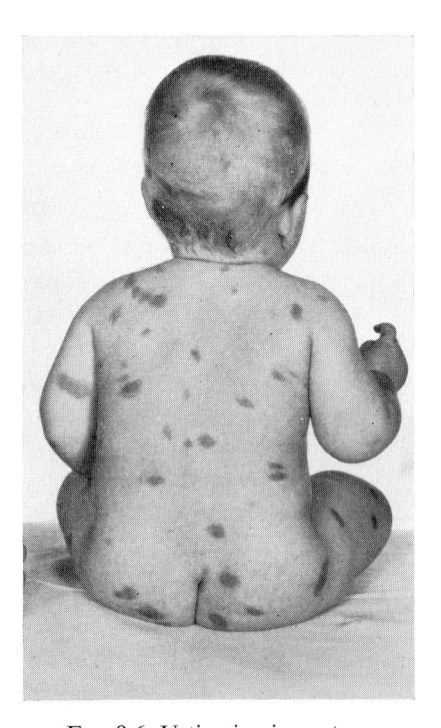

FIG. 9.6. Urticaria pigmentosa.

occurrence of the disorder in uni-ovular twins and in members of successive generations suggests that a gene may be responsible in some cases.

Histopathology. Apart from an increase in the number of melanocytes in the basal layer overlying the lesion in the dermis, little change is to be seen in the epidermis, unless vesicles are present. The basal cells may contain increased amounts of pigment. The characteristic mast cell accumulations are found in the upper and middle thirds of the dermis.

Differential Diagnosis. The congenital presence or early onset of the yellow or brownish lesions which produce weals on rubbing (Darier's sign) are unmistakable in the typical case. Certain types of xanthoma may be difficult to distinguish especially when the lesions are few in number, or even solitary, and the diagnosis can only be established after a biopsy specimen has been examined. Rarely, both cell types may be present in the same lesion.

Prognosis. The lesions nearly always disappear at or before puberty, usually without trace, but pigmented or atrophic scars may remain in a few cases. Spontaneous fractures may occur with extensive bone involvement and a progressive malignant course may be followed in the very rarest case.

Treatment. Most cases require no treatment but anti-pruritic remedies will be needed when itching is a troublesome feature, or excessive histamine release leads to collapse through transient hypotension. Blistering is usually confined to the early lesions, but exceptionally may persist until late in childhood, mild antiseptic applications will usually prevent sepsis.

VII. Vascular Anomalies Involving the Skin

Malformations and other anomalies involving the skin vessels are common, ranking second only to pigmented naevi in frequency. They may occur as solitary lesions or there may be a number of them. The anomaly is usually confined to the vascular and associated connective tissue elements of the skin, but sometimes other structures and tissues may be involved in the dysplastic process. Numerous so-called syndromes have been described with various permutations and combinations of vascular and other abnormalities which may be present in the same individual. Unfortunately, this has not always been to the advantage of our understanding of the disorders described, and a great deal of confusion has arisen because authors have failed to recognize that the alleged syndrome they describe is merely a variant of another, or that the association between the vascular lesions and other anomalies may be purely fortuitous, each having developed quite independently of the other. Some vascular anomalies, such as the strawberry mark (3 per cent of normal babies bear them), are so common that it is not surprising to find that they are present in the same individual with another, quite independent anomaly such as polydactyly. On the other hand, certain syndromes are truly such and we find that two or more anomalies 'run together' which is the literal meaning in Greek from which the word is

Y

derived. Good examples of such true syndromes include the Sturge–Kalischer–Weber (encaphalo-trigemino-angiomatosis), the Klippel–Trénaunay syndrome (telangiectatic hypertrophy of a limb) and that of Hippel and Lindau (angiomatosis of the retina and subtentorial meninges).

The vascular system, especially the minute vessels, is highly plastic during the development of the individual, both in order to accommodate for growth and for the the disappearance of transient structures such as the ductus arterious. Capillaries are capable of budding whenever the local inhibiting influence is removed, as in wound healing, and telangiectasia is not an uncommon feature of many skin disorders acquired during later life. Out-sprouting is a feature of capillary behaviour during growth and seems to occur as a result of the metabolic demands of the growing structures.

We have little understanding of the processes which lie behind the various congenital vascular anomalies met with in practice; their sporadic occurrence and the relative rarity of familial incidence point to epigenetic accidents rather than mutant genes as the causal factors: much has yet to be learned about these.

TELANGIECTASIA

Naevus arachneus (*spider naevus*)
This is an extremely common vascular lesion which may appear at any age and is sometimes present at birth. It is usually solitary but may be multiple with the face and hands as the sites of predilection; these lesions are less common on the upper trunk and very rare on the lower limbs. The appearance is unmistakable, resembling the arthropod whose name it bears. Treatment is simple: the lesion may be destroyed by diathermy. Multiple 'spiders' in older patients may be manifestations of liver disease or pregnancy, and they may appear with oestrogen therapy.

Hereditary Haemorrhagic Telangiectasis (*Osler–Rendu–Weber disease*)
The disorder is an inherited familial anomaly, affecting both sexes equally, and is characterized by the appearance of linear, punctate and/or spider angiomata on the face, buccal mucosa, lips, tongue, hands and elsewhere. The lesions may be present at birth, but more often they appear during childhood and adolescence and may not do so until much later in life. Involvement of visceral epithelial surfaces may lead to

haematuria, haematemesis, or haemoptysis. Frequent epistaxis is the common presenting symptom in childhood.

Genetics. The condition is transmitted as an autosomal dominant trait.

Progress and Treatment. The prognosis is usually good, but anaemia may result from repeated blood loss and transfusion may be an urgent lifesaving measure in certain severe cases.

Haemangiomas (Strawberry Marks)

Cavernous haemangiomas are the commonest vascular tumours met with in infancy and childhood but virtually all of these lesions are hamartomas and not true neoplasms. Haemangiomas may be classified as (1) capillary angioma or naevus flammeus, which appears as a flat or slightly raised vascular lesion, consisting of a plexus of dilated capillaries situated in the more superficial part of the dermis; (2) the cavernous haemangioma, a raised conspicuous lesion resembling a mulberry or strawberry; and (3) mixed lesions with involvement of deeper structures, including the muscle and at times the bone and often leading either to local gigantism or atrophy of the affected region.

Pathogenesis. Haemangiomas arise as a result of maldevelopment of angioblastic tissue, which for some reason has become sequestrated from the rest of the normally developing local vasculature. The *Anlage* of the angiomas is a bundle of solid endothelial cords derived from mesenchyme, some of which hollow out to acquire lumina and form capillaries. These capillaries may end blindly or they may sprout and anastomose; around some mesenchymal connective tissue cells multiply and differentiate so as to form the muscular and elastic coats of arteries or the corresponding structures in veins; the fate of any given vessel being normally determined by local circulatory hydrodynamics. The vessels comprising the vascular lesion may, however, differentiate irrespective of the needs of the tissue in which they find themselves, but many remain as larger or smaller endothelial lined spaces, giving to the lesion some of the properties of erectile tissues found in the penis or the nipple, well seen in the increase in prominence and turgidity of the lesion when the baby cries. The cavernous haemangiomata often have a single large afferent and efferent channel through which blood enters and leaves the lesion. It is important to realize that, although the angioma may increase in size as the infant gets older, it does not 'grow' in the sense that a cancer or a true neoplasm does. It should also be borne in mind that the vascular channels through which the blood flows in a cavernous haemangioma may have been laid down well before the infant's birth, but, for some reason at present not well understood, blood often does not enter until some time after birth and the gradual opening up and filling of the cavernous spaces during the subsequent weeks gives rise to the appearance of growth: in other words many cavernous haemangiomas are strictly congenital and are present at birth, but they may not be visible then because they are not yet filled with blood.

Nuchal Naevus Flammeus (Unna's Naevus)
This is probably the commonest of the vascular naevi and is situated on the nape of the neck where it is visible at birth. It has been estimated to occur in as many as 60 per cent of babies; it may disappear or decrease in size, and is usually of no cosmetic consequence.

Superficial Capillary Haemangiomas (Stork-bites)
These are often present at birth and usually involve one or more of the following sites: the forehead, especially the glabella, the eyelids, cheeks and temples on the face, but similar pale red areas may be found on the neck, abdomen and elsewhere. They invariably 'disappear' spontaneously, probably as a result of 'maturation' of the vessel, so that it is fully capable of responding to vasoactive stimuli.

Naevus Flammeus (Port Wine Stain)
Port wine stains of various sizes and shapes are not uncommon, and are always present at birth. They are usually flat, red or purplish macular lesions, but are sometimes slightly raised; very occasionally keratotic changes develop on the surface. Some capillary naevi are associated with vascular anomalies in tissues other than the skin: e.g. the meninges in the Sturge–Weber syndrome. It is unfortunate that such a high proportion of port wine stains occur on the face where they often produce conspicuous disfigurement with serious psychological disturbance in the sensitive or unstable patient. Young children may shun the company of their fellows when they become aware of their plight. The management and treatment of conspicuous port wine stains calls for much tact and sympathy on the practitioner's part, but excellent cosmetic disguise is now available, and children soon learn to apply the preparations very effectively.

Treatment. There is still no really satisfactory treatment for port wine

ABNORMALITIES OF THE SKIN 329

stains as there is no effective means of obliterating the dilated and atonic capillaries which make up the lesion and render it so conspicuous, without at the same time damaging the adjacent epidermis, so that scarring results; this scarring may be even more disfiguring than the untreated lesion, grafting too has limited value for the same reason.

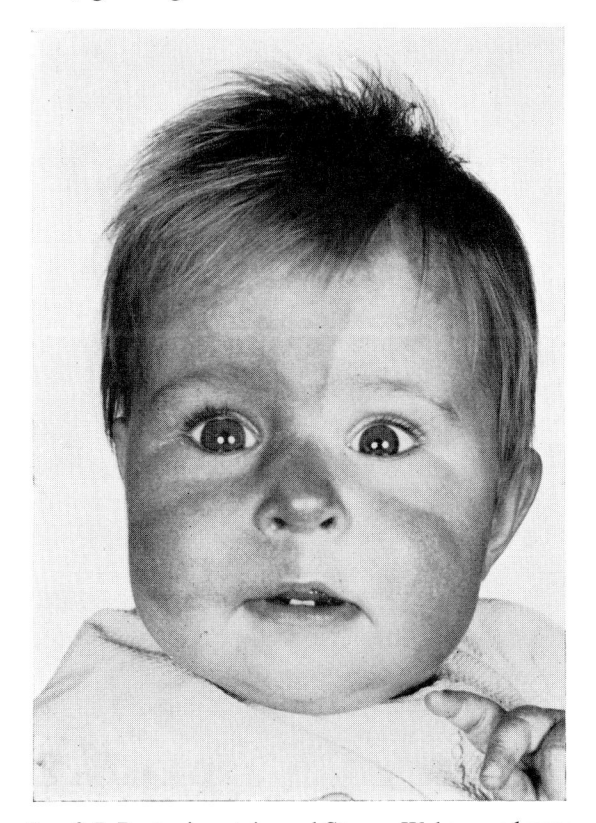

Fig. 9.7. Port wine stain and Sturge–Weber syndrome.

Dermabrasion by wire brush and sandpapers has been tried, and freezing the lesions with carbon dioxide snow or liquid nitrogen has occasionally produced some paling of the lesion without scarring, but the results are not very satisfactory. A variable degree of paling can be produced by repeated painting of the lesion with Thorium X 1,000–1,500 e.s.u. per ml in varnish. This radioactive decay product of radium has a half-life of 3–6 days and emits alpha particles which have low penetrating power but may reach the endothelium or surrounding tissue and produce an inflammatory reaction sufficient to obliterate the vessel. Promising results are being obtained from other radioactive isotopes such as ^{32}P (radiophosphorus) which may be impregnated into polythene or other plaques. Grenz rays have a certain favour in the United States; British experience is limited but competent radiotherapists do not consider them to have any advantage over other and more reliable forms of radiation therapy.

Most of the less extensive port wine stains can be successfully disguised by the application of an appropriately tinted cosmetic cream or powder. The practitioner should always encourage parents and child to disregard the lesion as far as possible and thus prevent the development of a neurosis about it. Young girls soon learn to use cosmetics, with excellent results.

Cavernous Haemangiomas (Strawberry Marks)
Cavernous haemangiomas or strawberry marks have been recognized since antiquity and are usually referred to by the laity as 'birth marks'. They were long referred to as *maculae maternae* or 'mother marks' and were attributed to the force of the 'Mother's Fancy' as Daniel Turner put it in his *De Morbis Cutaneis*, the first treatise in English devoted to skin disease. This belief has not yet died out and mothers sometimes link the lesion on baby's skin with an injury that they may have sustained during pregnancy, especially if it involved the same region: a frightening experience may also be blamed, and some mothers feel guilty at having brought a disfigured child into the world. Since nearly all of these lesions are likely to disappear spontaneously without leaving a trace, as was recognized by Bateman and Abernethy at the beginning of the last century, the parents' fears can usually be put to rest and emphatic assurance may be given as to the good prognosis and excellent cosmetic result which usually follows spontaneous involution of these haemangiomas.

Strawberry marks are solitary as a rule, but two or more may be present. They are not usually visible at birth but make their appearance soon after; beginning as a small red fleck, the lesion increases in size and becomes elevated. It reaches its maximum size between the fourth and sixth month, resembling in size, colour and shape a mulberry or cultivated strawberry. Relatively few of these exceed the size of a cultivated strawberry but occasionally the anomaly involves quite extensive areas and the whole surface of a limb or one side of the face and neck may be involved. Such cases are fortunately rare, but size alone is no bar to spontaneous involution; I have seen spontaneous involution occur in an extensive lesion involving the whole of the left leg, both buttocks, the lower abdomen and the upper part of the baby's right thigh; extensive facial lesions often involute very quickly.

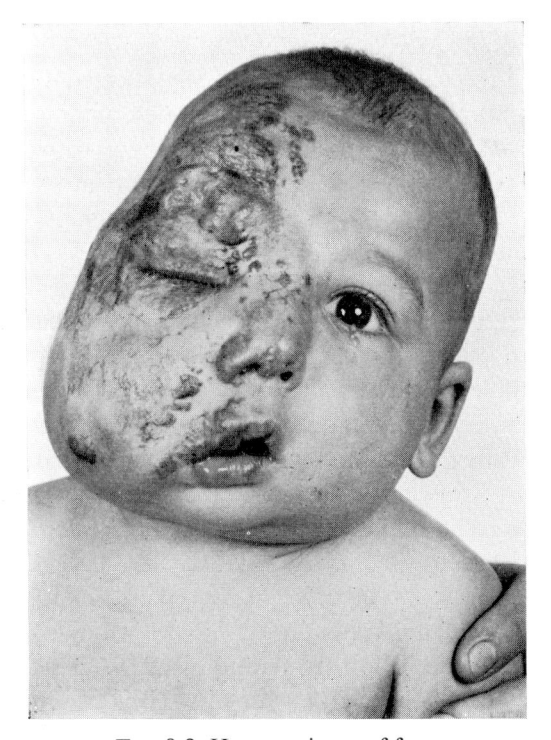

FIG. 9.8. Haemangioma of face.

The first sign of spontaneous involution is the paling of several pinhead areas on its surface. This paling corresponds with the closing down and complete disappearance of endothelial-lined blood spaces forming the lesion, which gradually becomes flatter and flabbier and eventually disappears entirely.

Natural History of Strawberry Marks. Girls are three times more likely to bear these lesions than boys, and the head and neck are the regions most affected. Cavernous haemangiomas have been found in every tissue and organ, except cartilage and cornea, but are more likely to be found in the skin than anywhere else.

Strawberry marks, one or more of which will be found in 3 per cent of all infants, may be present at birth, but more often make their appearance during the first 3 or 4 weeks of life. The maximum size is reached by the sixth month and thereafter the lesion remains stationary for a variable period before involution sets in. This occurs before the third birthday in approximately 60 per cent of the affected children, and of the remainder most will have lost their strawberry marks by their fifth birthday.

Aetiology. All races, it appears, are equally affected, but there is little evidence that mutant genes play any part in determining their origin. It has been suggested that there might be a connection between infection of the mother with Asian influenza during the first trimester of pregnancy and an increased incidence of cavernous haemangiomas has been observed in the offspring of such mothers.

Histopathology. The structure of these lesions varies somewhat, with endothelial-lined blood spaces predominating. Capillaries and small muscular coated vessels may also be present, but it is rare to find fully developed blood vessels, either venous or arterial. The lesion appears to be composed largely of immature vasoformative tissue to which their remarkable tendency to spontaneous involution may be due.

Complications. Strawberry naevi are liable to ulcerate, particularly extensive lesions and those situated in the napkin area or those involving moist mucosal surfaces such as the vulva or lips. Ulceration is far less frequent than might be expected, and is usually trivial, producing a small encrusted erosion with a marked propensity for healing. The appearance of such ulcers may speed up the involution of the angioma, but is undesirable because of the resultant scarring. A second type of ulceration is also met with, in which there is a more extensive and deeper erosion of the lesion; often leading to almost total destruction of the lesion and a correspondingly poor cosmetic result because of the large scar. Haemorrhage is a rare complication and is nearly always due to mechanical injury, but injudicious and unnecessary treatment by freezing with carbon dioxide snow or by electrocautery may also be followed by haemorrhage. Malignant change never occurs in strawberry marks and parents may need to be reassured on this, as there is a popular misconception that these lesions may turn into cancers; but cancer has followed treatment with radium and other sources of ionizing radiations.

Treatment. No treatment should be needed for the overwhelming majority of these lesions and they should be allowed to involve spontaneously. Infection and ulceration can be prevented by careful attention

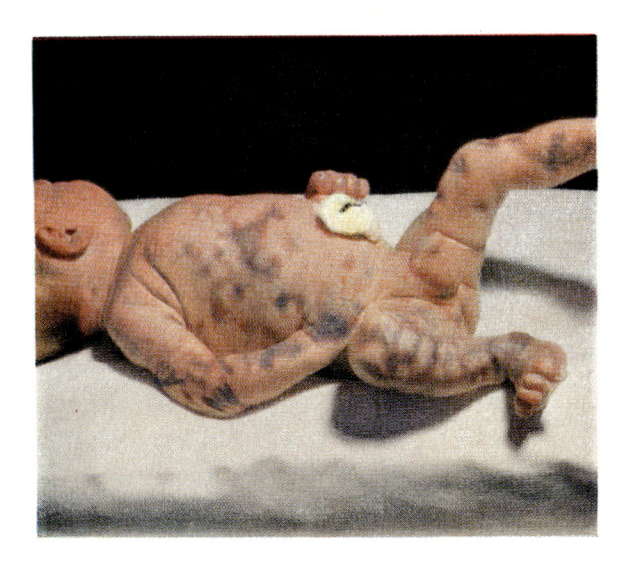

FIG. 9.9. Widespread haemangiomatosis with varicosities.

to lesions at sites where these are likely. Thus the prevention of chaffing and prompt treatment of any rash in the napkin area will render ulceration less likely: aureomycin cream or 'Tyroderm' is useful in preventing sepsis, but ulceration may proceed relentlessly until the lesion has been replaced by scar tissue in a certain number of cases. Haemorrhage, when it occurs merely requires compression and the catastrophic bleeds mentioned in older works are rarely seen nowadays. Radiotherapy is unsatisfactory because of the risk of radiodermatitis. Various methods of freezing have been tried but there is an inevitable risk of scarring when the lesion is of any size. The injection of sclerosing solutions has justifiably fallen into disuse; it is painful and often ineffective. The electrocautery almost invariably produces scarring and when misused on large lesions produces a brisk haemorrhage. There remains only one satisfactory method of dealing radically with strawberry marks; viz. careful surgical excision under general anaesthetic; it should be reserved for the more extensive lesions, when the help of a competent plastic surgeon should be sought, or the rare case where the mother is subjected to comment because of a very conspicuous lesion on her child's face and she is becoming psychologically disturbed by the situation.

It is important to inform parents (and health workers) about the natural history of these lesions and thus save mothers from unnecessary anxiety about the lesions themselves and also protect them from pressure by ill-informed relatives who are keen to 'get something done' to the lesion.

Syndromes Involving Strawberry Naevi

A number of syndromes have been recognized in which strawberry naevi occur in association with congenital anomalies of other structures. Of these, Maffucci's syndrome is the most striking, with multiple cavernous haemangiomas of skin, lips, bones and viscera and with prominent varices as well as enchondromata of many of the bones.

Cavernous haemangiomas may also be found in liver, spleen, kidneys, gut, endocrine glands, lungs, brain, etc; in short, in every structure which has vessels in it.

Lymphangiomas

Lymphangiomas are fortunately far less frequent than haemangiomas, as they are less likely to undergo spontaneous involution and are often difficult surgical problems. The cavernous variety is the commonest and is nearly always found on the head or neck. The tongue is not an uncommon site. A distinguishing feature of cutaneous lymphangiomas is the presence of numerous papules and vesicles produced by the dilated lymph channels. Most lesions are best left alone.

Mixed Angiomata
Mixed haemangiomatous and lymphangiomatous lesions are not rare, but their true nature may not be determined until a biopsy has been done.

ABNORMALITIES OF THE CONNECTIVE TISSUES AND DERMIS

Cutis Laxa Congenita (Generalized Elastosis)
Cutis laxa or dermatomegaly is a generalized disease affecting the elastic fibres throughout the body. The skin is enlarged and loose, and hangs in great folds, resembling the analogous condition met with in bloodhounds. The skin at birth is often abnormally wrinkled and gives the affected child a preternaturally aged look; the condition tends to worsen with advancing years.

Aetiology. The condition is known to result from the action of a mutant gene.

Genetics. That the disorder is inherited is now beyond doubt, but it is not clear whether it is transmitted as an incomplete autosomal dominant or as an autosomal recessive trait.

Histopathology. There is generalized reduction both in number and size of the elastic fibres in all tissues and organs.

Pathogenesis. It has been suggested that the lesions result from excess of circulating elastase over its inhibitor (pancreatic elastase inhibitor) which is diminished. Copper also acts as an elastase inhibitor and copper deficiency may present as cutis laxa in certain animals; serum copper has been found to be low in some cases and there is excess of the metal in the urine.

Differential Diagnosis. Cutis hyperelastica (Ehlers–Danlos syndrome) should present no difficulty as the hyperelasticity in Ehlers–Danlos syndrome can easily be demonstrated by picking up the skin which will then stand up in folds.

Complications. Because of the universal involvement of elastic tissue emphysema, aneurysms, cardiomegaly and intestinal diverticula may also be met.

Treatment. Mild cases require no treatment, but more severe cases will need the help of a skilled and experienced plastic surgeon.

Cutis Hyperelastica (Ehlers–Danlos Syndrome)

The Ehlers–Danlos syndrome is characterized by increased elasticity of the skin with gross hyperextensibility of the joints and an increased fragility of the blood vessels with consequent tendency to form haematoma after minor injury. More serious spontaneous haemorrhage occurs in certain variants.

Aetiology. The disorder is known to be a defect in mesenchyme which is gene controlled.

Genetics. Several independent clinico-genetic variants have now been recognized each due to a single mutant gene. Inheritance differs, some cases result from autosomal dominant gene, others show recessive transmission.

Histopathology. The collagenous tissue is reduced with atrophy of the collagen bundles, whereas the elastic tissue is normal or increased.

Differential Diagnosis. See cutis laxa, above.

Progress. Some forms improve with age—premature death from cerebral or other haemorrhage may occur.

Treatment. None is known—injury should be avoided.

Pseudoxanthoma Elasticum

Pseudoxanthoma elasticum is a rare mesodermal defect of genetic origin and occasional familial incidence in which flat, yellowish plaques begin to appear symmetrically in the skin of the flexures, sides of neck, upper and inner thighs and elsewhere. The elastic tissue in other organs, especially the vessels of the eye, brain, heart and gut are involved with consequent risk of serious haemorrhage. The association of skin and retinal lesions (angioid streaks) constitute the so-called Gronblad–Stradberg syndrome.

Aetiology. This is disputed but there does appear to be an alteration in the elastic tissue throughout the body, which shows an increased resistance to the enzyme elastase.

Genetics. The disorder is inherited as an autosomal recessive, or in some families as a dominant, suggesting that more than one gene is concerned and this may be reflected in the clinical picture and prognosis.

Histopathology. The affected areas of skin show circumscribed areas in which the elastic fibres are swollen and degenerate. There are no foam cells but calcium deposition has been observed.

Differential Diagnosis. The skin is never hyperelastic so that it can be distinguished from cutis hyperelastica, whilst the histological findings (absence of foam cells) serve to distinguish it from true xanthomatous conditions.

Prognosis. Usually benign, but in some cases with more extensive vascular and retinal involvement may develop aneurysm, hypertension, angina pectoris, retinal and other haemorrhages, leading to blindness or death in early adult life; in these patients it is likely that a different gene is involved controlling a more fundamental metabolic process.

Poikiloderma Congenitale
Poikiloderma congenitale is a very rare congenital abnormality, principally affecting girls, which begins with swelling and redness of the hands, feet, cheeks and buttocks, with later involvement of other regions. The redness is succeeded by irregular patches of brown pigmentation and crusts may appear over bony points later in childhood. Hair is sparse and may be lacking from eyebrows and elsewhere. Dental defects are usual. There is stunting of growth and the affected skin may undergo epitheliomatous change. Familial occurrence has been noted but the genetics of the disorder are not known. It has to be differentiated from Rothmund's syndrome and xeroderma pigmentosum.

Hereditary Oedema of Legs (*Milroy's Disease*)
There are two types of hereditary oedema of the lower limbs, one of which is congenital. In both types the swelling first appears in the foot and may progress until it reaches the ankle, knee or groin, where it ends abruptly at one or other of these joints. One or both legs may be affected. The swelling is firm with only the slightest pitting after prolonged pressure and there is no change in the colour of the skin in the affected limb.

Aetiology. The exact cause is unknown. There have been various theories in which congenital malformation of the lymphatics, venous or lymphatic obstruction, and arterial vasomotor defects have been invoked to account for the swelling. A disturbance in the development of the mesoderm of the leg is the most likely cause.

Genetics. The disorder is transmitted as an irregular dominant, but the gene shows variable expressivity. Sporadic cases may represent fresh mutations. The late or tardive type of Milroy's disease shows a similar mode of transmission.

Differential Diagnosis. Naevoid hemihypertrophy and congenital sclerodema will have to be differentiated. Symmetrical peripheral

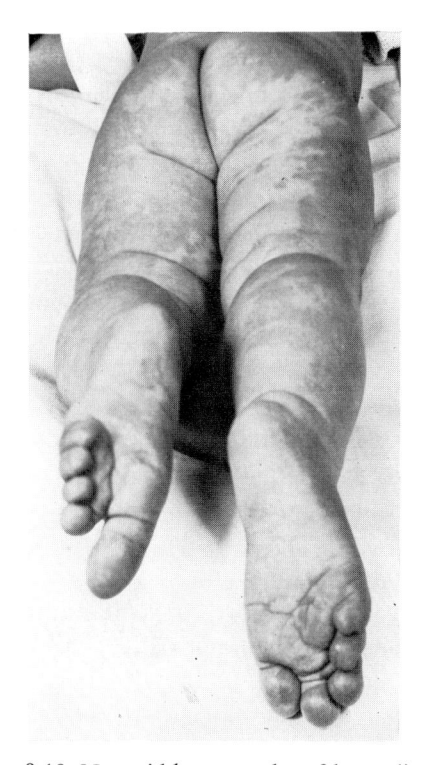

FIG. 9.10. Naevoid hypertrophy of lower limbs.

oedema of the limbs seen in Turner's syndrome affects upper as well as lower limbs.

Associated Conditions. Various other congenital abnormalities, including spina bifida, congenital heart disease, and neuropsychiatric disturbances, have been described in association with Milroy's disease.

Treatment
Bandaging of affected limb: corticosteroids may help.

Congenital Anomalies of the Nails

Congenital anomalies of the nails are not uncommon: they are sometimes found alone, but more often in association with one or more malformations of the epidermis and adnexa. However, care should be exercised before concluding that a given nail change is related to another cutaneous lesion merely because they occur together. Our knowledge of nail growth and the factors influencing it is still very meagre, since it has not, as yet, attracted the attention or interest that hair growth has for the biologist and the study of normal and pathological nail growth in man has largely been neglected by pathologist and dermatologist alike. It is not surprising, therefore, to find that a rich and seemingly erudite nomenclature has been accumulated to describe the anomalies and dystrophies which may affect the nails, a nomenclature unfortunately largely devoid of morphological or physiological foundation. It is probably true that in no other branch of dermatology is it more difficult to be certain whether a given nail change is the result of a disease process or merely a morphological variant. Many nail changes can be produced by more than one cause, thus clubbing may be a congenital familial character of no other significance or it may signify the presence of serious disease in the lungs, heart, or liver, and the practitioner should always bear this in mind.

Anonychia (Absence of Nails)
Total absence of the nails is a rare congenital anomaly and it may be associated with alopecia: one family has been reported in which anonychia was confined to the thumbs. Anonychia may be due to failure of the nail matrix to develop, to atrophy of the growing zone, or to overgrowth of the hyponychium (nail bed).

Nails may be lacking from one or more digits in dystrophic epidermolysis bullosa at birth, and nails are sometimes shed in congenital syphilis. However, in these disorders, the nails will usually regrow although there is a tendency in severe epidermolysis bullosa for the nails to be permanently lost.

Anonychia may form part of congenital ectodermal dysplasia.

There is no treatment.

Atrophy of the Nails
In congenital atrophy, the nails may show both atrophic and hyper-

trophic changes, as might be expected when disordered growth occurs in different parts of the nail matrix and hyponychium. The condition is often gene-controlled and families have been recorded in which the anomaly occurred in all the females: in another the transmission of the trait was principally through the females.

Congenital atrophy of the nails may occur in association with other anomalies such as congenital ectodermal defect, pachyonychia and alopecia.

Shedding of the Nails (Onychomadesis)
Spontaneous shedding of the nail plate which begins proximally and ultimately leads to loss of the nails is due to the gradual failure of the nail matrix to produce keratin. Familial incidence has been described.

Onychauxis (Thickening of Nails)
Congenital thickening of the nails due to overgrowth may occur as an isolated anomaly or in association with a number of congenital and hereditary disorders, including pachyonychia congenita, keratosis palmo-plantaris and Darier's disease.

Onychogryphosis of all Nails
Onychogryphosis affecting all of the nails is a very rare congenital anomaly inherited as a simple dominant. The more severely affected nails may have to be avulsed and the nail matrix destroyed.

Gigantism of Nails
Gigantism of the nails may occur as part of the gigantism seen in some cases of Von Recklinghausen's disease or in the gigantism of a digit seen in naevoid (haemangiectatic) hypertrophy of a limb (Klippel–Trénaunay syndrome).

Micronychia
Congenital micronychia is an anomaly which may affect one or many digits and is probably more common than reports in the literature would lead one to suspect. I have found it to affect the nail of the great toe more frequently than any other, except possibly the little toenail which in some families seems about to be lost. It may be part of the syndrome of congenital ectodermal dysplasia.

Racket Nail

Racket nail is an unusual anomaly which accompanies the so-called 'pouce en raquette' or short wide thumb, which itself is a hereditary condition transmitted as a simple Mendelian dominant. The anomaly is often unilateral and the contrast between the short wide nail on the affected thumb and that on the normal thumb is quite striking and conspicuous.

Nail Changes in Congenital Clubbing of Digits

Congenital familial clubbing is another anomaly which is probably of more frequent occurrence than the literature would lead one to suspect. It may affect one or two digits and should carefully be distinguished from acquired clubbing.

Koilonychia (Spoon-nails)

Koilonychia is another anomaly of the nail which may be congenital. The nails are thin and concave from side to side and only the fingers are affected as a rule, although severe koilonychia affecting the great toenails of several members of a family has been reported.

Supernumerary Nails and Polydactylia

Nails, usually small and atrophic, may occur on the tips of supernumerary digits, where the nail rudiment may resemble a wart.

Pterygium

Pterygium is the abnormal adhesion of the epidermis overlying the nail fold to the nail plate or the persistence of the eponychium after birth. It can easily be removed by cutting with scissors.

Leuconychia

Leuconychia may present in one of three forms: (1) punctuate, in which white spots are present in the nail plate; (2) striate, in which white bands are present; or (3) totalis, in which the whole nail plate is white. Leuconychia is due to imperfect keratinization. Mitchell (1953) failed to find any white spots in the newborn but by 3 months they were frequently found. Striate leuconychia may be analogous with vitiligo. Total leuconychia is often hereditary and is usually inherited as a simple dominant.

Pachyonychia Congenita

Marked thickening of the nails is seen as part of several congenital hereditary anomalies which include symmetrical keratoses of the hands and feet, buccal leukoplakia, follicular keratoses especially round the great joints, as well as corneal dyskeratosis often leading to blindness and alopecia. The disorders are transmitted by an autosomal dominant gene. The nails are thickened, opaque and longitudinally ridged as a result of the cornification anomaly in which horny cells are produced by the nail matrix, leading to a very characteristic wedge-shaped thickening of the nail plate. There is often an associated congenital alopecia and epidermal cysts have been found in one kindred.

Congenital Anomalies of the Hair

Anomalies of the hair are not uncommon and are usually present at birth or appear soon after, which should emphasize their genetic or developmental origin. The hair and nails are both adnexae of the epidermis and are therefore derived from the ectoderm. It is no surprise, therefore, to find that most serious hereditary skin maladies are associated with anomalies of the hair and nails, especially when the gene concerned exerts its effect before the stage of major organogenesis in embryonic development is passed. It is important, however, to bear in mind that later differentiation renders the hair follicle independent of the epidermis and that anomalies can arise which are limited to the hair alone.

A large number of congenital and inheritable anomalies of the hair have been reported in man, in striking contrast to the situation in the lower mammals, which exhibit relatively few hair anomalies. Most of the anomalies are very rare and have usually appeared in association with some other defect, an association which may be coincidental rather than aetiological, and calls for careful evaluation by the observer, if he is to avoid attributing a spurious relationship between the hair anomaly and other defects.

As elsewhere in the skin, the anomaly may vary considerably in severity. Thus hair loss may be total, due to failure of the hair follicle to develop or the follicle may produce poor quality hair which is fine and brittle; and then eventually fail to produce a hair of any kind, as in some cases of congenital hypotrichea.

Most attention has been paid to scalp hair because of its predominant cosmetic significance, but defects of the eyelashes and eyebrows are also important, and nearly always accompany the scalp hair anomalies.

Congenital Alopecia

Congenital alopecia may be either partial or complete. Absence of hair may be the only anomaly or the alopecia may be associated with other defects as in congenital ectodermal dysplasia, pachyonychia congenita, harlequin foetus, the more severe forms of ichthyosiform erythroderma and the like. Congenital absence of the hair is not at all rare and exhibits more than one type of inheritance; the trait may be transmitted as a sex-linked recessive limited to males, or as simple recessive. Dominant inheritance is a feature of congenital alopecia in pachyonychia congenita and congenital ectodermal defect.

Localized congenital alopecia may be found in linear naevi affecting the hairy scalp.

Associated defects include those of the teeth, absence of teeth, cataracts and other ocular changes, polydactyly, syndactyly, oligophrenia, sensory defects anhidrosis, as well as neuro-psychiatric disorders, all indicating a greater or lesser degree of disturbance of ectodermal development.

Hypotrichosis

Hypotrichosis is more common than total alopecia and is seen as an isolated anomaly or in association with the defects mentioned above. In this condition, the follicles produce hair of inferior quality and there is a tendency as the patient grows older for the follicle to cease producing hair altogether. Inheritance is similar to that for complete absence of the hair.

Hypertrichosis

Hypertrichosis, or overgrowth of the hair, usually on the limbs, is nearly always present at birth, but becomes longer and more conspicuous as the child grows older. Hypertrichosis may occur elsewhere and I have seen hypertrichosis of the vulva in a baby girl which was not associated with precocious puberty. Many pigmented naevi also exhibit hypertrichosis, some being quite extensive and covering the lower part of the trunk and thighs. Oligophrenia and hypertrichosis may be associated.

Universal hypertrichosis, in which the whole of the body, including the face and limbs, but sparing the palms and soles, becomes covered by a more or less downy silken coat, is a rare anomaly. Familial cases have been reported (Cockayne 1933). Extensive hypertrichosis of the face may occur and such subjects have later earned their living by appearing in circuses and travelling shows. The proprietary depilatories are very effective in dealing with hypertrichosis, even in the newborn, but overgrowth of hair in the external auditory meatus may require surgical excision of the meatal skin.

Monilethrix (Beaded Hair)
Monilethrix is a congenital anomaly, frequently hereditary, which is characterized by the presence of bead-like swellings alternating with atrophic constrictions in the hair. The hairs break off at these constrictions, producing alopecia. Keratosis pilaris is often present and another feature is the disorderly way in which the hair grows; the normal whorls are not formed and hairs may be found side by side growing in opposite directions.

Genetics. Inheritance tends to be dominant but sporadic cases occur. Dark hair seems to be linked with the anomaly. Spontaneous improvement has been reported and may occur during adolescence.

Pili Annulati (Ringed Hair)
This is an unusual condition of the hair in which it presents a banded appearance when viewed by reflected light. It may be mistaken for monilethrix but can easily be distinguished from the latter by viewing the hair in transmitted light when the 'white areas' will be seen to be dark. That it is more than a simple optical effect due to a slight structural change in the hair fibre which causes reflection of the light from the surface is shown by the frequent occurrence of increased fragility of the affected hairs. It is inherited as a dominant with incomplete penetrance.

Pili Torti (Twisted Hair)
Pili torti is a rare congenital anomaly which affects the hair on the scalp and eyebrows and sometimes elsewhere. The affected hairs are twisted through an angle of 180° on their long axis, as a result of which they are liable to break and alopecia is produced. Fractures take place at different levels in adjacent hairs giving rise to a picture very like that of monilethrix with which it may be confused. Microscopic examination will establish the diagnosis at once, but it should be remembered that monilethrix, pili torti and pili annulati can be present simultaneously in the same scalp, suggesting that the developmental defect in all three may be closely similar. Pili torti is usually sporadic in occurrence but

when gene-controlled the trait behaves as an incomplete dominant.

Trichorrhexis Nodosa

This is a fairly rare anomaly characterized by a mechanical weakness in the hair shaft which develops partial fractures at intervals to form the nodes. Under the microscope, the shaft presents the appearance of bundles of twigs impacted in each other. The hairs tend to break at the nodes but marked alopecia is not very common. It is a disorder of adult life rather than childhood although familial cases have been reported by Touraine.

Distichiasis

This is a rare anomaly involving the eyelashes, in which a second row develops posteriorly in line with the ducts of the meibomian glands, and may lead to chronic blepharitis or conjunctival irritation.

Hypertrichosis and Spina Bifida Occulta

Hypertrichosis is not uncommonly associated with spina bifida in the lumbo-sacral region where it often presents the appearance of a satyr's or faun's tail. Such cases should always be fully investigated neurologically, as diastematomyelia may be associated with the spina bifida.

CONGENITAL FISTULAE AND SINUSES INVOLVING THE SKIN

During the course of embryonic life, the surface of the body undergoes considerable folding and invagination at certain sites in association with the development of structures such as the external ear, the eyelids, lips, nose, mouth, bronchial clefts, umbilicus, perineum and coccyx. It is clear that at these sites there is the possibility that incomplete closure or other malformation may occur and produce fistulae, clefts, cysts, or merely trivial dimples in the skin. A large variety of these lesions have been recorded in the literature but only the more frequent or important need mention here. Fistulae are particularly liable to become infected and therefore need excision, apart from any cosmetic reason; glands are often present in the vestigial strictures and these, too, may become infected and give rise in turn to fistulae. The treatment, in every case in which it is desirable, is complete surgical removal, especially when cysts are present, because there is evidence that carcinoma is more likely to develop in such lesions. The surgeon should make sure of the full extent of the lesion by appropriate preoperative radiological investigation because the ramifications of some of these lesions are intricate and extensive. Most lesions, however, are inconspicuous and will not require treatment unless infection supervenes.

Anomalies of the external ear are fairly common, ranging from complete absence of the auricle to minor pits or depressions representing the cutaneous end of a congenital pre-auricular fistula. Skin tags may present as fleshy growths situated on the cheek in front of the ear, and represent heterotopic ear tissue; they may contain cartilage. Tags are easy to remove surgically, but the other abnormalities may require expert help from the plastic surgeon if a reasonable cosmetic result is to be obtained.

Fistulae occur on the dorsum of the nose and upper lip and labial commissures. Those on the nose are more important as they often extend deeply and penetrate between the nasal bones. They arise through faulty development of the supranasal sulcus and demand surgical treatment since infection is liable to be recurrent. They may contain hair and discharge blood and pus from time to time.

Pilonidal sinuses and cysts may be found at several sites, but give rise to little trouble until the terminal hair begins to grow into the skin of the lesion. The commonest site is the sacro-coccygeal region where they may be associated with spina bifida. Infection is liable to occur at any time and surgical treatment is the only satisfactory method of dealing with them, after the infection has been treated.

Cysts and fistulae around the anus and perineum are fairly common and may represent cloacal vestiges or failure of the perineal raphe to join. The more solid lesions, in the baby, may be mistaken for naevoid or haemangiomatous lesions.

Gross Congenital Defects in the Skin
The skin of the infant may appear as if it has been scooped out at birth, as a result of loss of subcutaneous tissue and muscle. There is sometimes a thin layer of unkeratinized skin overlying the defects, which vary very much in size, shape and number, and may occur at any site. Sometimes there is no skin covering the defect at all. The vertex is most commonly affected where lesions tend to be small and circular. All tend to heal by scarring. When associated with other anomalies trisomy should be suspected, especially of D group chromosomes.

Aetiology. The cause remains uncertain; amniotic adhesions used to be blamed in the older literature, but it is likely that the adhesions and skin defect have a common cause, rather than that one causes the other.

Treatment. Skin grafting may be necessary in a number of cases.

Congenital Cicatrices

Linear constrictions may affect the extremities and especially the digits. The part looks as if a tight ligature has been tied around it, and there may be some outward bulging of the limb, above and below the cicatrix. Spontaneous amputation of a limb or part of a limb may occur.

Congenital Amazia (*Absence of Nipples and Breasts*)

Congenital absence of nipples and breasts is extremely rare and may be hereditary. It may occur as the earliest (congenital) sign of progeria of the Hutchinson–Gilford type.

Polymastia and Polythelia (*Accessory Breasts and Nipples*)

Accessory nipples (polythely) are fairly frequent developmental anomalies and are usually to be found distributed along the so-called 'milk-ridge'. They may vary in number from one to several and are usually paired. The extra breasts may have normal breast tissue and may be functional during pregnancy. Polythely is not uncommon in the lower primates. The anomaly may be purely developmental in origin but polymastia has been shown to be an inheritable condition both in man and in the sheep.

Pachyonychia Congenita

There are several inherited conditions in which thickening of the nail plate forms a prominent part of the clinical picture. The form first described by Jadassohn is characterized by thickening of the nail plates of all the digits of the hands and feet present at or soon after birth associated with other anomalies. These include recurrent blistering and hyperkeratosis of the soles, keratosis pilaris involving the skin of the front of the upper end of the tibiae and over the median, certain dental anomalies, buccal, especially lingual leucokeratosis and occasionally ocular and hair defects. An unusual feature is recurrent progressive blistering around the mouth and nose due to infection by herpes simplex virus.

Aetiology. Manifestations are due to mutation of a single gene.

Genetics. The gene responsible is borne on one of the autosomal chromosomes, and transmitted as a dominant, with complete penetrance but variable expressivity.

Complications. Nil serious, unless cataract occurs.
Prognosis. Blistering tends to get less.
Treatment. Prevent infection.

5-iodo-dioxyuridine, applied every 90 minutes or so during waking hours in first 1000 days, will prevent spread of herpes virus and shorten attack.

THE MOUTH

The principal congenital anomalies of the mouth and buccal mucosa include:

Astomia or Absence of the Mouth
This anomaly is due to complete fusion of the upper and lower lips and is sometimes found in Cyclopean and other monsters; it is usually incompatible with life, but may be analogous with imperforate anus.

Macrostomia
Macrostomia results from incomplete fusion of the mandibular and maxillary processes of the developing embryo. Plastic surgery gives good results.

Aglossia (absence of the tongue) and *Microglossia* are very rare developmental errors.

Ankyloglossia (or tongue tie) may be complete or partial; the tongue is more or less firmly anchored to the floor of the mouth. Treatment is usually unnecessary but in the most marked instances consists in incision of the frenum.

Macroglossia. Congenital enlargement of the tongue is a rare anomaly which may occur as an isolated abnormality or may be seen in cretins and infantile myxoedema. One-half of the tongue may be enlarged in hemihypertrophy and lymphangioma may produce considerable enlargement of the organ. Treatment is surgical.

Cleft, or Bifid Tongue is another very rare anomaly.

Scrotal Tongue, characterized by extensive fissuring of the surface, is a fairly common and harmless condition.

Median Rhomboid Glossitis is a developmental error due to failure of the lateral halves of the tongue to fuse together before the tuberculum impar. It is usually unnoticed until later life and is quite benign.

Geographical Tongue (*Glossitis Areata Exfoliativum*). This may be congenital and familial. It is characterized by a continuously changing picture in which areas of the surface of the tongue exfoliate. The anomaly is due to thickening of the filiform papillae and hypertrophy of the lingual epithelium. The lesions appear as round or oval papules, sharply defined, yellowish or red in colour, and varying in size from that of a lentil to that of a penny. The lesions tend to spread peripherally *en cocarde* and to clear in the centre, usually within 8 or 10 days. The condition is harmless but persistent and no treatment is of any avail.

Melanoglossia (*black tongue*) may be a racial character.

CONGENITAL DENTAL ANOMALIES

The commonest dental anomaly present at birth is premature eruption of one or more of the deciduous teeth; usually the mandibular incisors. Many congenital anomalies are associated with disorders in the development of the deciduous teeth but the dental changes will, of course, not be seen until the teeth appear. Defects in the teeth are seen especially in congenital ectodermal dysplasia, where all types of dental defect, ranging from complete anodontia to mild dysplasia of one or more teeth, may be seen. Radiography of the infant's jaws may be helpful in establishing the diagnosis in conditions where gross dental defect is a prominent feature of the anomaly.

SELECTED REFERENCES

APLEY J. (1944) Familial tuberose sclerosis with calcification. *Brain* **67**, 258
BOWERS R.E., GRAHAM E.A. & TOMLINSON K.M. (1960) The natural history of the strawberry naevus. *Arch. Dermat.* **82**, 662
BROCQ L.A.J. (1902) Les parapsoriasis. *Ann. Dermat. Syph.* (4 ser.) **3**, 313–433
COCKAYNE E.A. (1933) *Inherited Abnormalities of the Skin.* O.U.P.
DARIER J. (1909) *Précis de Dermatologie.* Paris: Masson
HELLIER F.F. (1950) Hereditary koilonychia. *Brit. J. Dermat.* **62**, 213
MITCHELL J.C. (1953) Clinical study of leukonychia. *Brit. J. Dermat.* **65**, 121
MONTAGNA W. (1962) *The Structure and Function of the Skin*, 2nd edn. New York: Acad. Press

MOYNAHAN E.J. (1956) Baldness. *Med. Press* **236,** 87
ORMSBY O.S. & MONTGOMERY H. (1954) *Diseases of the Skin*, 8th edn. London: Kimpton
PERLMAN H.H. (1960) *Pediatric Dermatology*. Chicago Year Book Pub.
PILLSBURY D.M., SHELLEY W.B. & KLIGMAN A.M. (1956) *Dermatology*. Philadelphia: Saunders
ROBERTS J.A.F. (1970) *An Introduction to Medical Genetics*, 4th edn. O.U.P.
RONCHESE F. (1951) Peculiar nail anomalies. *Arch. Dermat. Syph.* **63,** 545
ROOK A. (ed) (1960) *Progress in the Biological Sciences in Relation to Dermatology*. C.U.P.
ROTHMAN S. *et al.* (1954) *The Physiology and Biochemistry of the Skin*. Univ. Chicago Press
SCHONFELD W.H.P. (1947) *Lehrbuch der Haut und Geschlechtskrankheiten*, 4th edn. Stuttgart: Thieme
SIMPSON J.R. (1959) The natural history of cavernous haemangioma. *Lancet* **2,** 1057
SUTTON R.L. (1958) *Diseases of the Skin*, 11th edn. St. Louis: Mosley
SCHUERMANN H. (1958) *Krankheiten der Mundschleimhaut und der Lippen*. Munich: Urban & Schwartzenburg
STERN C. (1960) *Principles of Human Genetics*, 2nd edn. San Francisco and London: Freeman
THOMPSON S. (1936) Poikiloderma congenitale. *Brit. J. Dermat.* **48,** 221
TOURAINE A. (1955) *L'Hérédité en Médicine*. Paris: Masson
TURPIN R. (ed) (1955) *La Progenese*. Paris: Masson
WADDINGTON C.H. (1956) *Principles of Embryology*. N.Y.: Allen & Unwin
WILLIER B.H., WEISS P.A. & HAMBURGER V. (ed.) (1955) *Analysis of Development*. Philadelphia: Saunders
WILLIS R.A. (1958) *The Borderland of Embryology and Pathology*. London: Butterworths
WILLIS R.A. (1960) *The Pathology of Tumours*, 2nd edn. London: Butterworths
ZUMKELLER R. (1957) A propos de la fréquence et de la hérédité du naevus vasculosus nuchae (Unna). *J. Génét. hum.* **6,** 1

10

Special Syndromes

A. WHITE FRANKLIN

INTRODUCTION

The term syndrome is difficult to define and by prefixing the adjective special the task is made no easier. Sorsby writes that syndromes 'bring together a mass of apparently disconnected anomalies', that is anomalies that are neither of one organ nor of one system, nor even necessarily of one embryonic layer. That there is a connection between the anomalies is shown only by their repeated occurrence together in single individuals, in siblings or in members of one family. The establishment of a new syndrome helps to identify aetiological agents and to illuminate prognosis. Sometimes new forms of preventive and curative treatment follow.

In this chapter the syndromes described are special in the sense that some abnormality is noted at birth or in the early weeks or months of life. This can be linked with other anomalies of greater or less seriousness because the association is known to form part of a recognized syndrome. The selection is arbitrary and includes some which are no more than coincidental combinations of single components. New syndromes may result from mutations, or they may be produced by drugs or diseases which affect the foetus through the mother. The discovery of a common factor, especially of aetiology, may link up syndromes hitherto regarded as unrelated. The current intensive revealing work on chromosomes and on kinships replaces the hunt for syphilis and alcohol conducted unavailingly by our forbears. The study of aminoacid metabolism, enzymes and lysosomes has shown how abnormalities may be produced. Electron microscopy has revealed the fault in cutis laxa and in osteogenesis imperfecta. The new techniques sound a challenge: these syndromes, experiments of nature as they are, must be recognized and studied so that the knowledge gained may help, if not the patient himself, then perhaps the generations of the future.

Clinical diagnosis in the newborn period is difficult. Examination of the nervous system or of the retina needs much patience and even more skill in interpretation. Urine specimens require special collection and are not ordinarily taken if the baby seems to be normal and well. A number of congenital defects, especially of brain, heart and urogenital tract, may give rise to no notable clinical symptoms or signs in the newborn period. It is therefore valuable to have as many correlations as possible, so that one finding draws attention to the presence of a silent and concealed abnormality for no better reason than that the two are sometimes found together. The low-set ears of Potter's facies mark the need for special study of the urogenital tract just as in a mongol baby (Down's syndrome) the heart must be most carefully examined.

The disadvantage in clinical practice is that too much knowledge can be a dangerous thing. The folly of stressing to the mother of the eczematous baby the risk of later asthma is well known. The management of the family with the problem of a mongol baby is made no easier because of the knowledge of the baby's future which is often given by one look at the face when the head has been delivered. The expectation that he will share the tragic fate of his relations as he grows in awareness, places great strain upon the child who suffers from an incapacitating familial disorder. There is a moral contained in the report in a case of suicide ending a life of painful apprehension in the fifth generation of Von Recklinghausen's syndrome.

The physician whose duty it is to reveal to the parents that the new baby has a serious defect carries a heavy responsibility. His policy is bound to be influenced by the method of presentation, whether there is a known family history, whether there has already been an affected sibling or whether he recognizes the condition on clinical grounds alone as something new and unforeseen. He would do well to take account of his knowledge of the quality and character of the parents and of the stability of their marriage. The presence of externally obvious anomalies should be revealed early to both parents, perhaps to the father first with the understanding that he or the doctor will tell the wife at once or with only a short interval.

Where dwarfism is certain, or if severe mental or physical handicap is obvious to the doctor but not known to the parents, discretion is necessary. Parents can withstand the shock of revelation more easily after they have recovered a little from the emotional stress of childbirth and when they have some experience of their new baby, who has had time to establish its own personality. The doctor must not give way to his own grief at what has happened. This danger is less for the paediatrician, to whom the family is often previously unknown, than for the obstetrician or the family doctor who is more deeply involved and who sometimes feels that through the birth of the abnormal baby he has failed to keep faith with the mother who has put herself, her pregnancy and her delivery into his hands. When the doctor feels, and this should never be the case, that the living baby would be better dead, he is in no state to discuss the case at all with the parents. Resentment expressed in word or attitude to the bearer of bad tidings should be met with patience and compassion although much later the doctor may need to show impatience to shock the parents out of self-pity and into sympathy with their own afflicted baby.

Many parents need genetic counselling and all need unhurried consultation at which they can be given a programme of treatment and the opportunity to discuss their anxieties.

The First Arch Syndrome

Developmental failure of bones and of soft tissues of the face have been described under various names and exist in various combinations. In 1900 Treacher-Collins described two cases with 'catarrhal ophthalmia', both having 'a shallow notch in the margin of each lower lid, a short distance from the external canthus. . . . In direction they (the lids) tend to slope downwards and outwards. Their appearance suggests, at first, an inaccurately united wound across the edge of the lid.' He observed also 'an unusual want of prominence of the malar bones'.

Pierre Robin in 1926 drew attention to 'dysmorphosis of the facio-cranio-vertebral skeleton' which he had been studying for many years and in which hypotrophy of the mandible causing glossoptosis produced feeding difficulty, failure to thrive and periodic attacks of asphyxia.

In 1944 Franceschetti and Zwahlen reported two cases of a new syndrome for which they suggested the name 'mandibulofacial dysostosis.' The characteristics were: (1) eyelids sloping downwards with coloboma of upper and lower lids; (2) hypoplasia of cheek bones and of lower jaw; (3) aural malformation; (4) macrostomia with blind fistulae between mouth and ear; (5) abnormality of position of teeth and of growth of hair, and an ogival palate.

McKenzie and Craig have attempted the synthesis of these varied clinical entities into one group—the first arch syndrome. The rational link is a foetal vascular anomaly depriving the first visceral arch of its blood supply, which comes mainly from the stapedial artery, between the third and the fifth weeks and so between the disappearance of the first aortic arch of the full development of the external carotid artery. Hövels has ranged a whole series of anomalies from simple outward and downward obliquity of the palpebral fissures to complete agnathia, but McKenzie would add congenital deaf-mutism due to absence of incus and stapes and hypertelorism, using Waardenburg's syndrome, perhaps mistakenly (see below), as a connecting link.

Whatever the merits of McKenzies' concept the clinical observer noting any one of the features of the first arch syndrome would be well advised to study carefully the anatomy of the face, the disposition of the orbits and palpebral fissures, the mandible and its angle, the external ears, the palate, to make sure of the patency of the nose and at a later stage to satisfy himself about hearing. A family history will be present in some cases. Other anomalies of the skeleton and in some cases mental retardation may complicate the picture. Any one of the anomalies included may occur by itself.

Mandibulo-facial Dysostosis—Hallermann–Streiff syndrome
The diagnosis depends on facial appearance, the eyes slanted downwards with a notch at the junction of the inner two-thirds and the outer third, eyelashes being scanty in the medial third of both lids. Malar bones lack prominence, the chin is receding, the angle of the lower jaw obtuse. The tongue is large and held to the back of the mouth. The ears are large, low-set and floppy from deficient cartilage.

The main symptom at first is feeding difficulty. Breast-or bottle-feeding may be prevented owing to an inability to suck, and tube or spoon feeding may be needed for the first month or 6 weeks. Vomiting, slow weight-gain, respiratory infection and cyanotic attacks are complicating hazards.

At post-mortem the zygoma and the zygomatic process of the temporal bone are defective or absent, while the masseters are attached to a ridge on the maxilla.

Six cases of this condition were discussed by Franceschetti and Klein in 1949, with a full review of the literature.

The condition is determined by an autosomal dominant gene with variable manifestation.

Mandibulo-facial dysostosis in association with ocular changes and areas of alopecia forms Hallermann–Streiff syndrome. The nose is beaked and the face bird-like. Micro-cornea and occasionally glaucoma are present with congenital cataracts that may rupture spontaneously and be absorbed. Palpebral fissures are anti-mongoloid. The mouth is very small, maxillae hypoplastic and dentition anomalous, teeth being present sometimes at birth. The child is small in stature and there is sexual immaturity. Aminoaciduria has been reported. Cases are sporadic and there is no evidence that this is a genetically determined disorder.

Micrognathia
A receding mandible is commonly found in the newborn. Pierre Robin has given as a critical figure a mandible more than 1 cm behind the maxilla. The frenulum of the tongue is attached far back so that the tip easily somersaults into the pharynx causing respiratory obstruction, cyanotic and apnoeic attacks, and a constant feeding difficulty. A cleft soft palate is often present. Marked retraction of the lower ribs and of the suprasternal notch with obvious respiratory effort and difficulty, is associated with a tendency to acute respiratory infection, in some cases a cause of death. Attempts to suture the tip of the tongue to the cheek usually fail, nursing, and especially feeding, in the prone position, with the ready use of antibiotics to combat infection, allows survival and weight gain; natural improvement with the development of a good lower jaw then follows in many cases.

Micrognathia is found in syndromes other than that of the first arch, notably in Möbius syndrome, in gonadal dysgenesis, in intra-uterine dwarfism and in a trisomy 17 or 18 described in 1960 by Edwards and his colleagues. Hanhart has described an association between extreme micrognathia and absence of hands or digits. The ears were set low in his two female patients.

Microstomia
Failure of division of the first branchial arch may lead to defective development of the mandible associated with abnormality of shape, size and position of the external ears. Extreme forms are incompatible with life. In less severely affected cases the jaws may be fused, the temporo-mandibular joints imperfect, and the compressed tongue may obstruct

respiration so that tracheostomy is required. Feeding is extremely difficult. Despite a poor prognosis in view of the breathing and feeding problems, attempts should be made to help such babies in the hopes of surgical relief at a later age.

Potter has drawn attention to the association of *macrostomia* with a dermoid tumour at the limbus involving the cornea.

Auricular Atresia
Microtia
Looking at abnormalities of the skull and face from the otologist's point of view Nager and de Reynier tabulated six groups of 'dyscephalies' associated with ear involvement: (1) dyscephaly from synostosis of cranial sutures; (2) acrocephaly–syndactyly; (3) cranio-cleido-dysostosis; (4) dysostosis-cranio-facialis with abnormalities of fingers and toes; (5) dysostosis facialis (usually called mandibulo-facial); (6) mandibular, in which mandibular hypoplasia was found with atresia of the external auditory meatus and a deformed pinna.

The fact that a similar aural lesion has been found under all these different conditions cannot be taken as evidence that they share an aetiological agent, nor that the manner of inheritance is the same. On the other hand microtia does form part of the thalidomide syndrome in combination with phocomelia and congenital anomalies of the gut (see below). It must be remembered also that atresia of the ear occurs without any other abnormality.

Posterior Choanal Atresia
It would seem wise to establish the patency of the posterior choanae in all cases where an element of the first arch syndrome is present, despite the rarity of the association. Breathing and feeding difficulties are likely to be present in the syndrome and are bound to occur with bilateral obstruction of the nares, since newborn babies and infants are usually unable to breathe regularly through the mouth. Two simple clinical tests will quickly establish the diagnosis. When the edge of a *cold* microscope slide is rested on the upper lip a puff of condensed moisture should normally be seen opposite each nostril. Auscultation of the chest during marked respiratory effort will yield breath sounds while the baby's mouth is open; with the mouth closed chest movements continue in auscultatory silence. The passage of a catheter through the nostril will

be obstructed and a few drops of radio-opaque oil instilled through the catheter will be seen by X-ray not to enter the nasopharynx.

Little except a nasal discharge may indicate the commoner unilateral case. Both sporadic and familial cases are on record. Besides other elements of the first arch syndrome, associated congenital anomalies include high arched palate, facial asymmetry, polydactyly and coloboma of the iris.

Hypertelorism, Waardenburg's Syndrome, Hereditary nerve deafness

An increasing number of syndromes is being described in which deafness plays a part. Fortunately the screening of infants for hearing defect is widely practised, with especial attention to babies exposed to hyperbilirubinaemia and rubella virus. About 1 in 6000 of the population may be expected to have a hereditary hearing defect, half of them without recognized complications. In the other half associations have been established with defects in the metabolism and transport of amino-acids (tyrosine, proline and methionine), with albinism, gargoylism, Tay Sachs, with nephropathies (see below), with skeletal defects in Klippel–Feil and Albers–Schonberg disease.

Another skeletal defect in which deafness is common is hypertelorism, first described by Greig and due to overgrowth of the lesser wings of the sphenoid giving a wide interocular distance and a broad root to the nose. Cleft lip and palate, mandibular asymmetry, microphthalmos and mental retardation were found among Greig's patients.

Waardenburg has described a hereditary syndrome of congenital perceptive deafness, a white forelock, heterochromia and an abnormal facies, the root of the nose appearing broader than normal. At first regarded as a form of hypertelorism, this is now recognized as being due to an abnormal fold of skin on either side of the nose, widening the bridge and reducing the amount of visible sclerotic. Fisch collected eighty-one cases, selecting thirty-five for careful analysis. The hearing defect may amount to total deafness or may be limited to the lower and middle ranges with normal high-tone hearing. Unilateral deafness is usually moderate, while in bilateral cases only one ear may be totally deaf. The degree of deafness varies among the relatives. In one child who died, ear and brain studies which were carried out showed an absence of the organ of Corti in the cochlear canal with atrophy of the spiral ganglion and nerve. The auditory pathway was intact. The white forelock in the middle or just to one side of the centre of the forehead may form a thick, well-outlined lock or may occur as a few white strands. The heterochromia of the iris consists of one brown with one persistent blue eye, or of partial brown pigmentation in both blue eyes. Fisch has noticed a similarity of profile in his cases with a depressed nasal bridge, sometimes a metopic suture, and a massive lower jaw. Nasal infections are frequent.

In some families there is dappled, part-brown, part-pigmented skin. One girl had congenital atresia of the lower part of the oesophagus which Fisch suggests as a possible cause of the wasting and early infant deaths recorded in a few of the affected families.

The Tongue
Aglossia—Macroglossia
Fulford has reviewed twelve cases of complete absence of the tongue. Aglossia was associated with harelip twice, complete cleft palate three times, but more interestingly with syndactyly twice and with partial adactyly twice. The disability is described as not very great after the first 3 months, but bottle feeding is necessary as gravity has to serve instead of active compression of the teat or nipple.

A protruded tongue of normal size should first arouse suspicion of mongolism (Down's syndrome), but, in the absence of supporting features, of cretinism. A large or protruded tongue in the neonatal period may be the only clinical evidence of thyroid deficiency for many weeks; it is also found in chondro-osteodystrophy. Gross enlargement of the tongue (macroglossia) is occasionally found in otherwise normal babies. Difficulty with feeding and with speech, and later malocclusion of the jaws, are to be expected. Lymphangioma and rhabdomyoma have been described, and in some cases excision of part of the tongue is necessary for the baby's comfort.

Acrocephaly–Syndactyly
Oxycephaly, turricephaly—hypertelorism—craniosynostosis.
Abnormalities of the shape of the skull are extremely common at the time of birth. Careful observation over a period of time is needed for a true assessment of their meaning. Moulding with considerable over-riding along the sagittal suture may take many days to disappear and during this time the skull circumference may change little so that there is a fear of scaphocephaly from premature synostosis. The use of standard growth curves for the interpretation of skull circumference and of skull

x-rays to show premature synostosis, while revealing abnormalities in some cases, can cause unnecessary anxiety, especially with too rigid an application of standards, inaccurate measurement and poor quality x-rays.

The severe forms of deformity are named: (1) acrocephaly, when the skull comes to a point in the region of the anterior fontanelle; (2) turricephaly or oxycephaly, when the vertex is domed; (3) scaphocephaly, when the skull is narrow and elongated with a ridge along the sagittal suture; (4) plagiocephaly, when there is a marked asymmetry.

These deformities are due to premature cranial synostosis which may affect any of the sutures. Those most commonly fusing are the sagittal (scaphocephaly) and the coronal (oxycephaly). Despite the marked skull deformity there may be no symptoms or increased intracranial pressure may give rise to headaches and convulsions. Eye symptoms include divergent squint, papilloedema, optic atrophy with some visual failure in about half the cases or even blindness and, rarely, cataract. Proptosis may in extreme form cause subluxation of the eyeballs. Skull x-rays show extreme digital markings.

Another correlation is with a beaked nose, hypoplasia of the maxilla and abnormalities of the extremities. Park and Powers confirmed Apert's findings in 1907 and Crouzon's in 1912 and established as an entity the association of acrocephaly and syndactyly.

Achondroplasia (Parrot 1878)
This skeletal defect has received much attention in recent years and observations, largely by Lamy and Maroteaux in Paris, have added greatly to the differential diagnosis of the short-limbed neonate. Classical achondroplasia remains a distinct entity. A general disorder of ossification in cartilage, it is not associated with defects in other systems. The occurrence is estimated at 1 in 10,000 livebirths, and the cause is believed to be a mutant gene (autosomal dominant) in 90 per cent of families. Many die in the first year, but newer knowledge suggests that the high death and stillbirth rates may owe more to the other forms of short-limbed dwarfs than to true achondroplasia. The name hypochondroplasia has been suggested for a form of the defect of less severity and with a good expectancy of life.

The defect involves ossification in cartilage and leads to dwarfing because the limbs are short. An antenatal x-ray shows the typical short broad 'long' bones without the typical dumbell shape seen in the older survivors, although the epiphyses are somewhat expanded. The limbs may project away from the trunk in the same fashion as when the foetus is oedematous, because of the relative thickness of the soft tissues. At birth clinical recognition depends on noticing the short limbs, the mid-point in length of the baby being well above the umbilicus. The ends of the fingers do not reach as far as the great trochanters. The head appears relatively large. The lips are thick and the tongue protrudes in the early months. Palpation of the upper arms and the

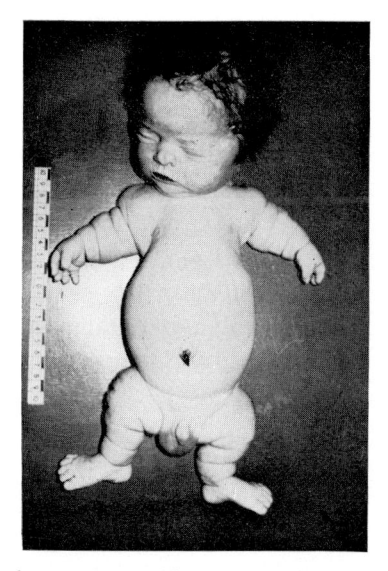

Fig. 10.1. Typical appearance of a baby with severe achondroplasia.

thighs shows the remarkable thickness of humerus and femur within; but the bones feel regular, and unlike the bones in osteogenesis imperfecta which is sometimes diagnosed as achondroplasia by the unwary. In these cases although the limbs appear short, the bones feel grossly irregular by reason of multiple healed intra-uterine fractures, as they are said to do in hypophosphatasia.

The hands of the achondroplastic are trident in form, the three middle fingers diverging from the hand. Limitation of movement at shoulders and elbows has been reported. The gait is a peculiar waddle with some lordosis and the older child can sit down on and rise from the ground with remarkable agility.

The ultimate height is limited so that the patient remains a dwarf. Intelligence and sexual maturity are expected to be normal. An achrondroplastic mother can bear a normal child, but delivery must be by Caesarean section.

Although no special association with other congenital defects exists, hypospadias, renal anomalies, spina bifida, aural defects and cleft palate have all been reported. In the lethal variety pulmonary hypoplasia occurs and survival is not usual.

The management of the parents in the neonatal period requires careful thought.

Thoracic dystrophy
This chondro-dystrophy affects especially the costo-chondral junctions preventing both rib growth and expansion of the thoracic cage. Death from asphyxia may occur within a few hours or, unless surgical enlargement is effective, at the latest early in the second year. Recently some, more mildly affected, have been shown to survive. The pelvis appears abnormal in two-thirds of the patients with short, squared iliac bones, deep sciatic notches and horizontal acetabulae. The skull is normal and the head of normal size. Inheritance is autosomal recessive.

Thanatophoric dwarfism
This lethal ($\theta\acute{a}\nu a\tau o\varsigma$ = death) condition, for which the mode of inheritance is still uncertain, is characterized by severe micromelia, a relatively large head, normal trunk length, narrow thorax and flattened vertebrae. Hydramnios is frequent, there is a preponderance of males and death results from respiratory distress. Histological studies show disorganization of endochondral bone formation, cartilage cells being in disorder in contrast to the orderly rows found in the classical achondroplastic who survives the perinatal period. It seems likely that some at least of the stillbirths labelled achondroplastic belonged to this group.

Diastrophic dwarfism
This, one of the first of the short-limbed neonates to be withdrawn from true achondroplasia, has an autosomal recessive inheritance. Head and face are normal in size and appearance. Intelligence is normal. Limbs are short, the defect distal rather than proximal, and thumbs and great toes are deformed. In infancy cystic swellings of the pinna recur leading to its later crumpling and calcifying. A scoliosis develops during infancy

and joints which are at first unduly lax are later deformed by contractures. The hips may dislocate. Cleft palate is occasionally present. X-rays show short long bones, delayed epiphyses with flattened and shortened metacarpals and metatarsals. Vertebrae appear normal. Eventual height is not expected to exceed 140 cm (56 in.).

Metatropic dwarfism
The newborn baby has a long trunk with short limbs giving a normal total length. The head appears normal. During growth the appearance which at birth resembles that of achondroplasia transforms to resemble that of Morquio's disease, the facies altering and the bones lengthening in relation to the trunk. A severe kyphoscoliosis rapidly develops. X-ray of the long bones shows widened metaphyses, the abnormality lessening with age. There are no abnormal muco-polysaccharides nor corneal opacities.

Cartilage–hair hypoplasia (McKusick)
It is now the practice to include this autosomal recessive disorder among the short-limbed dwarfs. Dwarfism is severe, hair is sparse, brittle and individual hairs lack pigment and are of small diameter. Cartilage cells are also sparse.

The reader is referred for further assistance in differential diagnosis of short-limbed dwarfs to two articles on thanatophoric dwarfism by Kaufman (1970) and to one on radiological differentiation by Geidion (1958), included in the list of references.

Marfan Syndrome
Arachnodactyly
To recognize arachnodactyly in a newborn baby by the length of the fingers and toes and limbs is problematical for most physicians. The older well-established case shows 'spider hands and feet' with a dolichocephalic skull, postural kyphosis with or without scoliosis, poor muscular development, little subcutaneous fat and excessive mobility of joints, a funnel or pigeon chest, a high patella and a high arched palate.

Measurements of body relationships are important in diagnosis. The span of the outstretched arms should be greater than the height and the distance from pelvis to heels should be longer than that from pubis to vertex. A metacarpal index based on the lengths and breadths of the metacarpals as measured in an x-ray gives the most accurate test. It would be interesting to apply these tests and the method described to newborn babies.

Defects of the eyes are found in about half the cases and include nystagmus, divergent squint, miosis, high myopia, strabismus and marked myopia. Coloboma, cataract, megalocornea, hydrophthalmos and tremulous iris also occur. The best-known lesion is dislocation or subluxation of the lens (ectopia lentis) due to a defective suspensory ligament, present in 55–60 per cent. Hypoplasia of the dilator muscles leads to poor mydriasis.

Cardiovascular disease is common and Sinclair in a study of forty cases found cardiovascular disease in fourteen. These authors point out that the lesions may fall into three groups. A true association exists with a congenital anomaly of the heart, such as an atrial septal defect, coarctation of the aorta or a patent ductus arteriosus. Secondary changes are described including dilation of the aortic valve ring, of sinuses of Valsalva, of the aortic arch and of the descending aorta. Total rupture of the aorta with or without a dissecting aneurysm is caused by a medio-necrosis and has been found in a 14-month-old baby. Valve cusp deformities result from myxomatous degeneration. The third group includes rheumatic heart disease, and myocarditis, conduction defects and arrhythmias of unknown aetiology.

Other associations are pulmonary hypoplasia (two- and one-lobed lungs) macroglossia, and large floppy ears lacking cartilage.

Congenital dislocation of the hip and habitual dislocation of the shoulder, patella and radio-ulnar joint, calcaneus deformities of the feet and spurring of the heels have all been noticed. Bone pain, especially in the hip, can be disabling, as can arthrogryposis with contracture of elbow or knee. In the urogenital tract genital hypoplasia, undescended testes, polycystic, ectopic and duplex kidneys have all been described. This widespread mesodermal anomaly is determined by an autosomal dominant mutant gene with variable manifestation.

Cranio-cleido-dysostosis
Examination of the neonatal skull sometimes reveals a wide deficit between the parietal bones, occupying two or three fingers'-breadths with a normal skull circumference. The common causes for such a finding are prematurity and the early stage of a later appearing hydrocephalus. Hypothyroidism and congenital syphilis are reputed additional causes. The examiner should always carefully investigate the

presence of clavicles, bearing in mind that there may be absence of all or part of one or both. In the absence of clavicles it may be possible to bring the shoulders together under the chin: this is not a disability and, indeed, may ease the delivery of the shoulders.

Cranio-cleido-dysostosis is a misleadingly limited name for this defect of ossification of the skull and clavicles, since often there is also a gap in the pubic symphysis; and developmental errors (delayed eruption, non-eruption and incomplete development) of the permanent teeth and of the mandible are common. Those affected are usually short of stature, with normal intelligence. Both sexes are equally involved.

Additional defects are coxa vara, and failure of fusion of the neural arches of dorsal and lumbar vertebrae. Hemi-vertebrae and partial or complete absence of the lower part of the sacrum and coccyx have been reported. The most striking x-ray change in the hands and feet is the presence of epiphyses at both ends of metacarpal and metatarsal bones.

Muscle abnormalities include absence of the clavicular portions of the trapezius, the sterno-mastoid and the pectoralis major. The condition is normally symptomless but pain and numbness in the ulnar area from pressure of the outer fragment of the clavicle on the brachial plexus has been reported.

Ossification continues late in life and the skull usually closes completely in the end. The mothers of the author's patients were diagnosed as having rickets in childhood (probably from what was thought to be delayed closure of the anterior fontanelle). A triangular depression with its apex emerging from beneath the hair margin in the middle of the forehead can sometimes be felt or seen when the mother herself lacks clavicles.

An autosomal dominant gene is responsible.

Osteogenesis Imperfecta
Fragilitas Ossium—Osteopsathyrosis—Lobstein, Vrolik Syndrome.
A hereditary liability of the bones to sustain repeated fracture without good external cause was first described by Ekman in 1788. It now seems certain that the syndrome described below is a single entity, often, although not always, lethal at birth or early in life in cases where the foetus has suffered multiple fractures, but compatible with a normal life span and improvement in the fragility of the bones in less severely affected individuals.

The prenatal case sustains multiple foetal fractures, perhaps as many as one hundred, recognizable in prenatal x-rays and at birth. Many of these are stillborn and many are sporadic cases. The survivors resemble achondroplastic dwarfs on account of their short extremities, but are readily distinguished by the easily felt surface irregularities of the bone resulting from healed fractures. The skull appears large and soft, the occiput sometimes resembling a membranous bag. In severe cases growth and weight gain are extremely slow. Death in infancy is likely. Survivors are dwarfed to a greater degree than can be explained by the fractures. The bone x-rays conform to the thick bone type described by Fairbank, who believes that the thickening is not entirely due to callus. Skull x-rays show that the occiput is poorly calcified or consists of a broken line of Wormian bones.

In the less severely affected, and in those who survive the early months of life, fractures are readily produced especially in the lower limbs, but although there is a peak incidence at between 2 and 3 years of age, the tendency is for the bones to strengthen with the passage of time. The bones heal rapidly, except in the subtrochanteric region of the femur. Prolonged immobilization, which increases osteoporosis, should be avoided although it is important to secure good position. The patients tend to be of slender habitus and small stature, and x-rays of cases presenting later show slender bones with a thin cortex.

In many the joints are lax, so that sprains are common, as is flat foot. The teeth may be irregular and small, and dentition delayed. Small cracks in the outer layer of the dentine cause the enamel to break and peel away, giving the teeth a greyish-brown, brown or yellowish colour (hereditary opalescent dentine).

Blue sclerotics are common and are seen in members of the family who have few fractures as well as in the lethal cases. The sclera are unusually translucent so that the choroid shows through. In some families typical in all other ways this sign is absent. In others some affected patients have normal sclerotics and some sclerotics of a Mediterranean blue, deeper than is ever seen in normal newborn babies, although theirs are bluer than those of older children. An arcus corneae is found in about 15 per cent of patients below 50 years, but there are no reliable observations about incidence in the early or lethal cases.

Deafness usually begins at between 20 and 30 years of age, and in Smars' survey affected 23 per cent of cases examined. In the group 50–59 years the incidence was 50 per cent. A tendency to easy bruising and to subcutaneous haemorrhages has been observed in many families, but not of a severe enough degree to need medical attention.

Follis has carefully studied connective tissue in osteogenesis imperfecta and has produced convincing evidence of a failure of reticulin to differentiate into mature collagen, leaving a thin layer of collagen of embryonic type in the corium, the sclera and the cornea. This peculiarity explains the thin skin and the thin blue sclera. Wounds of skin and fractures of bone heal normally.

Genetic studies support the action of autosomal dominant mutant genes, with some variation within families and more between families. There was no increase in mortality rate for either familial or sporadic cases over the age of 2 years, but the sporadic cases showed an excessive mortality during the first 2 years.

Fanconi's Anaemia, Congenital Aplastic Anaemia
Congenital anomalies of the skeleton associated with blood disorder (hypoplastic anaemia) have been reported under the general heading of Fanconi's syndrome. Although the blood dyscrasia characteristically appears in childhood, adolescence or young adult life, a few neonatal cases have been described with thrombocytopenia and an absence of megakaryocytes from the bone marrow with a variety of bony and some other abnormalities of development and are regarded as neonatal forms of the syndrome described by Fanconi in 1927.

It was E. Benjamin who in 1911 first identified the syndrome in three children. The features are a familial pernicious-like anaemia, skin pigmentation, a small head without mental defect, small stature, testicular hypoplasia, exaggerated tendon reflexes and a convergent squint. The associated anomalies recorded include webbed thumb without the first metacarpal bone, atresia of the auditory meatus, horseshoe kidney, absence of one kidney, right middle lobe hypoplasia, congenital heart disease and gynaecomastia. Beautyman's case had always bruised easily and had congenital dislocation of both hips. The parents were first cousins. Reinhold, Neumark, Lightwood and Carter, having studied one family and the previous reports, concluded that the condition was due to a recessive gene. They observe that although the skull circumference is small, being more than two standard deviations below normal, the shape of the skull is not like that in true microcephaly.

In some cases the leucocyte count has been extremely high on occasion with primitive cells in the peripheral blood. A link seems to exist between a complex genetic disorder of bone development, especially of radius and thumb, absence of megakaryocytes from bone marrow, anaemia and leukaemia. The obvious treatments by platelet transfusion splenectomy and steroid therapy have not yielded any good or permanent result. Androgens over long periods have diminished the need for blood transfusions, but although testosterone and oxymetholone have both been used, no clear line of treatment can yet be recommended. If the condition is due to an autosomal recessive gene, the time of action appears to be at 2 or 3 months of foetal life, the radii and the platelets beginning to develop between 6 and 8 weeks.

Klippel–Feil Syndrome
Apparent absence or extreme shortening of the neck, with a low hair line extending on to the back and with limited movement of the head on the shoulders, was described by Klippel and Feil in 1912. They thought that the cervical vertebrae were absent or were greatly reduced in number because the thoracic cage seemed in direct contact with the base of the skull. The clinical syndrome can be recognized at birth.

Bauman collected thirty cases adding six of his own and pointed out a number of extra features. He found an association with Sprengel's deformity (high position) of the scapula, torticollis and facial asymmetry. In some infant cases there is heavy breathing or shortness of breath, as if from respiratory obstruction, and there may be difficulty in feeding and in swallowing, although most cases are without such symptoms. Mirror movement (bimanual synkinesia) was observed in five of Bauman's six cases; movements of one hand were accompanied by the same movements of the other, so that the patient could not safely climb a ladder. Other neurological abnormalities reported include nystagmus, deaf-mutism and syringomyelia. Abnormal dentition, a lowered nipple line, micrognathia, cleft palate, hydrocephalus and congenital heart disease have also occurred, and the condition is found with both Möbius syndrome and pulmonary hypoplasia.

The essential lesions, evident in x-rays of the cervical spine, are gross structural irregularities of the vertebrae. Their number is always reduced, they assume abnormal shapes, and several appear to be fused together, some remaining as isolated hemivertebrae. There are fusion and deformities of the ribs, and cervical ribs are sometimes present.

Males and females are said to be equally affected. A positive family history has not been reported. Gilmour has suggested the Klippel–Feil syndrome is a mild form of iniencephaly that is compatible with extra-uterine life.

The condition is deforming and disabling, but only affects life when there are serious associated congenital anomalies.

Congenital Absence of the Sacrum

The physical appearance of the patient with absence of sacrum is characteristically a lack of prominence of the buttocks with no groove between them and with apparent wasting of the upper ends of the thighs. Digital examination of the rectum reveals soft tissues only and a startling absence of the expected bony prominences. An X-ray shows no sacral nor coccygeal shadows so that the iliac wings are near each other and the pelvic canal is narrow. The defect is not familial. The extreme form is found in sirenomelia (merman) and in other stillbirths associated with atresia of the rectum and anus and with anomalies of the urogenital tract. In some, life is possible, despite the considerable disabilities that follow orthopaedic and sphincter problems. Severe talipes, both equino-varus and calcaneovalgus, and congenital dislocation of the hips may require treatment, and weakness or even spastic paraplegia may prevent walking. There may be sensory and motor loss involving the sacral and lower lumbo-sacral plexus. Urinary and faecal incontinence are inevitable, and need the same careful handling as in cases of meningomyelo-cele. A watch for urinary infection by regular urine testing, with manual expression of the bladder and periodic exhibition of the appropriate antibiotic help to preserve renal function. The use of suppositories (Dulcolax) may prevent serious constipation and reduce the need for enemas and washouts.

Congenital Absence of Abdominal Muscles

The appearance of a baby with absent abdominal muscles is easily recognized. The skin is copiously wrinkled, the abdomen bulges with crying and as the gut distends, loops and peristalsis are well seen. Palpation reveals a thin wall with coils of gut and viscera too readily identified. The testicles are almost always undescended and remain intra-abdominal. The urachus is sometimes patent. Among some hundred recorded cases, only four or five are known to be females (the sex is not always stated).

The condition is serious because of the associated dangerous congenital defects, particularly in the genito-urinary (see Chapter 6, p. 228) and less commonly in the gastro-intestinal tracts. Abnormalities of the mesentery, mal-rotation and bowel atresia cause symptoms early in life so that any vomiting or appetite disturbance in the newborn period should be speedily investigated by x-ray studies of the abdomen for the diagnosis and relief of intestinal obstruction.

Abnormalities of the extremities include various forms of talipes, congenital dislocation of the hip, absence of parts of limbs, and both arthrogryposis and hypermotility of joints.

The muscles involved are most commonly the transverse abdominals, the rectus below the navel, the internal and the external obliques. Muscle fibres can be demonstrated microscopically near their attachments. The common presence of the gastro-intestinal and limb anomalies is more suggestive of a genetic origin though it is rare to find a second affected child in a family.

Purpura

Simple-Symptomatic—Wiskott–Aldrich syndrome—Haemangio-endothelioma.

Purpura appears commonly in the skin in the early hours or days of life and under many circumstances. It may follow pressure on the forehead or the presenting part. Sometimes there is associated thrombocytopenia as part of the rubella syndrome or as a result of foetal infection with cytomegalovirus.

Megakaryocytes may be absent from or much reduced in the bone marrow as the result of simple hypoplasia, congenital hypoplastic anaemia, congenital leukaemia, or severe infection.

In the majority of cases normal megakaryocytes are present, the mother's blood being affected by platelet agglutinins or by drugs which cross the placenta.

Wiskott–Aldrich Syndrome

Wiskott in 1937 first noted the association between eczema, thrombocytopenia and increased susceptibility to infection in three brothers. Aldrich, Steinberg and Campbell in 1954 studied a family of Dutch extraction which included forty male infants of whom sixteen died with this syndrome within the first 31 months of life indicating a sex-linked recessive inheritance. Gordon reported two cases in an English family, and black Americans have been affected.

Further accounts have extended the pathological features: haemorrhage occurs in the gastro-intestinal tract, skin, brain and adrenals, eczema remains important, infections include purulent otitis media, pneumonitis and meningitis. Hypo-aminoacidaemia has been reported in patients and in their clinically normal female siblings. Electron microscopy shows small, poorly granular platelets. Interest in reduced immunity production gives importance to the finding of lymphadenopathy, splenomegaly, thymic atrophy, lymphocyte depletion and reticulo-endothelial proliferation, as well as abnormal serum immunoglobulin levels, notably IgM. Recently malignant systemic reticulo-endotheliosis and lymphoma have been described in children with the syndrome. The clinical picture is remarkably constant, as is the relentless course to early death despite blood and platelets transfusions and steroid therapy.

Haemangio-endothelioma and thrombocytopenic purpura with bone changes

The syndrome was described by Kasabach and Merritt in 1940. A soft subcutaneous lump, often in the neck is noted at birth, with or without reddish staining of the overlying skin. Within a few weeks the lump suddenly enlarges as the result of haemorrhage, becomes plum-coloured and surrounded by a petechial rash. There may be severe anaemia; thrombocytopenia is present but the megakaryocytes in the marrow are normal. In the neck the resulting pressure may endanger life by suffocation. X-ray of contiguous bone may show rarefaction. The tumour, composed of atypical endothelial cells with little lining membrane, can infiltrate surrounding tissues, recur and metastasise.

Treatment by steroids or splenectomy is usually unsuccessful. When the acute crisis is over and the anaemia cured, the local lesion should be given a full course of radiotherapy. As the haemangio-endothelioma disappears, or within a few months, circulating platelets increase spontaneously. In some cases the bone structure gradually returns to normal, in others, possibly as the result of radiotherapy, the affected bone remains somewhat atrophic. In the author's oldest case fibrosarcomatous changes were found in biopsy of a tumour at the site of the original lesion at the age of 7 years. This resolved with further radiotherapy and he is alive and well at 22 years with a deformed right shoulder but full movement. A basal-celled carcinoma has appeared in the irradiated skin.

Kostmann's syndrome
Infantile genetic agranulocytosis.
Lethal and serious recurrent infections in families have been found to be due to defects in immunity production and there are many studies on the thymus, the lymphocytes and the immunoglobulins. A lethal form of agranulocytosis due to a single recessive gene has been reported in eighty-three children in eighteen families in Norbotten in Sweden by Kostmann. The illness was characterized by skin infection, boils or phlegmons, with fever and almost total lack of granulocytes in the peripheral blood. Marrow examination showed a retardation or block of maturation of myelopoietic cells. The disease is lethal, the infected areas indolent and without pus formation. Fourteen of Kostmann's affected patients died in the first 6 months. A baby seen by the author developed spreading ulceration of the skin round the umbilicus and died at 6 weeks of liver failure with multiple necrotic and calcified areas scattered through the liver. Marrow transplants might prolong life but hardly seem justifiable.

Potter's Facies
Potter, in conducting some 5000 peri-natal autopsies, found twenty instances of bilateral renal agenesis. There were seventeen males, and three females each lacking uterus and vagina. The lungs of all were hypoplastic. Other associated defects included sirenomelia (merman), hydrocephalus, arthrogryposis, spinal anomalies, absence of rectum and anus, duodenal atresia, malrotation of the gut and aortic and pulmonary atresia.

In time Potter found that she could often predict the presence of renal agenesis by a study of the face of which she gave the following description. There is increased space between the eyes, a prominent fold arising at the inner canthus which sweeps downwards and laterally below the eyes, unusual flattening of the nose and recession of the chin. The ears are large with decreased cartilage and are low-lying.

Potter's facies is a helpful guide clinically to the possible presence of renal tract anomalies. Hilson has described ears of peculiar shape in babies whose renal lesions are compatible with life, giving the descriptive titles of floppy, bat, folded, elfin and cockle-shell. The peculiarity both of ear shape and kidney may be unilateral. What constitutes a low-set ear has not been defined exactly, but the external auditory meatus lies close to or on a level with the angle of the mandible, a condition also found (p. 394) in some trisomies.

Aural–renal Syndromes
Sohar—Robin and Gardner—Alport.
A heredo-familial syndrome combining perceptive deafness, nephropathy and ocular changes (spherophakia) was first described by Sohar. Robin and Gardner found both familial glomerulonephritis and familial pyelonephritis. Williamson collected fourteen children in three families with Alport's syndrome, hereditary nephritis and perceptive deafness, considered to be dominant with sex-limitation to boys. Haematuria is common. An associated progressive peripheral polyneuropathy has also been described (Marin and Tyler).

Pendred's Syndrome
Deaf-mutism and goitre in two sisters of an Irish family living in Durham formed the subject of half a column in *The Lancet* by Pendred in 1896. Parents and siblings were normal. Russell Brain quoted five families, among whom were twelve cases of goitre with congenital deaf-mutism, and noted differences between these and twenty-six cases of goitre alone. Males and females are equally affected and the cases occur in one generation only. A more extensive survey of 113 cases in seventy-two families by Fraser, Morgan and Trotter supported these observations and demonstrated a recessive inheritance. The severity of the deafness varied from an extreme form to a condition helped by a hearing aid. High-tone deafness is characteristic and there is loss of vestibular function in some cases. Thould and Scowen in their series found that the goitre could present at birth or as late as at 27 years, while the deafness could be noted at any age up to 7 years. In their view the affected thyroid trapped iodine normally but through lack of peroxidase enzyme could not form thyroid hormone in the normal way. A lack of this hormone in the foetus could prevent the normal development of the cochlea. The association should always be borne in mind in infant or neonatal cases of simple goitre.

Metabolic Disorders with Osseous Dystrophy or Dwarfism
Ocular-cerebro-renal Dystrophy—Lowe's Syndrome—Marinesco–Sjögren Syndrome.
A small group of babies with cataracts or hydrophthalmos having symptoms and signs at or near birth include the ocular-cerebro-renal dystrophies with which the name of Lowe is associated and the possibly related familial syndromes of oligophrenia, cerebellar ataxia, cataract and abnormal calcium metabolism of Marinesco–Sjögren.

Lowe and colleagues described three patients with hydrophthalmos, two of whom had congenital cataracts with gross nystagmus. All were hyperactive, although fat, with flabby muscles and diminished tendon reflexes. Mental development was severely retarded. All had episodes of high and unexplained fever and two had soft bones. Renal ammonia production was said to be diminished, plasma CO_2 and pH were low and there was marked organic-aciduria. Debré reported a 2½-year-old boy with the same syndrome of mental backwardness, 'rickets', cataract and hydrophthalmos, and with albuminuria, aminoaciduria, hyperchloraemic acidosis and deficient renal ammonia production. The rickets improved with Shohl's solution and calciferol. The parents, who were healthy and unrelated, had a general aminoaciduria.

Bickel and Thursby-Pelham included, among three cases of aminoaciduria, one boy noticed at 4 months to have bilateral cataracts, who later showed marked dwarfism, with peculiar jerky movements of his very hypotonic limbs and rickets evident clinically and radiologically.

McCance and colleagues describe two brothers, the only children of unrelated English parents who had had one female stillbirth. Both brothers showed marked anorexia from birth with poor weight gain. General hypotonia was present together with visual defect, corneal opacities, nystagmus and slow mental progress. One had convulsions and died at 3 years 10 months with evidence of renal failure and the second died at 8 months probably also of renal failure, but with an acute diarrhoea. At post-mortem there were structural abnormalities of the brain, calcification in the kidneys, many glomeruli being underdeveloped. Testes were absent. The bones were normal. The 'total CO_2' in the serum was very low, the sodium low-normal, potassium above normal, phosphorus normal, and urea rose from a high level (0·080 to 0·100 per cent) to a terminal 0·270 per cent. The urine in life had always been sterile and highly acid. The severe hyperchloraemic acidosis was associated with a very defective renal ammonia production.

Neurologists are familiar in older patients with the heredofamilial combination of congenital cataract, oligophrenia, cerebellar ataxia, small stature, bone defects and abnormal calcium metabolism. Marinesco (Sjögren, 1949–50) found four affected children in a family born to two normal Roumanian peasants. Their ten pregnancies had resulted in one stillbirth, three who died in infancy, two normal children and the four patients. All four were dwarfed, mentally defective, with failing vision and cataracts becoming apparent at 3 years of age. Three had old rickets, serum calcium being low in two. A low serum calcium level was found in the father and one unaffected sibling. Sjögren recognized some cases in Sweden and the combination of bilateral congenital cataract, idiocy and cerebellar ataxia, but makes no reference to urine or blood chemistry.

McCance regards Lowe's cases as having had renal tubular acidosis, and writes that 'there is no evidence that their kidneys could not have produced NH_3 in normal measure if there had been any way of putting them under test by making the urine acid'. Careful chemical studies are essential when a baby has hydrophthalmos, cataract, or a family history of these conditions and of any neurological disorder resembling Marinesco–Sjögren syndrome, so that treatment to limit or to prevent cerebral damage might become available. Inborn errors of metabolism, already identified in aural–renal syndromes with or without ocular changes, include prolinaemia and homocystinaemia.

Laurence–Moon–Biedl Syndrome
Laurence–Bardet Syndrome
Laurence and Moon in 1866 described a family in which non-consanguineous parents had ten children of whom four were affected by 'retinitis pigmentosa' accompanied by general imperfections of development. These were dwarfism, flabbiness and very small genitalia. Visual acuity was reduced to one-fifth, although visual fields were undiminished. The fully developed syndrome consists of obesity, hypogenitalism, mental retardation, and retinal pigmentation with night blindness. Polydactyly was added by Bardet in 1920. Many of the patients are short in stature.

Cockayne and Sorsby and their colleagues have contributed greatly to modern knowledge of the syndrome. They have shown that consanguinity in parents is not constant, that direct inheritance of the full syndrome is unknown, but that one or more of the components occur in ascendants of the sibships showing the full syndrome, and that incomplete syndromes are acceptable.

Polydactyly is the only recognizable sign present at birth, a condition widespread through the animal kingdom and all races of mankind. One or more extremities may be involved and the extra tissue ranges 'from a small fibrous skin clad nodule without a bony centre to a fully developed digit'. In some families syndactyly or brachydactyly with dystrophy of the second phalanx also occurs, and the lesions, which are not always symmetrical, may vary in type and situation within the one family.

Obesity develops in the first 2 years in some cases, and it is then that the retinal examination is usually made which shows the abnormal pigmentation. The date of onset of nystagmus, loss of visual acuity, night blindness and pigmentation is difficult to learn from the published reports. In the male, testicles are undescended, but in some cases both male and female, sexual maturity may be attained late, and normal children have been born to affected women. Polydipsia is found in some, and the affected members of Laurence's original family are said later to have become paraplegic. Internal frontal exostosis causing severe headache has been found in some affected adults.

A number of syndromes made up of the components of Laurence–Moon–Biedl syndrome have been reported.

Associated congenital defects include hydrocephalus, oxycephaly, ptosis, facial palsy and deaf-mutism.

Inheritance of the syndrome is due to a recessive autosomal gene, and Fraser Roberts thinks that the variation in the clinical picture results probably from incomplete penetrance, despite the rarity of this phenomenon.

Brachydactyly

An elaborate classification of brachydactyly into five types is given by J. Bell in the fifth volume of Karl Pearson's *Treasury of Human Inheritance* (1951). Fingers and/or toes may be affected and any of the phalanges may be small, deformed or absent. The thumb may be double or short and broad. Metacarpals or metatarsals may be short. Although often a dominant the isolated defect is a limited handicap only, but in some kindreds and some varieties there is an association with more serious defects. This has led to the creation of more and more eponymous syndromes.

With Macular Coloboma (Bell type B)

Sorsby has reported such a family, a mother and five children all affected. Two children, like the non-consanguineous father, were normal. Horizontal nystagmus was present in all patients, who could only just see to read. This is transmitted as a simple autosomal dominant.

With Cardiac Arrhythmia (Tabatznik Syndrome): Stub Thumb (Bell type D)

A short broad terminal phalanx of thumbs and great toes associated with cardiac arrhythmia has been described by Tabatznik (McKusick 1966).

With Mental Retardation and Mandibulo-facial Dysostosis (Rubinstein–Taybi Syndrome)
Stub thumbs with radial deviation of the terminal phalanx and broad flattened great toes occur in association with mental retardation, antimongoloid slant of palpebral fissures, a high-arched palate and a beaked nose producing a facies reminiscent of Hallermann–Strieff syndrome. The skull is small and the occiput flattened. Unusual dermal patterns which may be diagnostic have been described (Padfield *et al.* 1969).

With nail dysplasia (Bass Syndrome)
Bass has noted an association between hypoplastic nails on all fingers and both second toes and absent middle phalanges of all fingers and the lateral four toes. The distal phalanges of the thumbs were duplicated. Inheritance is autosomal dominant with complete expressivity.

Marchesani Syndrome
Dwarfism and glaucoma may be associated with brachydactyly in the Marchesani syndrome. In 1939 Marchesani reported four patients with brachydactyly, spherophakia and glaucoma. Rosenthal and Kloepfer described four further cases in 1956 and collected twenty-seven in the literature. The fingers are short and stubby, stature is dwarfed and mentality handicapped in many. A curved little finger and wide *a.t.d.* angle have been reported. The lens is small and light, easily dislocated by trauma, and the curvature of both surfaces increased. Glaucoma is common. The syndrome is inherited as a recessive, but heterozygous carriers may show the wide *a.t.d.* angle and are shorter than other members of the family. In two families the gene was dominant.

Holt Oram Syndrome
Holt and Oram (1960) described four patients with bizarre arrhythmias and atrial septal defects in a kindred in which four generations were affected. The thumbs were in the same plane as the fingers with the terminal phalanges turned inwards. The thumbs may be absent or have three phalanges. Inheritance is autosomal dominant.

Lipo-chondro-dystrophy
Gargoyle (dysostosis multiplex, Hunter–Hurler—Sanfillipo–Scheie)

Morquio–Ullrich—Mucopolysaccharidosis—Mucolipidosis—Fucosidosis.

The recognition of a 'gargoyle' in the early days or weeks of a baby's life is beyond the skill of most physicians, depending as it does on a facies and on a lumbar kyphosis noted usually when the baby begins to sit. Yet in this familial disease, parents of a previous affected baby claim to know that the next is also affected soon after it has been born.

The classical gargoyle has a heavy unprepossessing face, with eyes rather widely spaced, prominent supra-orbital ridges and sometimes ridges along the suture lines and round the fontanelles. The nose is broad and flat with little bridge, and the tongue is large. Commonly the nose runs intractably; dentition is delayed and irregular. The birth weight is expected to be normal but slows down later, and, if dwarfism is present, results from the spinal abnormalities rather than shortness of the limbs. When the baby sits up, and this may be delayed because of increasing mental retardation, the characteristic angular kyphosis is seen. The abdomen becomes distended with marked enlargement of liver and spleen. Additional features are corneal clouding and deafness. Typical x-ray changes include a large shallow sella turcica, vertebral bodies with convex upper and lower surfaces and anterior beaking, abnormalities of shape and texture of many of the bones, and coxa valga with long femoral necks.

The prognosis is bad, physical and mental growth are seriously affected and an early death is expected. Among thirty-nine cases in the literature Keith found that nineteen had a cardiac death. Progressive cardiac enlargement with a systolic murmur of increasing intensity is associated with fibrous nodules at the free edges of the mitral valve, swollen vacuolated cells in the connective tissue of all the cardiac layers, and narrowing of the coronary arteries. There is no association with congenital heart disease.

Herndon attempted in 1954 to clarify genetic inheritance in a study of 247 gargoyles. Twenty-one males with a clear-cut X-linked recessive inheritance were markedly deaf, none had corneal clouding and only one-third were dwarfed. Corneal clouding and dwarfism with little deafness characterized an autosomal recessive group of ninety-six which included all the families of consanguineous parents.

Leroy (1966) reviewing fifty patients with Hurler–Hunter syndrome separated them into four phenotypes. Hunter's name is given to the condition from which Herndon's X-linked group suffered while the classical autosomal recessive type is named for Hurler. In both, mucopolysaccharide accumulates in the reticulo-endothelial cells of liver, spleen and bone marrow; the urine contains excess acid mucopolysaccharide and the clinical appearance conforms. A third group with Sanfilippos syndrome shows these features, but visceral and skeletal lesions are outweighed by those in the central nervous system. Some present with infant feeding problems and may at first be diagnosed as suffering from cerebral palsy. A fourth type (of Scheie) is recognized in adult life by excess urinary acid mucopolysaccharide excretion, the presenting symptom being clouding of the cornea. One such patient is included among Leroy's 50 with 8 of Sanfilippo, 19 of Hunter and 22 of Hurler types. Attention is drawn to the laxity of ligaments and of fascia so that umbilical and inguinal hernias are common and tend to recur after radical operation.

In *Morquio's* disease the face and skull are little affected but the spine and chest are severely deformed, the thorax short and broad with forward protrusion of the sternum, kyphosis and scoliosis. Enlargement of the joints, poor muscles and lax ligaments contribute to a waddling gait. Mentality is unaffected. Bitter and his colleagues (1966) list the critical radiological bony changes.

Clinical descriptions intermediate between classical gargoyles and classical Morquio's syndrome, which is sometimes called Morquio–Brailsford syndrome, have raised the question of the relationships between these syndromes. The skeletal peculiarities which underlie these descriptions seem now usually to be associated with defects of lipid and mucopolysaccharide metabolism. Accurate clinical or even radiological classification is unlikely to be possible. Chemical understanding awaits the successful result of current studies of lipid synthesis, storing and degradation. Meanwhile enzyme chemists are busily identifying abnormal levels of activity in some lysosomal enzymes, notably glucosaminidase, galactosidase and glucuronidase, which give some support to the idea that in this group of diseases the fault lies in lysosomal accumulations of different lipids. Van Hoof and Hers (1968) have found by electron microscopy enlargement of liver lysosomes in Hurler's and intermediate syndromes. Levels of α-L fucosidase were greatly raised in some livers, but when absent, fucose accumulated in all tissues. The name fucosidosis is suggested for this variant.

Whether accumulation results from excessive synthesis, a block in degradation or in excretory pathways, or an avidity of certain tissues for a particular lipid, cannot yet be said.

The effects on the skeleton have been described above. The other more variable elements in the syndromes are corneal opacities, deafness, mental defect, peripheral neuritis, hepato-splenomegaly and cardiac involvement and their occurrence depends upon which of the organs and tissues form the sites for lipid accumulation.

In classical gargoyles and in the intermediate form of Morquio's syndrome, sometimes called Morquio–Ullrich syndrome, but not in Morquio–Brailsford syndrome, the urine contains large quantities of the mucopolysaccharides, chondroitin sulphate B and heparitin sulphate. Manley and Hawksworth (1966) have described a fairly simple turbidity test for excess urinary mucopolysaccharide and an electrophoretic test, staining with Alcian blue.

Other findings include metachromatic granules in the lymphocytes. Similar coarse inclusions in fibroblasts in some gargoyle-like children with normal acidmucopolysaccharide urinary excretion and normal lysosomal enzymes have been studied by Spranger and Wiedemann (1969) under the diagnosis of mucolipidosis.

Maroteaux and Lamy (1965) had previously suggested that at least five different varieties of osteochondrodystrophy could be distinguished. In time cranio-facial changes and corneal clouding are added to the classical skeletal abnormalities and all patients are regarded as having a form of mucopolysaccharidosis. Hurler and Hunter's syndrome patients excrete chondroitin sulphate B and heparitin sulphate. Children with polydystrophic oligophrenia (which includes Sanfilippo's syndrome) excrete heparitin sulphate while those with polydystrophic dwarfism, excreting chondroitin sulphate B, seem to suffer from a variant of Hurler's disease. The fifth type, Morquio's disease, is regarded as a mucopolysaccharidosis excreting keratosulphate, although the authors mention one family with negative urine.

Should the view prove correct that it is specific inherited enzyme defects that interfere with lipid and mucopolysaccharide metabolism, the present clinical, radiological and biochemical tangles should cease to bedevil classification. New relationships are likely also to be established among a number of 'storage' diseases including Gaucher's, Tay–Sachs', Niemann–Pick's and Fabry's disease and metachromatic leukodystrophy.

Cornelia de Lange Syndrome
Typus Degenerativus Amstelodamensis
This form of severe mental retardation, first described in 1933, has

recently been reviewed by Schlesinger (1963). A characteristic facies has some resemblance to gargoylism, with bushy eyebrows, a low forehead, the nostrils tilted upwards with a long philtrum, low-set ears, an antimongoloid slant of palpebral fissure, a short neck and a low hair-line. The upper limbs are short with limitation of extension at the elbows. Defective hand development is common, the thumbs arising proximally. Congenital heart disease is associated. Aetiology is unknown, but may be by a dominant mutant. Falek (1966) has described the finding of an apparent translocation of the major portion of G chromosome on to A3 in a kindred including four affected children, all of whom had seizures, one normal parent and several immediate relatives. Opitz (1966) disputes the proposition that de Lange syndrome is a chromosomal disorder on the ground that fifty undoubted patients have a normal cytology.

Leprechaunism

Donohue in 1948 described under the title Dysendocrinism, a curious-looking female infant who died of an acute respiratory infection at $7\frac{1}{2}$ weeks. She was the first child of consanguineous parents who after two abortions had a normal girl, a normal boy, a miscarriage and then a second girl, similar in appearance to their first, who died at 10 weeks.

Summarizing their findings in the two siblings Donohue and Uchida suggested the name leprechaunism for a syndrome with these features: apparent cessation of foetal growth at 7 months; muscle wasting, emaciation and failure of neonatal growth; a typical elfin facies, the eyes widely spaced and prominent, the ears large and much fine hair on the face; enlargement of breasts and of clitoris; cystic enlargement of ovaries, islet cell hyperplasia in the pancreas, and abnormal histology of the thymus; normal adrenals; hypertrophy and calcification in the kidneys; foamy vacuolated cells and increased glycogen in the liver, which contains excess iron; multiple subcutaneous abscesses (possibly a chance complication).

Evans later reported two cases, both girls, one at least of whom sufficiently resembled Donohue's cases to justify the diagnosis. The second case had large ears, mammary enlargement which disappeared after methyltestosterone treatment, increased liver glycogen, large cystic ovaries and decreased bone age. Birth weight had been normal, she was thin but not wasted, the facies did not fit Donohue's description, and she was $2\frac{3}{4}$ years of age.

Discussing these cases Evans suggests that in leprechaunism there are congenital abnormalities of face, ears and ovaries, with excess oestrogen production. This causes hyperplasia of nipples, clitoris and labia minora, with slight increase in 17-ketosteroid excretion. A resulting decrease in pituitary growth hormone leads to wasting of soft tissues, delayed bone growth, increased insulin production and lack of response to hypoglycaemia.

Low Birthweight Dwarfism
Silver's and Russell's syndrome.
Dysmature and small-for-dates babies have been studied extensively because of their extra hazards, their perinatal morbidity and their liability to neurological disturbance. Exact definition of this state is difficult but for a term baby, a birthweight of 2·5 kg is highly suspicious, while a weight of 2·0 kg or less is diagnostic. Silver in 1953 noted a special facies in two low-birth-weight babies who showed asymmetry in the size of the limbs and who remained dwarfed. Russell in 1954 reported five such babies, some but not all with asymmetry. The face is triangular with a hypoplastic mandible at the apex, the philtrum of the upper lip is drawn upwards, the lips forming an inverted U. The nose is beaked and the bridge well-developed, merging into a prominent metopic suture. The chest is narrow and tubular, there is cubitus varus, incurved fifth fingers, some have short upper limbs. There are low values of subcutaneous fat and a relative lack of muscle. Syndactyly and *café-au-lait* skin patches have also been found. Chromosomes are normal, sex incidence equal, intelligence normal.

Some observers regard these two syndromes as essentially one. Tanner and Ham (1969) prefer to separate Silver's from Russell's syndrome on the basis of asymmetry of the limbs. Out of five of their six children with Silver's syndrome, assayed for growth hormone, one only was low. Two responded to growth hormone treatment.

Willi-Prader-Laurance Syndrome
Hypotonia, cryptorchidism, dwarfism, obesity, mental retardation and diabetes.
In 1956 Prader, Willi and their colleagues described some Swiss children who resembled each other in appearance and shared the abnormalities listed above. By 1961 fourteen Swiss children were known and Laurance reported six in England. The parents were non-consanguineous and, like

the siblings, healthy. The babies are floppy at birth and the males show very small external genitalia with small or impalpable testicles. Sucking is poor and general progress slow. Obesity is apparent at 3 or 4 years of age. Scoliosis affects some. Diabetes mellitus appears clinically in the second decade. No specific test is known, nor any treatment. The diagnosis should be considered in infancy when the baby is thought to be floppy or to have Werdnig–Hoffman's progressive spinal muscular atrophy. Chromosomes are normal and there is no evidence of genetic determination.

Familial Dysautonomia
Riley, Day and others in 1949 described five cases where defective lachrymation was observed in five children who showed symptoms of central autonomic dysfunction such as excessive sweating and salivation, and unstable blood pressure, rising particularly with anxiety. Symmetrical erythematous patches of variable duration appeared on the skin. One had presented a feeding problem from birth, one began with acute respiratory disease at 3 months and another with vomiting at 6 months. All were Jewish. In a second paper inheritance as an autosomal recessive was established and a study of the forty-eight known cases revealed significant dwarfing, postural hypotension with a fall of 10 to 60 mm Hg in systolic blood pressure from supine to erect position, variable neurological abnormalities including disturbed speech, deterioration in psychological test results over the years and inadequate adjustment to daily life. Other symptoms include cyclic vomiting, swallowing difficulty, recurrent bouts of respiratory infection, exaggerated fever, dehydration associated with excessive sweating and salivation, and a tendency to corneal ulceration and exposure keratitis from corneal hypaesthesia and defective lachrymation. In Liebman's case renal pelves and ureters were duplicated.

The majority of cases are Jewish, but one affected family are Quakers who go back ten generations on both sides. The diagnosis should be considered when there is absence of tears in an infant with swallowing difficulty, who presents a genuine feeding problem. A drop of 2·5 per cent methacholine produces conjunctival injection and rapid constriction of the pupil (confirmatory not pathognomonic).

Möbius Syndrome
Nuclear Agenesis—Congenital Facial Diplegia

Unilateral facial palsy is common as a temporary finding in the newborn, usually explained by intrapartum pressure on the facial nerve. Sometimes the face and the external ear appear deformed and squashed by the shoulder. Occasionally the palsy persists, and when there are other congenital abnormalities and especially when the facial palsy is bilateral, the diagnosis of Möbius syndrome becomes likely.

The essential features are: (1) unilateral or bilateral complete or incomplete facial weakness; (2) unilateral or bilateral loss of abduction of the eyes; (3) congenital anomalies of the extremities; additional possibilities are: (4) involvement of brachial musculature; and (5) other cranial nerve palsies.

Clinically the presence of bilateral facial palsy may escape notice in the early days, but careful observation of the face of a baby who is difficult to feed may show a lack of or a mask-like expression on crying and an incomplete closure of the eyelids in sleep. An abducens palsy also is difficult to identify at first. After a few months the expressionless face without a smile or a laugh and convergent strabismus which prevents the eyes from following a moving object are all too obvious, raising the fear of brain damage with mental retardation. Micrognathia, wasting of the tongue and web-neck with abnormalities of the cervical vertebrae (Klippel–Feil) are sometimes present. The limbs are affected at their distal extremities, the typical lesions being syndactyly, talipes and absence of some or all of the phalanges of hands or feet.

The peri-oral muscles are less affected than those round the eye, and in the course of years some improvement in both groups takes place. Aplasia or hypoplasia of the relevant muscles and of the nerves and muscles connected therewith has been established. Henderson reviewing sixty-one cases of facial diplegia found the sexes equally affected. In four instances two or more members of a family were affected. Six cases were diagnosed as mentally defective.

The possible mechanisms causing a combination of nuclear agenesis and distal lesions of the extremities are well discussed by Evans. Evans, sceptical of the idea of a primary nuclear agenesis, suggests that there may be some interference with the development of the muscles of the mandibular and hyoid arches. An interrelationship between muscles and nerve development has been demonstrated in arthrogryposis multiplex congenita by Fowler and J. R. Moore has suggested that Möbius syndrome may be a form of arthrogryposis limited to the muscles of the face (Richards 1953).

Sturge–Weber Syndrome
Encephalo-facial Angiomatosis
The characteristics of this syndrome are well known. First there is a simple naevus flammeus or red staining of the skin of the face, roughly in the area of distribution of the trigeminal nerve, always affecting the eyelids but extending on to the forehead or scalp or down on to the cheek and upper lip, usually unilateral, sometimes just crossing the midline, and sometimes affecting both sides of the face. Under this area there may be a thin mesh of veins, a meningeal angiomatosis, but this occurs only when the facial naevus involves the upper eyelid and/or the supra-orbital regions. The conjunctiva and the sclerotic may also be affected. Increased intra-ocular tension (buphthalmos) is found in many, including that originally reported by Sturge in 1879.

The naevus flammeus of characteristic distribution, and the buphthalmos (when present), are evident at birth. In the course of time other changes follow. Convulsions begin at a few months, are hemiplegic and lead to hemiparesis on the side opposite to the naevus. Mental development slows. At a later stage, and only exceptionally before the second year, the classical double-contoured gyriform shadows of cortical calcification are seen in x-rays of the skull. Later still, careful study reveals an homonymous hemianopia. Electro-encephalography shows electrical inactivity over the affected areas.

The condition is not familial and affects the sexes equally.

G. L. Alexander and R. M. Norman in their monograph have produced data which call for a reorientation of outlook by physicians in charge of early cases. There is good reason to believe that the epilepsy, the hemiplegia and the mental retardation which often appear in time in the natural evolution of the disease, are, at least in some cases, secondary and therefore perhaps preventable. They should no longer be regarded as essential to the diagnosis of the syndrome and for this reason the name of encephalo-facial angiomatosis approved by Parkes Weber is to be preferred.

Norman's careful histological studies suggest a progressive accumulation of calcium in the outer cortical layers not obviously related to the blood vessels. Cyanosis can be seen in the angiomatous areas at exploration and would be expected to affect tissue metabolism adversely. The increasing concretions may obliterate part of the capillary bed. There are also areas of 'neuronal devastation and gliosis' due to acute ischaemia, and if these are caused by the fits, preventive treatment, both medical and surgical, needs to be most carefully considered, especially as the angiomatous lesion seems highly epileptogenic. These studies suggest also that the typical stunted growth of the affected hemisphere is not due to prenatal malformation but rather to the effect of the vascular

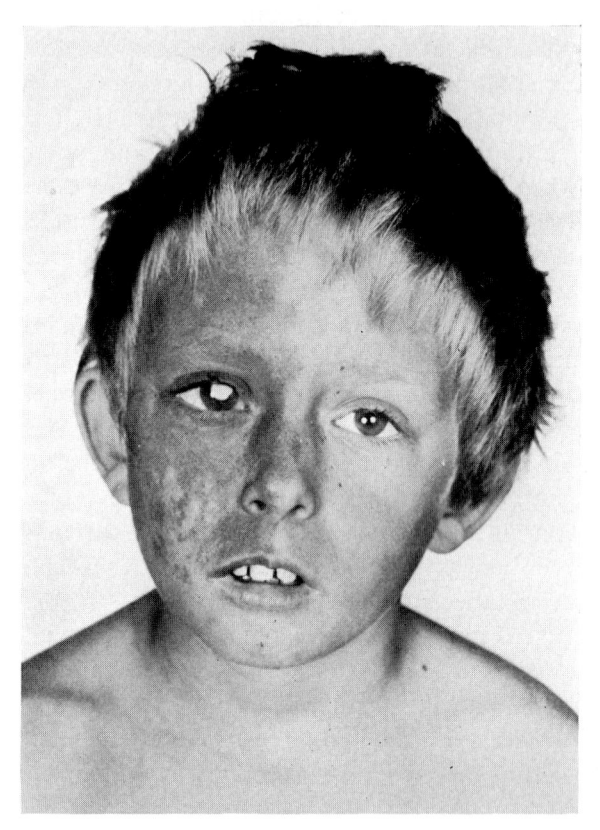

FIG. 10.2. Sturge–Weber syndrome. Capillary naevus in infracranial involvement—supra-orbital distribution is almost pathogenic. Eye involvement not rare.

anomaly. Alexander recommends confirming the meningeal involvement by exposure of a limited part of the cortex posteriorly of any infant exhibiting a naevus flammeus affecting the supra-ocular part of the face on one side. This must be done before the first fit, which may mean before the age of 3 months. He considers hemispherectomy to be too drastic a procedure and prefers selective lobectomy of affected areas.

Unfortunately dogmatism about the timing and the extent of surgical excision is not justified.

Tuberous Sclerosis
Epiloia, Bourneville's disease.
The classical triad making up this syndrome consists of adenoma sebaceum, seizures and mental handicap. The two latter are unlikely to be apparent at birth, but may become so during the first few months of infancy in association with depigmented patches in the skin. Such early evidence as there is depends on the presence of multiple 'adenomatas' which may be found in any organ or in the skin. Rhabdomyomas may affect the heart leading to cardiac enlargement and death. Bilateral enlargement of the kidneys has been found in the newborn; small whitish or grey nodules can be seen in the retina, and retinal haemorrhage and glaucoma may occur. Nodular growths in brain, responsible for convulsions, vary in size from a few millimetres to several centimetres, their dense fibrous matrix giving a cartilaginous consistency. Similar lesions are found in the spinal cord. The skin lesions include typical adenoma sebaceum in a butterfly area over the nose and cheeks, vitiligo, *café-au-lait* patches and a cuirass of thickened scaly, shagreen skin over the sternum. Incidence is estimated as 1 in 30,000 births and inheritance is autosomal dominant.

Thalidomide Syndrome
'The malformations that may be found in the extremities are legion', writes Potter, and some, for example polydactyly and syndactyly, have already been described. Their association with other and distant congenital defects as well as positive family studies strongly support a genetic origin. To argue on this account against environmental factors acting on the foetus would be foolhardy, and there is a strong probability that intra-uterine amputations through the amniotic coverings do occur. When they do, the circumstances must be exceptional, for it is inconceivable that the complex abnormalities described could be due to a process so direct and so simple. The named varieties are: amelia (totally absent limbs), ectromelia (total absence of a limb), micromelia (abnormally short limbs), phocomelia (small hands and feet attached to the trunk by a small single bone), hemimelia (normal proximal part with rudimentary distal part).

During 1961 and 1962 an alarming increase in severe malformation of the extremities, especially in Western Germany, led Lenz to suspect that a new popular and excellent tranquillizer and anti-emetic was responsible. It is now accepted that thalidomide (distaval, contergan) acting especially between the twenty-eighth and the forty-second days, even in a single dose can produce a devastating effect on the foetus. Phocomelia is the commonest result, usually bilateral and often symmetrical. The proximal parts of the limbs are the worst affected and may be absent. Radius, thumbs and some digits may be absent, and syndactyly and polydactyly occur. Malformed hips, various types of talipes and severe wrist deformities are common. The spine has been affected. Congenital anomalies also involve heart, urogenital and alimentary tracts. Some children have only microtia or congenital absence of the ear. A flat capillary naevus on the forehead, upper lip and tip of the nose with a flattened broad bridge gives a recognizable facies. Intelligence is unaffected. Perceptive deafness is not uncommon.

As in other instances of severe congenital deformities, it is essential that the parents should receive all the support and encouragement possible. Management of the affected child begins with as complete an assessment as possible of all the defects. Treatment should then be planned with the purpose of helping the child to develop its potentialities as far as possible and to achieve the maximum independence. This will call for the co-operation of paediatrician, orthopaedic surgeon, physiotherapist and limb-fitting centre.

The production of limb defects has been reported in newborn and stillborn rabbits after oral doses of thalidomide had been given to female rabbits daily from the eighth to the sixteenth day of pregnancy. It is said that similar defects have not been known to occur spontaneously.

It is not without interest that ectromelia has previously been attributed to the effect of maternal vitamin deficiency, nitrogen mustard, nucleic acid antagonists, carbon-monoxide poisoning and attempted suicide in early pregnancy.

Severe 'reduction deformities' of the limbs are still encountered in small numbers, but the 'epidemic' followed exactly the sale and distribution of thalidomide.

The thalidomide epidemic has focused attention on the possible dangers of drugs given to pregnant women, although unfortunately damage can be done before the woman knows that she is pregnant. It has also awakened the public conscience to the difficulties both physical and emotional associated with the birth of handicapped babies. The dangers of withholding information from parents, pretending that the baby has died and not allowing the mother to see her baby have all been highlighted. The one good result of what was otherwise an unrelieved tragedy has been the stimulation to greater and more appropriate efforts of all those, medical and lay, concerned with the supervision and care of the handicapped.

CONCLUSION

The object of a review of syndromes is to help in revealing abnormalities that would otherwise be concealed because unexpected. Clinical acumen is sharpened, special examinations made, laboratory tests performed. To some extent the future can be foretold and, not least, the risks of problems in future children can be assessed.

In certain circumstances other features of the history, besides the obvious one of hereditary or familial disorder, can put the doctor on his guard. Hydramnios is commonly present in congenital anomalies, particularly those causing oesophageal, duodenal or high intestinal obstruction. The congenital absence of one umbilical artery should also arouse suspicion. Benirschke and Bourne examining 1500 placentas found a single umbilical artery fifteen times, seven of the babies having some congenital anomaly. Perinatal autopsies show a higher association, since many of the anomalies, for example sirenomelia, are incompatible with survival.

The occurrence of maternal rubella in the first trimester, and perhaps vaccinia during the same period, increases the congenital malformation rate, as well as increasing the risk of miscarriage and still birth.

Testosterone-treated mothers have produced female pseudohermaphrodites, and thalidomide (Distaval)-induced deformities have been described. Large doses of x-rays for treatment may produce microcephaly; while relatively small diagnostic exposure of the whole foetus does increase somewhat the risk of leukaemia.

This gathering experience stresses the vulnerability of the foetus especially during the highly active organogenesis of the fourth to the twelfth weeks. This ought to lead doctors to the utmost caution in the use of drugs during pregnancy. Nevertheless it would be unwise to assume that these risks are evenly spread and that genetic or enzyme defects are not waiting to be exploited by these subtle forms of trauma. Certainly a review of the commoner syndromes can only serve to accentuate the importance of genetic constitution.

SELECTED REFERENCES

ALDRICH R.A., STEINBERG A.G. & CAMPBELL D.C. (1954) Pedigree demonstrating a sex-linked recessive condition characterized by draining ears, eczematoid dermatitis and bloody diarrhoea. *Pediatrics* **13**, 133

ALEXANDER G.L. (1961) The surgical treatment of Sturge-Weber syndrome, in *Hemiplegic Cerebral Palsy in Children and Adults*, Little Club Clinics No. 4, 138

ALEXANDER G.L. & NORMAN R.M. (1960) *The Sturge-Weber Syndrome*. Bristol: John Wright

APERT E. (1907) *Traité de Maladies Familiales et Maladies Congénitales*. Paris: Baillière.

BASS H.N. (1968) Familial absence of middle phalanges with nail dysplasia. *Pediatrics* **42**, 318

BAUMAN G.I. (1932) Absence of the cervical spine Klippel-Feil syndrome. *J. Amer. med. Ass.* **98**, 129

BEAUTYMAN W. (1951) A case of Fanconi's anaemia. *Arch. Dis. Childh.* **26**, 238

BENIRSCHKE K. & BOURNE G.L. (1960) The incidence and prognostic implication of congenital absence of one umbilical artery. *Amer. J. Obst. Gynec.* **79**, 251

BENJAMIN E. (1912) Über eine selbständige Form der Anamie im frühen Kindesalter. *Verh. Ges. Kinderheilk.* **28**, 119

BICKEL H. & THURSBY-PELHAM D.C. (1954) Hyperamino-aciduria in Lignac-Fanconi disease, in galactosaemia and in an obscure syndrome. *Arch. Dis. Childh.* **29**, 224

BITTER T., MUIR H., MITTWOEK V. & SCOTT J.D. (1966) Contribution to the differential diagnosis of Hurler's disease and forms of Morquio's syndrome. *J. Bone Jt. Surg.* **433**, 637

BRAIN, W. RUSSELL (1926) Heredity in simple goitre. *Quart. J. Med.* **20**, 303

COCKAYNE E.A., KRESTIN D. & SORSBY A. (1935) The Laurence-Moon Biedl syndrome. *Quart. J. Med.* **4**, 93

COLLINS E. TREACHER (1900) Case with symmetrical notches in the outer part of each lower lid and defective development of the malar bones. *Trans. Ophthalmol. Soc.* **20**, 190

CROUZON O. (1912) Dysostose cranio-faciale héréditaire. *Bull. Soc. Med. Hôp. Paris* **33**, 545

DEBRÉ R., ROYER P. & LESTRADET H. (1952) L'insuffisance tubulaire congénitale avec arrieration mentale, cataracte et glaucome. *Arch. franc. Pediat.* **12**, 337

DONOHUE W.L. & UCHIDA I. (1954) Leprechaunism. *J. Pediat.* **45**, 505

EAGLE J.F. & BARRETT G.S. (1950) Congenital deficiency of abdominal musculature; A syndrome with associated genito-urinary anomalies. *Pediatrics* **6**, 721

EMERY J.L., GORDON R.R., RENDLE-SHORT J., VARADI S. & WARRACH A.J.N. (1957) Congenital amegakaryocytic thrombocytopenia with congenital deformities and a leukemoid blood picture in the newborn. *Blood* **12**, 567

EVANS P.R. (1955) Leprechaunism. *Arch. Dis. Childh.* **30**, 479

EVANS P.R. (1955) Nuclear agenesis; Möbius' syndrome; the congenital facial diplegia syndrome. *Arch. Dis. Childh.* **30**, 237

FAIRBANK SIR T. (1951) *An Atlas of General Affections of the Skeleton*. Edinburgh: Livingstone.

FALEK A., SCHMIDT R. & GERVIS G.A. (1966) Familial de Lange syndrome with chromosome abnormalities. *Pediatrics* **37**, 92

FALLS H.F. & SCHULL W.J. (1960) Hallermann–Strieff syndrome, a dyscephaly with congenital cataracts and hypotrichosis. *Arch. Ophthalmol.* **63,** 409

FISCH L. (1959) Deafness as part of an hereditary syndrome. *J. Laryng.* **73,** 355

FRANCESCHETTI, A. & KLEIN D. (1949) The mandibulo-facial dysostosis; a new hereditary syndrome. *Acta ophthal.* **27,** 141

FRANCESCHETTI A. & ZWAHLEN P. (1944) Un syndrome nouveau; la dysostose mandibulo-faciale. *Bull. Acad. Suisse Sci. Med.* **1,** 60

FRANKLIN A.W. (1956) Two cases of haemangio-endothelioma with haemorrhage, thrombocytopenia and bone changes. *Proc. Roy. Soc. Med.* **49,** 595

FRASER G.R., MORGAN M.E. & TROTTER W.R. (1961) Sporadic goitre with congenital deafness (Pendred's syndrome). *Trans. IV Internat. goitre Conference,* p. 19. Pergamon Press

FRASER ROBERTS J.A. (1959) *An Introduction to Medical Genetics,* 2nd edn. London: O.U.P.

FULFORD G.E. (1956) Aglossia congenita. *Arch. Dis. Childh.* **31,** 400

GIEDION A. (1968) Thanatophoric dwarfism. *Helvet. Paediat. Acta* **23,** 175

GILMOUR J.R. (1941) The essential identity of the Klippel–Feil syndrome and iniencephaly. *J. Path. Bact.* **53,** 117

GILMOUR J.R. (1946) Amyoplasia congenita. *J. Path. Bact.* **58,** 675

GORDON R.R. (1960) Aldrich's syndrome: familial thrombocytopenia, eczema and infection. *Arch. Dis. Childh.* **35,** 259

GREIG D.M. (1924) Hypertelorism. *Edin. Med. J.* **31,** 560

HENDERSON J.L. (1939) The congenital facial diplegia syndrome: clinical features, pathology and aetiology (61 cases). *Brain* **62,** 381

HERNDON C.N. (1954) Gargoylism. *Res. Publ. Ass. nerv. ment. Dis.* **33,** 251

HILSON D. (1957) Malformation of ears as sign of malformation of genito-urinary tract. *Brit. med. J.* **2,** 785

HOLT M. & OZAM S. (1960) Familial heart disease with skeletal malformations. *Brit. Heart J.* **22,** 236

HÖVELS O. (1953) Zur Systematik der Misbildungen des 1. Visceralbogens unter besondere Berücksichtigung der Dysostosis mandibulo-facialis. *Z. Kinderheilk.* **73,** 532 and 568

HUNTER C. (1917) A rare disease in two brothers. *Proc. Roy. Soc. Med.* **10,** 104

KASABACH H.H. & MERRITT K.K. (1940) Caphillary emangioma with extensive purpura. *Amer. J. Dis. Child.* **59,** 1063

KAUFMAN R.L., RIMION D.L., MCALISTER W.H. & KISSANE J.M. (1970) Thanatophoric dwarfism. *Amer. J. Dis. Child.* **120,** 53

KEITH J.D., ROWE R.D. & VEAD P. (1958) *Heart Disease in Infancy and Childhood.* New York: Macmillan

KLIPPEL M. & FEIL A. (1912) Anomalie de la colonne vertebrale par absence des vertebres cervicales—Cage thoracique remontant jusqu'a la base du crâne. *Bull. Soc. anat. Paris* **14,** 185

KOSTMANN R. (1956) Infantile genetic agranulocytosis. *Acta Paediat. Scandinavica* **45,** supp. 105

LAURANCE B.M. (1967) Hypotonia, mental retardation, obesity, and cryptorchidism associated with dwarfism and diabetes in children. *Arch. Dis. Childh.* **42,** 126

LAURENCE J.Z. & MOON R.C. (1866) Four cases of 'retinitis pigmentosa' occurring in the same family, and accompanied by general imperfections of development. *Ophthal. Rev.* **2,** 32

LENZ W. (1961) Kindliche Misbildungen nach Medikamenteinnahme während der Gravidität? *Dtsch. med. Wschr.* **86,** 2555

LEROY J.G. & CROCKER A.C. (1966) Clinical definitions of the Hurler–Hunter phenotypes. *Amer. J. Dis. Child.* **112,** 518

LIEBMAN S.D. (1956) Ocular manifestations of Riley–Day syndrome, familial autonomic dysfunction. *Arch. Ophthal.* **56,** 719

LOWE C.U., TERREY M. & MACLACHLAN E.A. (1952) Organic-aciduria, decreased renal ammonia production, hydrophthalmos, and mental retardation. *Amer. J. Dis. Child.* **83,** 164

MANLEY G., HAWKSWORTH J. (1966) Diagnosis of Hurler's syndrome. *Arch. Dis. Childh.* **41,** 91

MARIN O.S.M. & TYLER H.R. (1961) Hereditary interstitial nephritis associated with polyneuropathy. *Neurology* **11,** 999

MAROTEAUX P. & LAMY M. (1965) Hurler's disease; Morquio's disease. *J. Pediat.* **67,** 312

MCCANCE R.A., MATHESON W.J., GRESHAM G.A. & ELKINGTON I.R. (1960) The cerebro-ocular-renal dystrophies: a new variant. *Arch. Dis. Childh.* **35,** 240

MCCUSICK V.A. (1966) *Mendelian Inheritance in Man*, p. 17. London: Heinemann

MCKENZIE J. (1958) Aetiology and treatment of congenital deaf mutism. *Brit. Med. J.* **2,** 201

MCKENZIE J. & CRAIG J. (1955) Mandibulo-facial dysostosis (Treacher Collins syndrome). *Arch. Dis. Childh.* **30,** 391

NAGER F.R. & DE REYNIER J.P. (1948) Dyscephalies associated with involvement of ears. *Practica Otorhinolaryngol.* **10,** Supp. 2

NORMAN R.M. (1958) Chapter 5 in *Neuropathology*, by J.G. Greenfield *et al.* London: Arnold

OPITZ J.M. (1966) de Lange syndrome. *Pediatrics* **37,** 1028

PADFIELD C.J., PARTINGTON M.W. & SIMPSON N.E. (1968) Rubinstein–Taybi syndrome. *Arch. Dis. Childh.* **43,** 94

PARK E.A. & POWERS G.F. (1920) Acrocephaly and scaphocephaly with symmetrically distributed malformations of the extremities: a study of the so-called 'acrocephalosyndactylism'. *Amer. J. Dis. Child.* **20,** 235

PENDRED V. (1896) Deaf mutism and goitre. *Lancet* **2,** 532

POTTER E.L. (1946) Bilateral renal agenesis. *J. Pediat.* **29,** 68

POTTER E.L. (1952) *Pathology of the Fetus and the Newborn.* Chicago: Year Book Publishers

REINHOLD J.D.L., NEWMARK E., LIGHTWOOD R. & CARTER C.O. (1952) Familial hypoplastic anaemia with congenital abnormalities (Fanconi's syndrome). *Blood* **7,** 915

RICHARDS R.N. (1953) The Möbius syndrome. *J. Bone Jt. Surg.* **35A,** 437

RILEY C.M., DAY R.L., GREELEY D.McL. & LANGFORD W.S. (1949) Central autonomic dysfunction with defective lacrimation. *Pediatrics* **3,** 468

ROBIN E.D. & GARDNER F.H. (1957) Hereditary factors in chronic Bright's disease—a study of two affected kindreds. *Trans. Ass. Amer. Phys.* **70,** 140

ROBIN P. (1934) Glossoptosis due to atresia and hypotrophy of the mandible. *Amer. J. Dis. Child.* **48,** 541

ROSENTHAL J.W. & KLOEPFER H.W. (1956) Spherophakia-Brachymorphia syndrome. *Arch. Ophthal.* **55,** 28

RUSSELL A. (1954) A syndrome of 'intra-uterine' dwarfism recognizable at birth (5 cases). *Proc. Roy. Soc. Med.* **47,** 1040

SCHAFFER A.F. (1960) *Diseases of the Newborn.* Philadelphia: Saunders
SCHLESINGER B., CLAYTON B., BODIAN M. & JONES E.V. (1963) Typus degen. amsteledamensis. *Arch. Dis. Childh.* **38**, 349
SELIGMAN S.A. (1961) Ectromelia. *Arch. Dis. Childh.* **36**, 658
SILVER H.K., KIYASU W., GEORGE J. & DEAMER W.C. (1953) Syndrome of congenital hemihypertrophy, shortness of stature and elevated urinary gonadotropins. *Pediatrics* **12**, 368
SINCLAIR R.J.G., KITCHIN A.H. & TURNER R.W.D. (1960) The Marfan syndrome. *Quart. J. Med.* **29**, 19
SJÖGREN T. (1947) Hereditary congenital spinocerebellar ataxia combined with cataract and oligophrenia. *Acta Psychiat.* Supp. **46**, 286
SMARS G. (1961) *Osteogenesis Imperfecta in Sweden.* Stockholm: Svenska
SOHAR, E. (1954) Renal disease, inner ear deafness, ocular changes. *Harefuah* **47**, 161
SOMERS G.F. (1962) Thalidomide and congenital abnormalities. *Lancet* **1**, 912
SORSBY A. (1935) Congenital coloboma of the macula. *Brit. J. Ophthal.* **19**, 65
SORSBY A., AVERY H. & COCKAYNE E.A. (1939) Obesity, hypogenitalism, mental retardation, polydactyly and retinal pigmentation. The Laurence-Moon-Biedl syndrome. *Quart. J. Med.* **8**, 51
SPIERS A.L. (1962) Thalidomide and congenital abnormalities. *Lancet* **1**, 303
SPRANGER I., WIEDEMANN H.R. (1969) Lipomucopolysaccharidosis; a second look. *Lancet* **2**, 270
STURGE W.A. (1879) A case of partial epilepsy, apparently due to a lesion of one of the vaso-motor centres of the brain. *Trans. Clin. Soc.* **12**, 162
TANNER J. & HAM T.J. (1969) Low birth weight dwarfs with asymmetry (Silver's syndrome): treatment with human growth hormone. *Arch. Dis. Childh.* **44**, 231
THOULD A.K. & SCOWEN E.F. (1961) The syndrome of congenital deafness and simple goitre. *Trans. IV Internat. Goitre Conf.*, p. 22. Pergamon Press
VAN HOOF F. & HERS H.G. (1968) The abnormalities of lysosomal enzymes in mucopolysaccharidoses. *European J. Biochem.* **7**, 34
WAARDENBURG P.J., FRANCESCHETTI A. & KLEIN D. (1961) *Genetics and Ophthalmology*, Oxford: Blackwell vol. 1, p. 386
WILLIAMSON D.A.J. (1961) Alport's syndrome of hereditary nephritis with deafness. *Lancet* **2**, 1321

II

Syndromes due to Chromosomal Abnormalities

A. P. NORMAN

The rapid and very recent increase in knowledge of chromosomal anomalies has made it possible to introduce some order into an account of the various clinical syndromes for which these are responsible. However, as Polani points out, whilst the majority of cases of a syndrome may show a given type of chromosomal change, others clinically indistinguishable may be caused by chromosomal changes of a different type. Further, a simple classification of autosomal anomalies by errors of number and errors of structure is not entirely satisfactory when dealing with the clinical aspects of these syndromes.

1. Klinefelters syndrome:
   a. XXY
   b. XXXY
   c. XXXXY
   d. XXYY
   e. XXY mosaics
   f. XX males
2. Turner's syndrome XO (or XXq)
3. XXX females
4. XXXX females
5. XY females; testicular feminisation syndrome
6. XYY males

FIG. 11.1. Sex chromosome abnormalities

The classification used in this chapter is based on that of Race and Sanger for sex chromosome anomalies (Fig. 11.1) and of Polani for autosomal anomalies (Fig. 11.2), both adapted from the first number of the *British Medical Bulletin* of 1969.

No attempt is made in the following pages to explain the way in

A. **Mainly numerical**
1. Down's syndrome
2. Patau's syndrome
3. Edward's syndrome
4. Other autosomal trisomies
5. Triploidy
6. In spontaneous abortion

B. **Mainly structural**
1. Deletions and duplications
2. Ring chromosomes

FIG. 11.2. Autosome anomalies.

which chromosomal anomalies can occur as this has already been done in the first chapter of this book, but a brief explanation of the symbolic designations used for the various karyotypes is given in Fig. 11.3.

	Examples
47, XY, G+	47 chromosomes XY sex chromosomes in G group, additional chromosome
46, XY inv (p+ q−)	46 chromosomes one X chromosomes normal one Y chromosomes with short arm longer than normal and long arm shorter than normal (the change being interpreted as a pericentric inversion)
45, XX, D−, G−(Dq Gq) +	45 chromosomes XX sex chromosomes D group one chromosome absent G group one chromosome absent Extra chromosome present formed from long arms of a D and of a G group chromosome
45, X/46XX/47, XXX	Mosaic with 3 cell lines containing one, two and three X chromosomes respectively.

FIG. 11.3. Symbolic designation of human karyotypes (adapted from (1969) *Brit. med. Bulletin* **21**, based on a system published in Conference on Standardization in Human Cytogenetics, Chicago 1966, published by National Foundation, New York).

Descriptions of the cytology have been kept to a minimum and accounts of the various genotypic possibilities greatly condensed on the understanding that the object is primarily to present a description of the clinical syndromes, organized on a basis of the known chromosomal changes. Conditions in which only a single or occasional finding of chromosomal abnormality have been reported, or syndromes which have been suggested on the recognition of very few cases, have been entirely omitted.

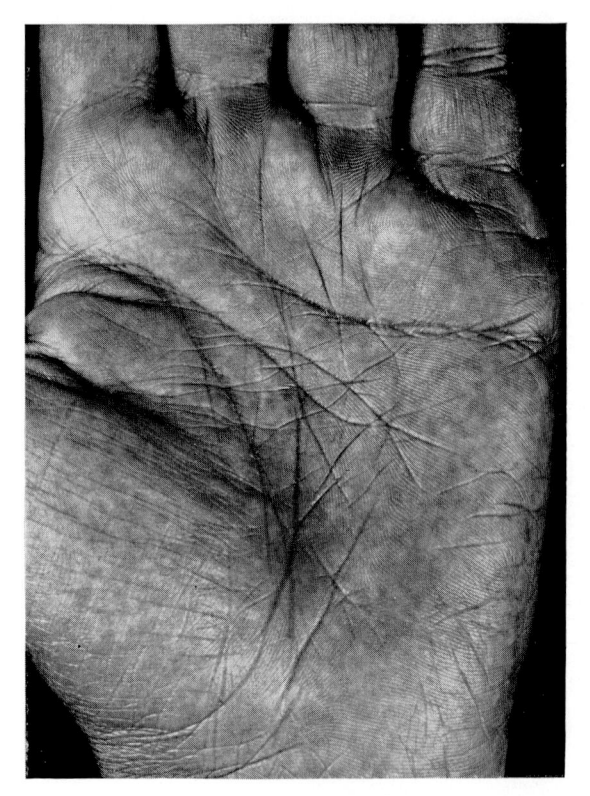

FIG. 11.4. Direct ultra-violet photograph of palm.

Two features to which reference is constantly made in descriptions of syndromes due to autosomal abnormalities are the dermatoglyphics and the position and shape of the ears. The appearance of the normal palmar ridges and lines as demonstrated by Penrose are shown in Fig. 11.4. These can be very difficult and indeed impossible to see in newborn infants, especially if premature; some form of lens is essential, but in the slightly older child an ordinary auriscope without the speculum is often adequate.

Abnormalities in the formation and shape of the ear are easily enough recognized but the expression 'low-set ears' is loosely used and may mean little unless qualified. The surface markings do not appear to have been defined in the standard textbooks of anatomy, but in most normal individuals the upper tip of the ear lies above a line drawn horizontally through the outer canthi of the eyes. The distance between the auditory meatus and the angle of the jaw is greatly diminished when the ear is 'low-set'.

Incidence

The incidence of chromosomal abnormalities in live-born infants is fortunately very low, but tends to be higher with greater maternal age; a recent survey from Edinburgh, of 3500 consecutive live-born males, revealed a chromosome abnormality in 20 cases, an incidence of 1 in 175. Twelve of these, of whom five had 47 XYY karyotype, showed no obvious external abnormality. Another recent survey from Athens, of 10,412 live-born infants, included 22 cases of trisomy 21, an incidence of 0·21 per cent, 3 cases of trisomy 18, and one case of trisomy 13–15.

Polani has recently discussed the frequency of chromosomal deviations from data available in a number of different studies and Table 11.1 summarizes his estimates of the incidence in surviving newborn infants.

It can be seen from these figures that apart from Down's syndrome, autosomal anomalies are an extremely uncommon cause of congenital abnormalities in live-born infants, whereas sex chromosome defects are considerably less rare.

SEX-CHROMOSOME ABNORMALITIES

KLINEFELTER'S SYNDROME, 47 XXY

An extra X chromosome in a male, due to non-disjunction resulting from the failure in meiosis of the two X chromosomes to separate so that the nucleus of one of the zygotes is given two X chomosomes, is the cause of Klinefelter's syndrome. The extra X may come from either parent. The chromosome distribution is then XXY, but may be XXXY or even XXXXY. There is some evidence of maternal age effect in XXY cases.

TABLE 11.1
Frequency of autosomal anomalies in surviving newborn infants (male and female)

TRISOMIES	Frequency
Down's syndrome	1/660
Edward's syndrome	1/6700 ±
Patau's syndrome	1/7600 ±
STRUCTURAL DELETIONS (Cri du chat syndrome)	
Deletion 5	1/50,000–1/100,000
Deletion 4	1/300,000 (?)

Frequency of sex-chromosome anomalies in surviving newborn infants

XYY	1/700 males
XXY	1/700 males
XY/XXY	1/1400 males
XXX	1/1250 females
XO	1/2500 females
Others	1/3500 females (?)

Incidence

The incidence of Klinefelter's syndrome is estimated at 1·7 in 1000 live male births for England and Wales.

Clinical Findings

Klinefelter's syndrome is a variety of male hypogonadism in which the buccal smear is chromatin-positive, as it is in the normal female.

The diagnosis only becomes obvious after puberty although unusually small testes and penis might earlier arouse suspicions of the possibility. Neonatal cytological screening makes possible the identification of this and other sex chromosome abnormalities at birth but is at present hardly practicable for more than selected communities.

Intelligence is likely to be limited, but the degree to which this is so is uncertain; there is a higher incidence of Klinefelter's within mental subnormality hospitals than in the general population, but the majority of cases have an I.Q. of 50 or more.

Gynaecomastia is common, and fat deposition may be increased and female in distribution. The voice may be high-pitched. Fusion of the epiphyses is delayed, and growth continues longer than usual.

Turner's Syndrome

Gonadal dysgenesis—$45 \times O$, Bonnevie–Ullrich syndrome.
Females, chromatin-negative and lacking the second X chromosome, or the short arm of the X, comprise Turner's syndrome. Some may be mosaics or have the karyotype XX/XY or a similar one, in which the X is defective and inactive. There is no maternal age effect.

Incidence
The incidence of this condition at birth is probably about 1 in 2500 live female births; it is thought to be much commoner at conception but the early foetal mortality is very high.

Clinical Findings
The birth weight tends to be low, 2·5 kg or less; diagnosis is often possible at, or soon after, birth on account of oedema of the extremities; this pits on pressure and may be both marked and persistent. There is webbing of the neck, and loose skin folds at the back of the neck, These neck folds disappear towards the end of the first year and the webbing becomes more obvious. Micrognathia, epicanthus, and low-set ears have also been described. Short fourth metacarpals and hypoplasia of the nails are also a feature. There is cubitus valgus. The nipples are small and widely spaced. There may be a systolic cardiac murmur, loudest at the back, resulting from coarctation of the aorta; the femoral pulses will then be weak or absent.

The external genitalia are usually normal in appearance. Urinary tract and numerous other abnormalities have been described, including serous effusions not due to cardiac failure.

Autopsy Findings
Coarctation of the aorta may be found, but no satisfactory cause for the oedema of the extremities has been demonstrated; abnormal development of the lymphatic channels is postulated. No true gonad is present, the ovary being represented by a ridge of connective tissue in the

mesosalpinx, without any germinal elements although a few primordial follicles may be present.

Progress
In the older child a low hairline at the back of the head is characteristic. Secondary sexual characteristics do not develop, but pubic hair may appear. Height remains less than normal. Mental retardation, however, occurs only in a minority.

Cases of the Ullrich syndrome may closely resemble Turner's syndrome but have a normal karyotype with no deficiency of the X chromosome. They are chromatin-positive and have normal ovarian development.

Triplex X Females—XXX

Females with three or more X chromosomes occur more or less rarely. XXX females are estimated to have an incidence of about 1 per 1000 births. They are of normal appearance and usually of normal intelligence and are only picked up in the newborn period as the result of screening. Nothing, therefore, should or need be said to the parents about the chromosomal abnormality. In later life mental retardation or secondary amenorrhoea may lead to the diagnosis.

47 XYY Males

These are not recognizable in infancy and are only ascertained in the neonatal period as the result of chromosomal screening. There is a tendency for men of this karyotype to develop into tall, strong individuals of somewhat diminished intelligence. The possible risk of antisocial behaviour in later life is neither so definite nor so well understood that any measures can be taken to avoid it and there is as yet no good reason for informing parents of the abnormal chromosome pattern.

Testicular Feminization—XY

This condition is fully dealt with in Chapter 6.

MAINLY NUMERICAL AUTOSOME ANOMALIES

Down's Syndrome
Mongolism—G trisomy—trisomy 21

Down's syndrome, described by Langdon Down in 1866 and named by him Mongolian Idiocy, was recognized to be due to trisomy of chromosome E of the 21–22 group after Lejeune in 1959 had reported the presence of 47 chromosomes in this condition. A lesser number, especially those born to young mothers, are due to translocation (p. 15) and have the normal number (46) of chromosomes. One of these is, however, an abnormally large chromosome which may incorporate part of a third chromosome 21.

Incidence

The incidence of Down's syndrome is between 1·5 and 2·0 per thousand live-births (p. 2) in those countries where adequate diagnosis and records exist, but there is a marked maternal age effect and the risk of a woman bearing an affected child trebles after the age of 40, rising to an incidence of about 10 per 1000 after 45 years. The risk of the birth of another affected child to a woman who has already borne one is at least double the expected risk for her age, where the condition is due to trisomy. In those cases where the mother is 13–15:21 translocation carrier, the risk at conception is very high, perhaps one in four for each pregnancy; one in four is likely to be a carrier, and one in four perfectly normal; the remaining zygote is non-viable. There is intra-uterine loss of those with effective G trisomy, but the empirical risk of Down's syndrome appears to be between 1 in 5 and 1 in 10. If it is the father that is the translocation carrier the risk is less, unless he is the carrier of 21:22 chromosome fusion or an isochromosome 21, when the risk is perhaps again high.

Radiation and Virus Infection

There is evidence that radiation of the mother prior to conception may have a marginal effect as a predisposing cause of Down's syndrome. The possibility that the virus of infective hepatitis might be responsible for an increased incidence of Down's syndrome in the offspring of women who have developed infective hepatitis at about the time of conception has also been suggested but remains unconfirmed.

Leukaemia

It has been shown that there is an increased risk of leukaemia in children suffering from Down's syndrome. The leukaemia is usually acute, and no specific chromosomal change has been demonstrated apart from the 21 trisomy. However, in chronic leukaemia an abnormal small acrocentric chromosome has been reported, and this may originate through loss of material from the long arm of chromosome 21 or 22 and it is suggested that the same chromosomal material may be affected in both conditions.

Clinical Features

The average birth weight at term is 2·900 kg, almost 350 gm less than the normal.

The condition is usually recognized at birth or within a few hours in the more obvious instances, and in any case within a few days. The puffy appearance of the eyes in some normal babies after birth can wrongly arouse suspicion of Down's syndrome.

The notable floppiness and hypotonia of the baby may first suggest, especially to the mother, that the baby is not normal, together with the curious flatness of the face. The general appearance of the face is quite characteristic; broken down into its individual parts this consists in the rather small eyes with palpebral fissures sloping upwards and outwards and with an epicanthic fold running from the inner end of the orbital part of the upper eyelid and disappearing into the skin on the side of the nose The highest point of the upper lid is midway (Chapter 5, p. 150) and not, as is usual in Western races, at the junction of the inner one-third and outer two-thirds. The nose tends to be small and the bridge flat. The tongue is intermittently protruded but is of normal size and shape.

The skull is of less than normal circumference and the occiput is usually flat; a third (sagittal) fontanelle is palpable about 2·5 cm above the position of the posterior fontanelle in half the cases in the neonatal period. The ears are small, with deficient lobes and other abnormalities. Not obvious in infancy, but present in blue-eyed children, are Brushfield's spots (p. 175) small white spots in the iris; strabismus often occurs, myopia is common, and cataract may develop later.

The neck is broad and the shoulders sloping; this, with the flat back to the head, gives the typical appearance when seen from behind.

The hair is fine and silky and the skin soft; the peripheral circulation is poor.

SYNDROMES DUE TO CHROMOSOMAL ABNORMALITIES 401

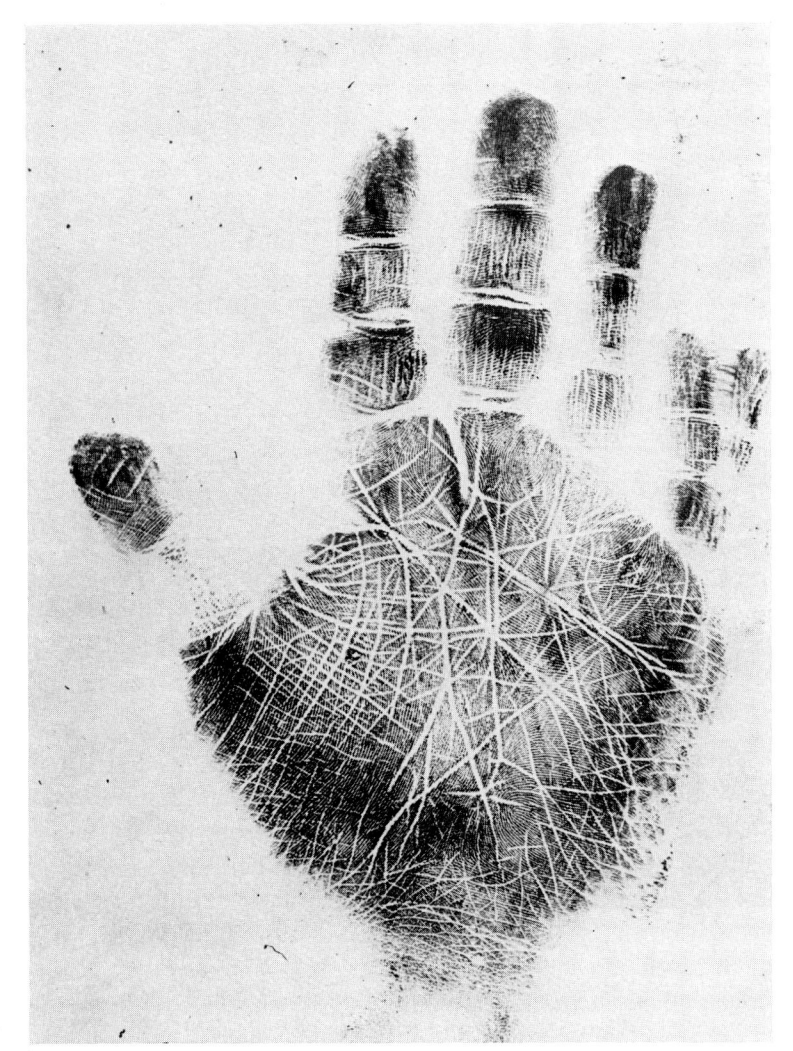

FIG. 11.5. Hand prints in a case of Down's syndrome showing the transverse crease.

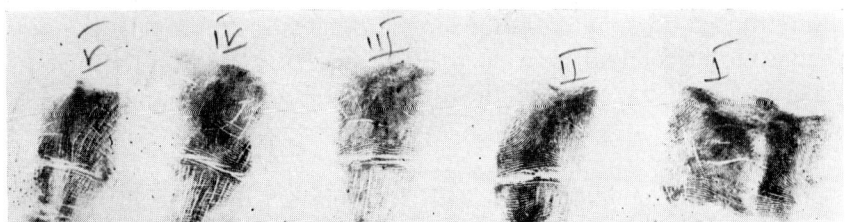

FIG. 11.6. Dermatoglyphics of the digits in a child with Down's syndrome.

The hands are short and broad, with a short and often incurved 5th finger; its 2nd phalanx is small or rudimentary in 40 per cent of cases. The fingers, too, are short and stubby. A single transverse palmar crease is present in 50 per cent of cases; this occurs normally in 10 per cent of people of European stock, and in a larger but unknown proportion of those of Asian origin. The foot has unusually wide separation between the great toe and the second toe with a deep longitudinal crease running down from it.

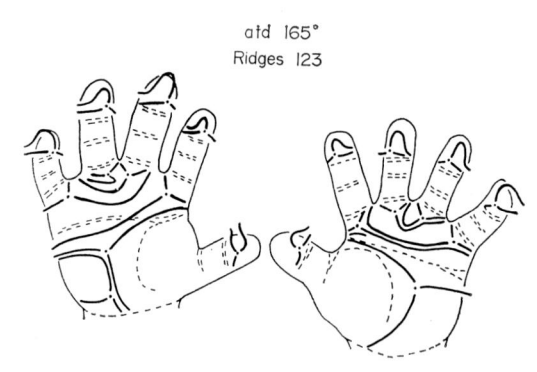

FIG. 11.7. Diagram of the dermatoglyphics in the hand of an infant with Down's syndrome.

The finger-tip ridges show more ulnar loops than whorls and the axial t triradius is displaced distally so that the angle between the lines drawn from the index finger triradius a and from the 5th finger triradius d to the axial triradius t is over 60°. Where there are two axial triradii the more distal one is used. In one out of ten normal palms the $a.t.d.$ angle is over 60°, but in Down's syndrome the mean angle is about 75°.

Congenital heart disease is common; atrial and ventricular septal defects are the most frequent lesions but cyanotic heart disease due to Fallot's tetralogy and Eisenmenger's complex is also common. Intestinal abnormalities are fairly frequent, especially oesophageal atresia with tracheo-oesophageal fistula and duodenal atresia. Hydramnios in the mother should indicate the necessity of excluding the first by passage of a gastric tube and the aspiration of acid gastric juice, and of the latter by a plain abdominal X-ray. Annular pancreas, malrotation of the gut, and imperforate anus have all been reported.

The external genitalia are usually hypoplastic; in males the penis is small or undescended; in females the vulva is poorly developed.

SYNDROMES DUE TO CHROMOSOMAL ABNORMALITIES 403

Autopsy

The brain in the newborn does not differ markedly in size from others at this age, but at later ages is definitely smaller. The frontal lobes, brain stem and cerebellum are particularly small, giving the brain a round

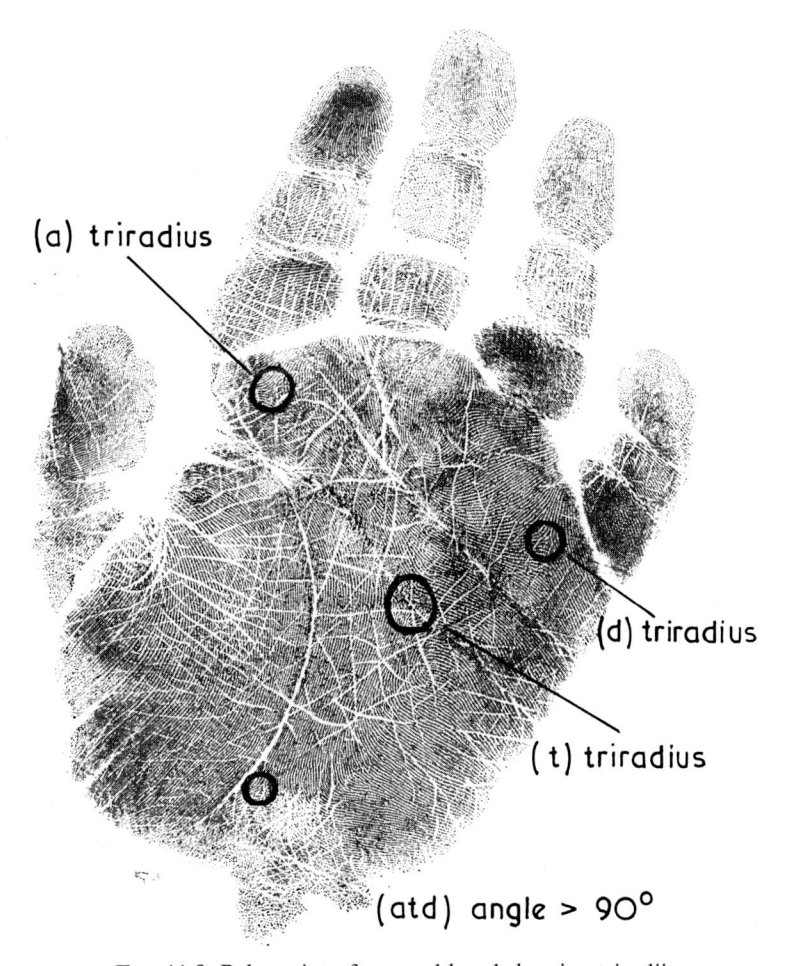

FIG. 11.8. Palm print of mongol hand showing triradii.

shape when viewed from above. Histological changes are indefinite, apart from heterotopias of the cerebellum; these are small nodules of cerebellar cells crossed by bundles of nerve fibres. Other findings are specific only to the various abnormalities that may be associated with Down's syndrome.

Radiology
In Down's syndrome characteristic radiological findings are demonstrable in the pelvis. These are: (1) Bilateral flattening of the lower edges of the ilium, measured quantitatively as the acetabular angle; (2) bilateral widening and flaring of the iliac wings measured quantitatively as the iliac angle.

Biochemistry
Blood 5-hydroxytryptamine (5HT) concentration is decreased in newborn and older children with Down's syndrome. This deficiency may reflect decreased production elsewhere in the body and perhaps in the central nervous system, but could be due to defective platelet uptake of 5HT. Treatment with 5-hydroxytryptophan, the metabolic precursor of 5HT, has been shown to decrease the degree of hypotonia. Serum tryptophan levels are normal in Down's syndrome and on feeding tryptophan to these children, unlike normal controls, no rise in circulating 5HT occurs unless pyridoxine is given simultaneously.

Progress
Abortions and stillbirths are probably common in all trisomies, and the mortality for live-born autosomal trisomies is high. In trisomy 21 death in the newborn period is usually due to heart disease or atresia in some part of the digestive tract. Excluding deaths in the neonatal period the life expectancy rose from 9 to 18 years between 1932 and 1963 and is certainly much greater now.

Intelligence is greatly limited, but developmental quotients in the first year of life tend to be in the region of 70 compared to a normal of 100. The ultimate intelligence quotient reached is variously estimated to average between 30 and 50 but social ability is greater than intelligence.

PATAU'S SYNDROME—TRISOMY 13–15—D TRISOMY

In 1960, Patau described a syndrome displaying anomalies of the face, hands, and feet in which there is a trisomy of the D 1 chromosome of the 13–15 group; other chromosomal abnormalities may occasionally be responsible, but sometimes no chromosomal abnormality at all has been demonstrated. Autoradiography shows the extra chromosome in this trisomy to be late in synthesizing D.N.A. as is typical of chromosome No. 13 in the D group. It is probable that the majority of cases arise as the result of the primary non-disjunction during gametogenesis. Maternal age at conception may have some effect, the mean

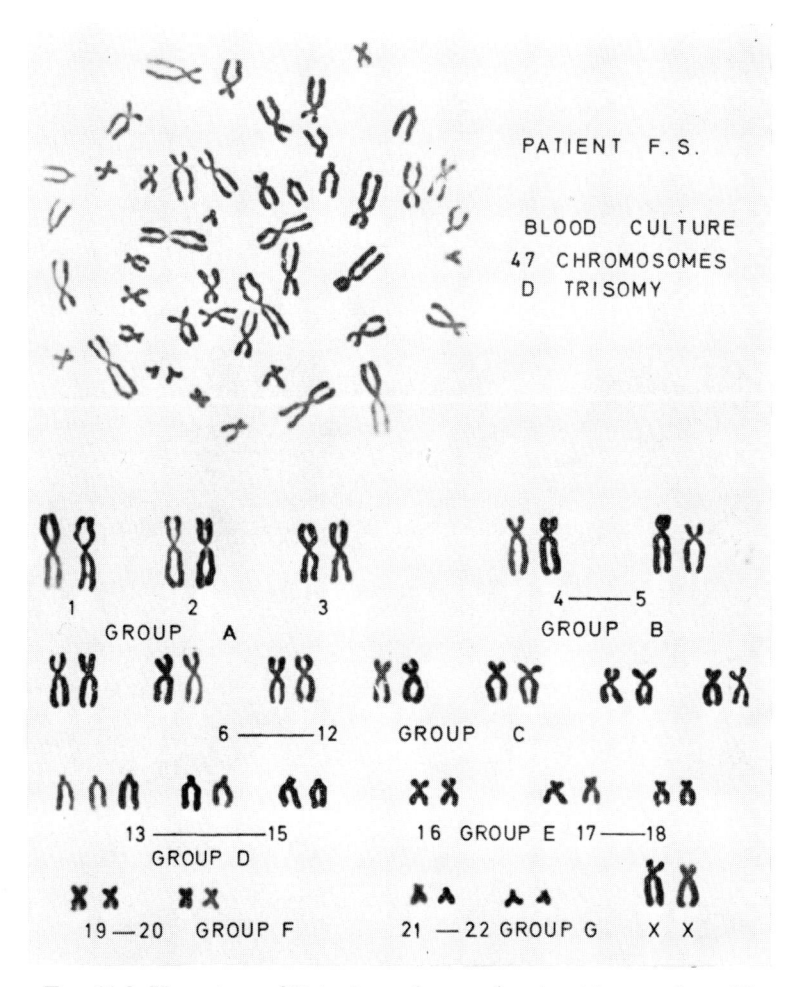

Fig. 11.9. Karyotype of Patau's syndrome, showing trisomy of no. 13 chromosome of D group.

being at least 31 years in place of the mean for England and Wales of about 27 years. It is possible that some cases of Patau's syndrome independent of maternal age may be due to other causes such as mosaicism in a parent.

DD

Incidence
This has variously been estimated to be between 1 in 7000 and 1 in 9000 live-births with equal numbers of males and females.

Clinical Findings
Birth size is small, the average weight being 2·600 kg. The head is small,

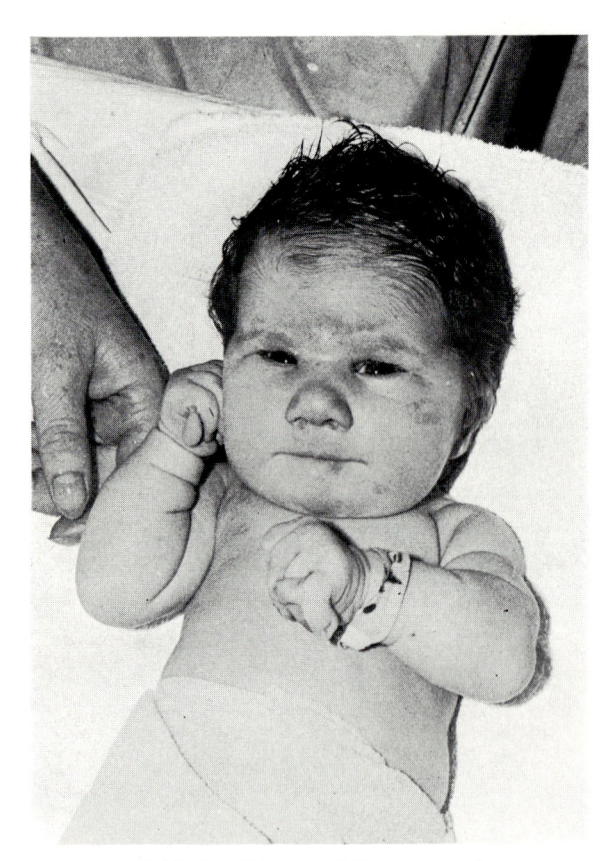

FIG. 11.10. A mild case of Patau's syndrome.

and the neck is short. The nose is large, with a bulbous tip and the mouth large. There is microphthalmia and hypertelorism, with an eye defect of some sort in most cases and colobomata of the iris in about a third of the cases; epicanthic folds are fairly usual. Scalp defects may be present. Micrognathia is invariable. Hare lip and cleft palate occur in about three out of four cases. The ears are low-set and malformed. Polydactyly is frequent and the nails are unusually long and convex. There is an over-riding index finger and all the fingers show flexion deformities with axial deviation. The ridge pattern on the thumbs characteristically shows radial loops, and on the finger tips radial loops and arches. The axial *t* triradius is displaced distally with an obtuse *a.t.d.* angle, and there is a single palmar crease in more than half the cases.

Cardiovascular anomalies are commonly present as are abnormalities of the external genitalia, with undescended testicles in the male.

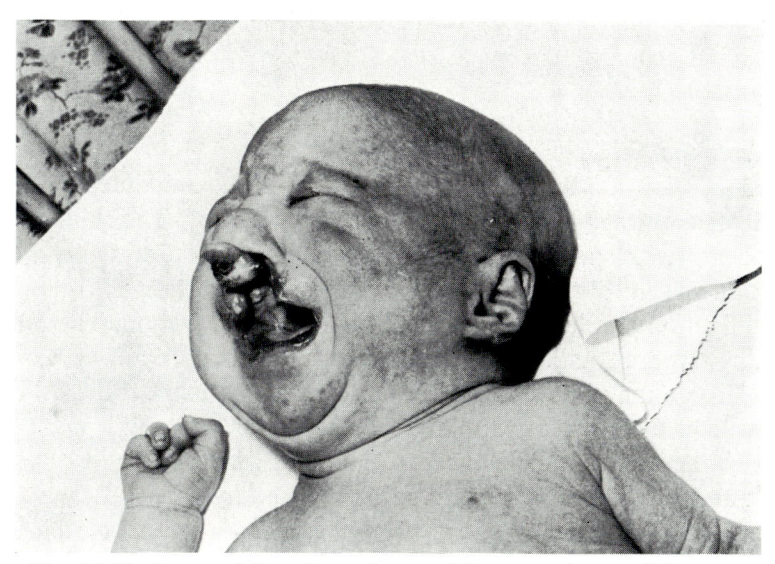

FIG. 11.11. A case of Patau's syndrome with severe abnormalities.

Autopsy Findings
The brain may superficially appear normal, but abnormalities of the prosencephalon with absence of the major commissures and hypoplasia of the cerebellum are common. There may be a cerebral holosphere and single ventricle; the olfactory bulbs are often absent and the optic nerves small. In the heart, ventricular and atrial septal defects and patency of the ductus arteriosus are found in about half the cases.

A renal abnormality is present in about half, polycystic kidneys being the most frequent anomaly. In females a bicornuate uterus may be present, in males undescended testes are usual and the penis is small.

Edwards Syndrome—Trisomy 18—E Trisomy

This syndrome, with abnormalities of the skull, ears and extremities, was separately described by Edwards and by Patau in 1960. It was identified as due to primary trisomy of chromosome 18 of the E group in most cases, but mosaics and other abnormalities have been demonstrated, and in some instances no chromosomal abnormality has been found. The maternal age is above the average, with a mean of 32 years.

Incidence
Estimates of the frequency vary between 1 in 3500 and 1 in 6500, with four times as many females as males, possibly because of higher male foetal mortality.

Clinical Findings
Pregnancy is often complicated by hydramnios, and the placenta is small. The average birth weight is low, about 2200 g. The skull is long and narrow, with a prominent occiput; the ears are malformed and their position low and abnormal. The eyes are narrow and there is epicanthus; apart from microphthalmos, eye defects are not common. The mouth and the jaw are small. Clefts of lip and palate occur in a fourth of the cases. There may be webbing of the neck and an extra roll of skin at the nape of the neck. The thumb may be rudimentary and is implanted distally, the index and ring fingers overlapping and the great toe is often short and dorsiflexed. The fingernails may be hypoplastic. The ridge pattern characteristically shows simple arches on most or all of the fingertips, with crease abnormalities and some distal displacement of the axial triradius *t*.

Talipes calcaneo valgus is common and the calcaneus bone itself very prominent. The chest is short and broad, the sternum short, and the nipples hypoplastic.

Progress
Developmental retardation is usual and severe and other neurological defects occur. The affected baby fails to thrive and remains feeble and hypotonic, death usually occurring within a year, and mostly by 3 months of age.

Autopsy Findings
Macroscopic changes in the brain are not usual, but histological findings

SYNDROMES DUE TO CHROMOSOMAL ABNORMALITIES 409

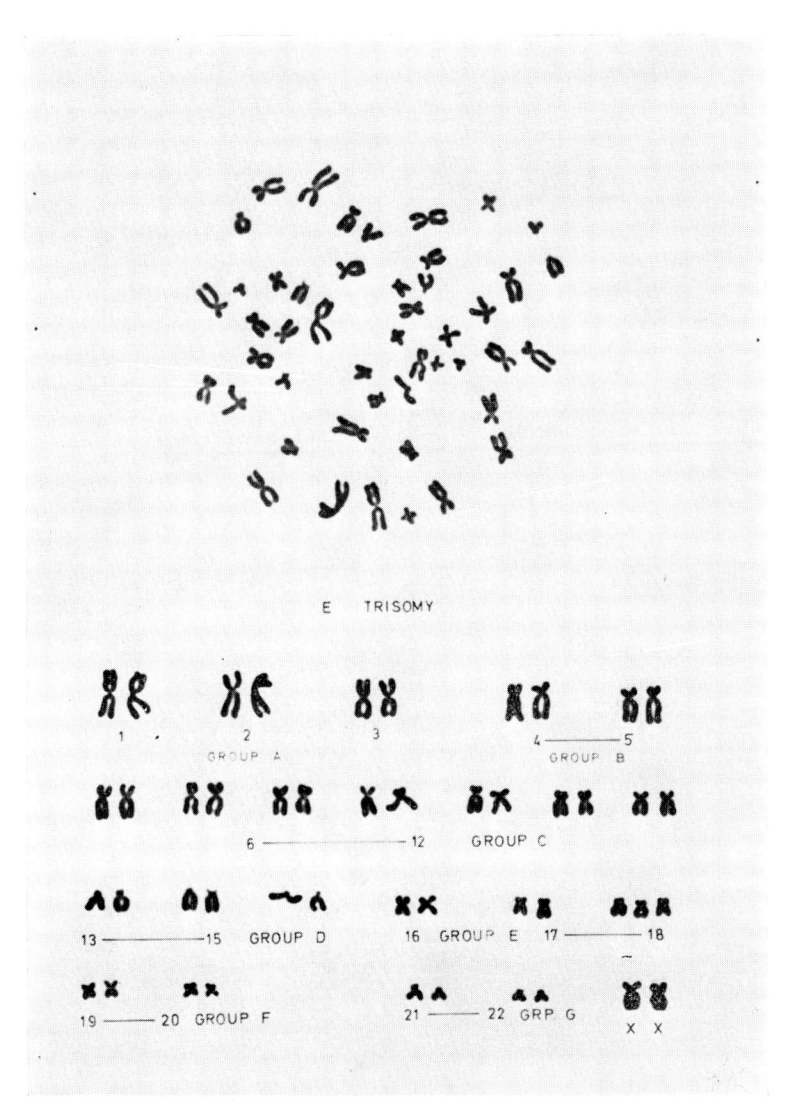

Fig. 11.12. Karyotype in Edward's syndrome showing trisomy of chromosome 18 of E group.

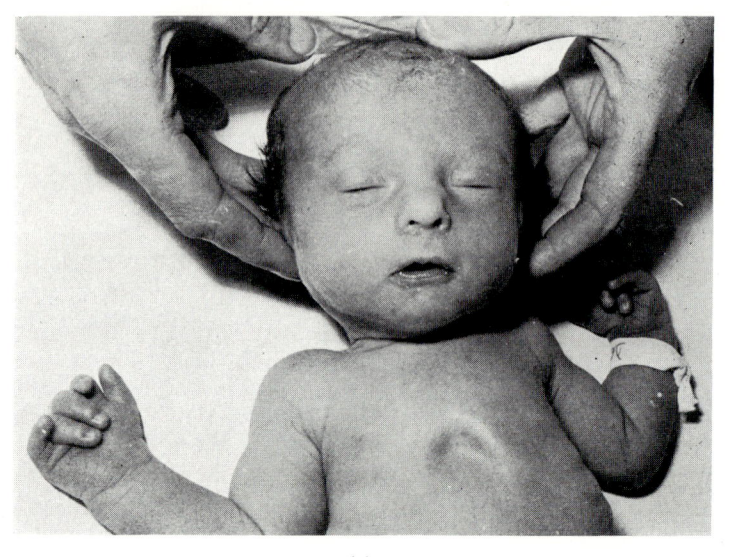

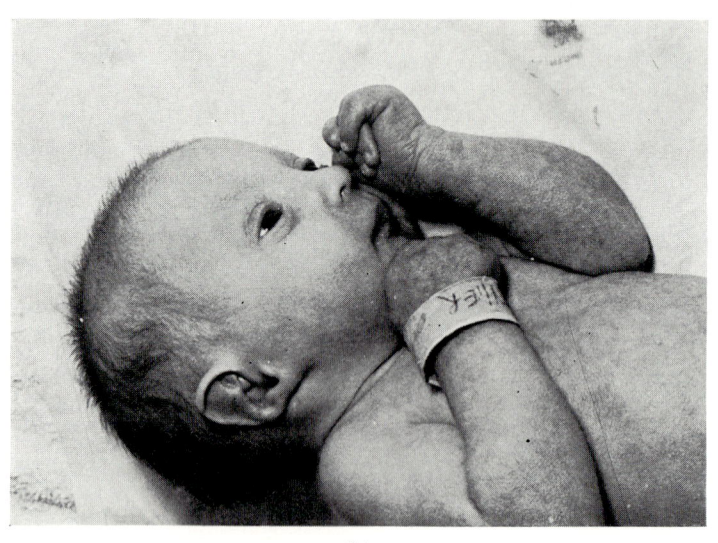

FIG. 11.13 (a and b). Photograph of a baby with Edward's syndrom showing the characteristic appearance.

of heterotopia are common in the cerebellum. Meningomyelocele has also been described.

Cardiovascular abnormalities are present in almost every case, principally septal defects, patency of ductus arteriosus and coarctation of the aorta.

Renal abnormalities, especially cystic kidneys, hydronephrosis, and horse-shoe kidney are common. Malrotation of the intestine, Meckel's diverticulum and even pyloric stenosis may be present.

Spontaneous Abortion

Chromosomal abnormalities are found in about 40 per cent of early spontaneous abortions. About 45 per cent of these are autosomal trisomies, 20 per cent are triploids, and 7 per cent mosaics. The frequency of chromosomal abnormalities is three times higher in the first trimester as second trimester, and nine times higher in malformed embryos than normal foetuses.

Other Autosomal Trisomies

Trisomies other than those described above have been reported, but no definite pattern of clinical features has emerged to form a definite syndrome; nor has the nature of the extra autosome been clearly defined and confirmed.

Triploidy

Diploid–triploid mosaics or chimaeras have been reported with a variety of anomalies; several have had hemiatrophy or congenital asymmetry, many syndactyly and a number are externally intersexual. None had cardiac anomalies but all were severely mentally retarded. The abnormal triploid cells were found on fibroblast culture, only normal diploid cells being seen in blood cultures.

MAINLY STRUCTURAL AUTOSOME ANOMALIES

Deletions

Deletions of short arm of B group chromosome (Bp −) Cri-du-chat syndrome.

This condition is probably usually due to deletion of the short arm of a B group chromosome, thought generally to be a no. 5 chromosome. It is possible that deficiency of material from an arm of a no. 4 chromosome of the B group may give rise to a similar but distinct and more severe variant of the syndrome.

The syndrome is very rare, with a possible incidence of 1 in 50,000 to 1 in 100,000; about two-thirds of reported cases are females. There is no parental age effect.

Clinical Features

The name of the syndrome arises from the feeble cry of an affected infant, which is like the mewing of a kitten in distress. It is this which is most distinctive. The birth weight is below the normal. There is a small head with a round face, epicanthus, downward- and outward-slanting palpebral fissures and some hypertelorism. The eyes have large prominent corneas, and coloboma of the iris may be present. There may be true microcephaly. The baby is usually limp and hypotonic and there is severe developmental retardation and delay in growth. On the fingertips arches and whorls are chiefly present and the t triradius is displaced distally.

The no. 4 chromosome deletion type has marked hypertelorism, a prominent glabella, ptosis, carp-like mouth, cleft palate, mildine scalp defects, abnormalities of nails and of carpal bone ossification.

DELETIONS OF SHORT ARM OF E GROUP CHROMOSOME (Ep −)

Very few, not more than thirty, instances of this condition have so far been reported, but as it may resemble the Bonnevie–Ulrich syndrome it may be commoner than it would seem.

Morphologically the cause appears to be deletion of the short arm of a no. 18 chromosome (18p −). Several cases have been transmitted through a mother with chromosomal defects and in almost all cases there is advanced maternal age; the mean maternal age being 34 years.

Clinical Findings

The bridge of the nose is flat, the jaw small and the ears large; there is hypertelorism, epicanthus and congenital ptosis. In the Bonnevie–Ulrich type there is a redundant fold of skin at the back of the neck.

Severe brain abnormalities may be found at autopsy but other organs are not affected. Mental retardation is usual.

Deletions of Long Arm of E Group Chromosome (Eq−)

A small number of cases of a syndrome attributed to deletion of the long arm of chromosome no. 18, have been described. In a few instances, one or other of the parents have also had some chromosomal abnormality. Birth weight is low, the baby microcephalic with hypoplasia of the naso-maxillary region, deep-set eyes and prominent forehead and jaw. The mouth is shaped like that of a carp, but cleft lip and palate may occur. The helix and antihelix of the ear are prominent, and the external auditory meatus stenosed or atretic. Dimples are present on elbows, shoulders, knees and knuckles. The fingers are long and tapering and the dermatoglyphics on the fingertips show an excess of whorls. Cardiac abnormalities may be present. Mental retardation of a very severe degree is invariable except for mosaics, but death in infancy is not usual.

Deletions of Other Chromosomes

Other deletions have been recorded without any definite symptom complex being associated.

RING CHROMOSOMES

Ring-chromosome formation, deletions or monosomy of a G-group autosome. Anti-mongolism.
Deletion of part of the long arm of a G-group autosome (Gq−) which has been shown to be no. 21, was first described by Lejeune in 1964 who suggested that it was the reverse of Down's syndrome. The name 'anti-mongolism' was later given to it. Parental age is not increased and no other aetiological factors are known.

Clinical Features
The palpebral fissures slope downwards and outwards in contrast to the upward and outward slant of Down's syndrome. The nose is long and prominent, the skull elongated with a small jaw and large ears. Muscle

tone is increased and vomiting, suggestive of hypertrophic pyloric stenosis, is common.

The fingertip ridge pattern shows simple arches with a proximally placed t triradius and an absent c.

SELECTED REFERENCES

BAIRD P.A. & MILLER J.R. (1968) Epidemiological aspects of Down's syndrome. *Brit. J. Prev. Soc. Med.* **22**, 81

BAZELON M. & PAINE R.S. (1967) Reversal of hypotonia in infants with Down's syndrome by administration of 5-hydroxy tryptophen. *Lancet* **1**, 1130

CAFFEY J. & ROSS S. (1956) Mongolism during early infancy; diagnostic changes in the pelvic bones. *Pediatrics* **17**, 642

EDWARDS J.H., HARNDEN D.G., CAMERON A.H., CROSSE V.M. & WOLFF O.H. (1960) A new trisomic syndrome. *Lancet* **1**, 787

GORDON R.R., O'NEILL E.M. (1969) Turner's infantile phenotype. *Brit. med. J.* **1**, 483

JACOBSON C.B. & BARTER R.H. (1967) Cytogenetic aspects of habitual abortion. *Amer. J. Obstet. Gynec.* **97**, 666

LEJEUNE J., GAUTHIER M. & TURPIN R. (1959), Les chromosomes humains en culture de tissus. *C.R. acad. Sci. Paris*, **248**, 602

PANTELAKIS S.N., CHRYSSOSTOMIDOU O., ALEXIOU D., VALAES T. & DOXIADIS S.A. (1970) Sex chromatin and chromosome abnormalities among 10,412 liveborn babies. *Arch. Dis. Childh.* **45**, 87

PARE C.M.B. (1968) 5-Hydroxyindoles in phenylketonuric and non-phenylketonuric mental defectives. *Adv. Pharmacol.* **6B**, 159

PASSARGE E., TRUE C.W., SUEOKA W.T., BAUMGARTNER N.R. & KEER K.R. (1966) Malformations of the central nervous system in trisomy 18 syndrome. *J. Pediat.* **69**, 771

PATAU K., SMITH D.W., THERMAN E., INHORN S.L. & WAGNER H.P. (1960) Multiple congenital anomalies caused by an extra autosome. *Lancet* **1**, 790

PENROSE L.S. (1963) Finger prints, palms and chromosomes. *Nature* **4871**, 923

PENROSE L.S. & SMITH G.F. (1966). *Down's Anomaly.* London: Churchill

POLANI P.E. (1967) Chromosome anomalies and the brain. *Guy's Hospital Reports* **116**, 365

POLANI P.E. (1969) Autosomal imbalance and its syndromes, excluding Down's. *Brit. med. Bull.* **1**, 81

POLANI P.E. (1970) The incidence of chromosomal malformations. *Proc. Roy. Soc. Med.* **63**, 50

RACE R.R. & SANGER R. (1969) Xg and sex chromosome abnormalities. *Brit. med. bull.* **1**, 99

RATCLIFFE S., STEWART A., MELVILLE M., JACOBS P. & KEAY A. J. (1970) Chromosome studies on 3500 newborn male infants. *Lancet* **1**, 121

SIGLER A.T., LILIENFELD A.M., COHEN B.H. & WESTLAKE J.E. (1965) Radiation exposure in parents of children with mongolism—Down's syndrome. *Bull. Johns Hopkins Hosp.* **117**, 374

TAYLOR A.I. (1967) Patau's, Edwards, and Cri du-chat syndrome. *Devel. Med. Child. Neurol.* **9,** 78
TAYLOR A.I. (1968) Autosomal trisomy syndromes. *J. med. Genet.* **5,** 227
WARKANY J., PASSARGE E. & SMITH L.B. (1966) Congenital malformations in autosoal trisomy syndromes. *Amer. J. Dis. Child.* **112,** 502
WOLTENHOLME G.E.W. & PORTER R. (eds.) (1967) *Mongolism.* Ciba Foundation Study Group. No. 25. London: Churchill

Index

Abiotrophies 181
Abdominal distension 247-8
Abdominal muscles, absent 228
Acanthosis nigricans 317-18
Acetabular insufficiency, unilateral 277
Acetyl methyl choline in heart failure 129
Achondroplasia 358-60
  dominant genes 17
Acrocephaly 80
Acrocephalosyndactyly, see Apert's syndrome
Adenoma sebaceum, see Sclerosis, tuberous
Adenomatous dysplasia of the lung 95-6
Adrenal cortical hyperplasia, associated with pseudohermaphroditism 215, 216
Adrenal hyperplasia, congenital, causing intersex, genetics 19
Adrenal tumours, in newborn 220
Aetiology of malformations 6-24
Aglossia 357
Albers-Schonberg's disease (marble bones) 257
Albinism 316-17
  histopathology, prognosis, treatment 317
  ocular features 197
Alimentary tract, duplication 250-1
  classification 250
  Meckel's diverticulum 251
  presentation 250
Alkaline hypophosphatasia 256

Alopecia, congenital 342
Alport's syndrome 138
Amaurotic family idiocy, see Tay-Sach's disease
Amazia, congenital 346
Aminoacid metabolism, anomalies, ocular features 196-7
Amyoplasia congenita, see Arthrogryposis multiplex congenita
Amyotonia congenita 259-60
  bad prognosis 260
  good prognosis 260
  symptomatic 260-1
Anaemia, congenital aplastic, see Fanconi's anaemia
Anencephaly
  aetiology 28
  associated conditions 27
  birth order and maternal age effect 10
  familial recurrence 27-8
  geographic variation 27
  incidence 2, 3, 25
  management 27
  pathology 26-7
  sex ratio 26
Angiofibromatosis, see Sclerosis, tuberous
Angiography in hydrocephalus 61
Angiomata, ophthalmic 154-5
Angiomatosis of retina and subtentorial meninges 326
Aniridia 163-4
  dominant genes 18
Ankle and foot, anomalies 282-7
Ankyloblepharon 150-1

416

Ankyloglossia 347
Anonychia 338
Anophthalmos 156
Anoxia, and cataract 170
Antibiotic therapy in heart failure 127–8
Anti-mongol syndrome, chromosome mutation 16
Anuria 221
Anus, in ectopia vesicae 207–8
Anus and rectum
 abnormalities 251–4
  classification 251–2
  covered anus 253, 254
  ectopic anus 253–4
Aortic arch, transverse, atresia 107
Aortic valve atresia 107
 with mitral atresia 107
 with mitral hypoplasia 107
Apert's syndrome 18, 81, 357
 dominant genes 18
 ocular features 193
Aqueduct stenosis, genetics 19
Aqueduct of Sylvius malformations 52–3
Arachnodactyly 361
 and ectopia lentis 166
Arm, abnormalities 272–4
Arnold–Chiari malformation 53–5
 associated anomalies 53
 myeloceles in 31
Arrhythmias, cardiac
 in newborn 124–5
 treatment 128
Arrhythmias, cardiac, see also individual anomalies
Arteries, great, transposition 104–6
 cyanosis 104
 treatment 105–6
Arteriovenous fistulae, congenital 262–3
Arthrogryposis 273
Arthrogryposis multiplex congenita 261–2
Astomia 347
Association for Spina Bifida and Hydrocephalus 46
Atresia of fourth ventricle exit foramina 55
Auditory canal, external, atresia 135–7

Aural-renal syndrome 371
Auricles, abnormalities 133–4
Auricular atresia 355–7
Auricular flutter, digitalis in 129
Autosomes, anomalies 399–414
 in surviving newborn infants, frequency 396
 see also Chromosomes, Genes and individual anomalies

Barlow's test 276
Biliary atresia 241–3
 diagnosis 241
 treatment 241–2
Birth marks, see Haemangiomas
Birth order and maternal/paternal age effects 10
Bladder, distension in newborn 220–1
 diverticula 226
 duplication 226
 ectopia vesicae 204–8
 incontinence, disorders 220–1
 see also Genito-urinary system
Blepharophimosis 150
Blistering
 epidermal anomalies 300–3
 other causes 303–4
Bloch–Sylberger anomaly, see Incontinentia pigmenti
Blount's disease 281
Bourneville's disease, see Sclerosis, tuberous
Brachial plexus, lesions 273–4
Brachycephaly 80
Brachydactyly 374
 with cardiac arrhythmia 374–5
 dominant genes 17
 with macular coloboma 374
 with mental retardation and mandibulo-facial dysostosis 375
 with nail dysplasia 375
Brain
 anencephaly 26–8
 cebocephaly 28–9
 cyclopia 28–9
 iniencephaly 28
 microcephaly acrania 28
 destructive lesions 74–8

Breasts and nipples
  absence 346
  accessory 346
Bronchi, anomalies 89

Calcaneo-valgus foot 286
Calcium deficiency and cataract 270
Carbohydrate metabolism, anomalies, ocular features 197
Cardiac development 100
Cardiac malformations, incidence 2, 3
  see also individual anomalies
Cardio-auditory syndrome of Jervell & Lange–Nielson 138
Cardiomegaly as presenting sign 121–2
Cardiothoracic system, abnormalities 87–130
Cardiovascular system, anomalies 98–104
Cartilage-hair hypoplasia 361
Cataract
  associated syndromes 174–5
  congenital 167–8
    dominant genes 18
    incidence 6
  developmental
    polar 168–9
    sutural 169
  and Down's syndrome (mongolism) 175
  due to maternal infections 171–4
  due to nutritional disturbances 169–71
  hereditary 169
  lamellar (zonular) 169–71
    causes and treatment 170–1
  nuclear (cataracta centralis pulverulenta) 169
  postnatal
    galactosaemia 174
    in premature infants 174
    and toxoplasmosis 173
Catarrhal ophthalmia 352
Cebocephaly 28–9
Central nervous system, abnormalities 25–86
  frequency of malformations 2
Cerebrospinal fluid examination in hydrocephalus 60

Cervical rib 266
Cervico-oculo-acoustic syndrome 138
Chiari malformation, in meningocele 34
Chlorthiazide in heart failure 127
Choanal atresia, posterior 141–2, 355–6
Chondrodystrophy, and perceptive deafness 138
Chordee, in hypospadias 203
Chorioretinitis
  intra-uterine 177
  and tuberculosis 179
Choroid
  coloboma 158
  and retina, abnormalities 175–81
Choroideraemia 181
Chromatin, sex, in intersex states 213, 218–19
Chromosome mutations 11–16, 19
  autosomal non-disjunction 11–13
  chromosome non-disjunction 14
  classification 392–5
  counselling 21–2
  in cyclopia and cebocephaly 29
  and deafness 138
  deletions 411–13
  frequency 396
  incidence 395
  and intersex states 213–15
  mosaicism 16–17
  point or gene, associated malformations 17–19
  in pseudohermaphroditism 217
  ring 413–14
  syndromes due to 392–415
  translocations 15–16
  triple X females 398
  triple X syndromes 213
  47 XYY males 398
Cicatrices, congenital 346
Circumcision and congenital phimosis 200
Clavicle, congenital pseudarthrosis 273
Cleft lip and cleft palate 231–6
  feeding 232
  genetics 236
  incidence 2, 3, 4
  in Pierre-Robin syndrome 232
  speech therapy 235
  treatment 233–5

Cleft lip and palate (*cont.*)
  types 231–2
Cleft palate, incidence 4
Cleidocranial dysostosis 83–4
  dominant genes 17
Club foot, *see* Talipes equino-varus
Cockayne's syndrome 138
Cogan's syndrome 138
Coloboma 152
  and cyclopia 156
  disc 159
  iris 163
    choroid and retina 158–59
  lens 165–6
  macula 175–6
Congenital dislocation of the hip, *see* Hip
Conradi's syndrome, genetics 19
Constriction rings 263
Contracture
  fifth finger 271
  fifth toe 283
Cor biloculare 107–9
Cor triloculare 107–9
Cornea
  abnormalities 160–3
  opacities, congenital 162
Cornelia de Lange syndrome 378–9
Coronary artery, left, anomalous origin 122
Corpus callosum
  aetiology 73–4
  agenesis 72–4
    and chromosome abnormality 74
    features and diagnosis 72
    pathology 72–3
  associated with hydrocephalus 72
Cortical hyperostosis, infantile 258
Cortisone, in pseudohermaphroditism 216
Counselling
  genetic, principles 20–3
  malformations of mixed aetiology 22–3
  psychological principles 23
Coxa vara, congenital 278
Coxsackie virus infection during pregnancy and heart malformation 10
Cranio-cleido dystosis 17, 83–4, 362–3

Cranio-facial dystosis (Crouzon's disease) 81, 194
  dominant genes 17
  see also Mandibulo-facial dystosis
Craniostenosis, treatment 81
Craniosynostosis 357
  aetiology 79
  features 79–81
  treatment 81
Cranium bifidum 46–8
Cranium bifidum occultum 46
Cretinism, endemic and perceptive deafness 138
Cri-du-chat syndrome 411–12
  chromosome mutation 16
Crouzon's disease 17, 81, 194
Cryptophthalmos 150
Cutis hyperelastica (Ehlers–Danlos syndrome) 335
Cutis laxa congenita (generalized elastosis) 334–5
Cyanosis, cardiac malformations causing 104–30
  see also individual headings, e.g. Transposition, Cor biloculare
  in congenital heart disease 99–104
    due to abnormal forms of haemoglobin 101–2
    due to abnormal amount of reduced haemoglobin 102–4
  differential 115
  from left ventricular failure produced by acyanotic lesions 114–15
Cyclopia 28–9, 155–9
Cyst(s)
  bronchogenic 93
    multiple 94–5
    solitary 93–4
      differential diagnosis 94
  dermoid, mediastinal 92
    orbital 183
  iris 165
  laryngeal, congenital 144
  mediastinal, treatment 93
  neurenteric canal 90
Cystic diasease of the kidneys 223–4
Cystinosis (Fanconi's syndrome) 257
  ocular features 196
Cytomegalic inclusion disease 178

Cytomegalic virus infection in pregnancy, and malformation 9

Dandy–Walker syndrome 55
　with cystic kidneys, genetics 19
Deafness 137–40
　congenital conductive 139
　congenital perceptive 137–9
　　hereditary factors 137
　detection 139–40
　genetics 18
　nerve, hereditary 356–7
　in Waardenburg's syndrome 82
Death, in infancy, and congenital malformations 3
Deltoid, absence, part or all 273
Dental anomalies 348
Dermatoglyphics, in chromosome abnormalities 394–5
　in Down's syndrome 401–2
Dermis
　and connective tissues, abnormalities 334–44
　embryology 292
Dermoid
　conjunctival 160
　cysts, orbital 183
　limbal 159
　nasal 141
　spinal 48–50
Dextrocardia 123–5
Diabetes, effect on malformation rate 8
Diaphyseal achlasis (multiple exostosis) 257
Digitalis, in heart failure 126
Digits, anomalies 270–2
Diphallus 209
Disc
　coloboma 159
　optic, normal and abnormal 181–2
Distichiasis 154, 344
Diuretics in heart failure 127
Diverticulum
　development 91
　of left ventricle 123
Djerine–Sottas syndrome and perceptive deafness 138
Dolichocephaly 80

Down's syndrome (mongolism) 399–404
　associated with cataract 174, 175
　autopsy 403
　biochemistry 404
　chromosome mutations 15–16
　clinical features 400
　dermatoglyphics in 401–2
　genetic influences 7
　incidence 2, 3, 6, 399
　incidence of congenital heart disease 99
　leukaemia in 400
　maternal age effect 10
　progress 404
　radiation and virus infection 399–400
　radiology 404
　with epicanthus with ptosis 150
Drainage, pulmonary venous, total anomalous 112–14
Duane's retraction syndrome 188–9
　and perceptive deafness 138
Dwarfism
　cartilage-hair hypoplasia 361
　diastrophic 360
　　genetics 18
　low birthweight 380
　metatropic 361
　thanatophoric 360
Dysautonomia, familiar 381
Dyskeratosis, congenital, genetics 19
Dysostosis multiplex, see Gargoylism
Dystrophy, thoracic 360

Ears
　in chromosome abnormalities 394–5
　embryology 131–3
　external 133–7
　nose and throat abnormalities 131–46
　see also Auricles and individual anomalies
Ebstein's malformation 114, 115
Echoencephalography in hydrocephalus 62
Ectodermal dysplasia
　congenital 299–300
　　associated with cataract 175
　　dominant genes 18

Ectopia cordis 123
Ectopia lentis 166
Ectopia vesicae
  complications 207–8
  and epispadias 204–8
  herniae in 204
  incontinence 204
  treatment 206–8
  vaginal orifice in 204
Ectrodactyly, dominant genes 18
Edwards syndrome 408–11
  autopsy 408–11
  clinical findings 408
  incidence 408
  progress 408
  spontaneous abortion 411
Ehlers–Danlos syndrome, *see* Cutis hyperelastica
Elastosis, generalized, *see* Cutis laxa congenita
Elbow
  bony ankylosis 273
  dislocation 272
    recurrent 273
Electrocardiogram
  in hydrocephalus 67
  interpretation 125
Ellis-van Creveld syndrome, genetics 19
Embryotoxon 162
Emphysema, lobar obstructive 97
Encephalocele
  cranial 47–8
    prognosis and treatment 48
Encephalo-facial angiomatosis, *see* Stürge–Weber syndrome
Encephalography in hydrocephalus 61
Encephalo - trigemino - angiomatosis 326
Endocardial fibroelastosis 122
  primary, cardiac failure in 121
Entropion 151–2
Environmental influences 7, 8
Environment/genetic influences 19–20
Epiblepharon 151
Epicanthus 148–50
  with ptosis 150
  simple 150
  treatment 150

Epidermis
  anomalies 293–303
    associated with blistering 300–3
  embryology 289–90
Epidermodysplasia verruciformis 299
Epidermolysis bullosa group of disorders 300–3
  dystrophica (dominant) 302
  gravior 303
  gravis 302
  mitis 302
  genetics 18
  Letali's (Herlitz) 303
  localised to soles 301
Epilepsy, associated with neurofibromatosis 311
Epiloia, *see* Sclerosis, tuberous
Epiphysial dysplasia, punctate, associated with cataract 175
Epispadias and ectopia vesicae 204–8
Erb's paralysis 274
Erythroderma, bullous congenital ichthyosiformis 303–4
Ethacrynic acid, in heart failure 127
Exomphalos 243–4
Exostosis, multiple, *see* Diaphyseal achlasis
Eyes
  abnormalities 147–98
  examination methods and results 147–8
  in full-term infants 185
  vascular system 184–7
    abnormalities 186–7
Eyelids, abnormalities 148–55

Face
  abnormalities 352–5
  asymmetry 264
  first arch syndrome 352–3
Faecal incontinence, in myelocele 44
Failure
  cardiac 119–21
    congenital anomalies causing 120–1
    surgery in 128
    treatment 126–9
    see also Ventricular failure

EE

Fallot, tetrad, and pulmonary atresia 109–10, 116
Fanconi's anaemia 365–6
   genetics 19
Fanconi's syndrome, *see* Cystinosis
Femur
   anomalies 274
   short 278
Fibroblastic tumours 262
Fibula
   abnormal length 279
   absence 280
Fingers, anomalies 270–2
First arch syndrome 352–3
Fistulae, arteriovenous, congenital 262–3
   aural, congenital 135
   collaural 135
   lacrimal, congenital 191
   pre-helicine, incidence 5
   and sinuses involving the skin 344–7
   urinary, at umbilicus 226
Flat feet 287
Floppy baby (amyotonia congenita) 259
Foetus, vulnerability 387
Foot and ankle 282–7
   congenital amputations 282
Fragilitas ossium, *see* Osteogenesis imperfecta
Frusemide, in heart failure 127
Fucosidosis 376–8

Galactosaemia, and postnatal cataracts 174
Gargoylism 375–8
   ocular features 195–6
Gastro-intestinal system, abnormalities 230–55
   duplications 90–2
Gene autosomal dominant in cleido-cranial dysostosis 83–4
   and megalocornea 161
   in Waardenburg's syndrome 82
   autosomal recessive, counselling 21–2
   malformations 18–19
   and megalocornea 161
   dominant, and epicanthus 148

mutant, dominant and congenital joint laxity 259
and osteogenesis imperfecta 258
Genetic determination of malformation 6, 7–23
Genetic/environmental influences 19–20
Genito-urinary system
   abnormalities 199–229
      early diagnosis 199
      external 199–219
      internal 219–28
Genu-recurvatum 281
Genu varum 281
Gigantism 262
   nails 339
Glaucoma
   congenital (buphthalmos) 189–91
      clinical features 190
      genetics 18
      treatment 190–1
Glial remnants 187
Gliosis of the aqueduct 57
Globe, abnormalities 155–60
Glossitis areata exfoliativum 348
Glossitis, median rhomboid 347–8
Glycogen storage disease 122
Goitre and deafness 139
Great vessels, incidence of malformation 4
Gronblad-Stradberg syndrome 335

Haemangioma-endothelioma, and thrombocytopenic purpura with bone changes 369
Haemangio-lipomata 262
Haemangiomas (strawberry marks) 327–8
   associated syndromes 333
   cavernous 330–3
      complications 332
      histopathology 332
      natural history 331–2
      spontaneous involution 330–1
      treatment 332–3
   laryngeal or tracheal 145
   and lymphangiomas, mixed 334
   specific capillary (stork bites) 328

Haematocolpos 212
Haemoglobin, abnormal, in cyanosis of congenital heart disease 101–4
Hair, anomalies 341–4
  beaded 343
  and hair follicle, embryology 290–1
  ringed 343
  twisted 343–4
Hallermann–Streiff syndrome 353–4
Hallux valgus 283
Hamartoma, lung 97–8
Hand, anomalies 269–72
  club, radial 271
  congenital amputation 270–1
  deformities, genetics 272
Hanlon's atrial septostomy 106
Harelip with or without cleft palate 235
Hearing defects, incidence 6
Hearing tests in children 140
Heart block, congenital 124
Heart disease
  congenital, aetiology 99
    cyanosis 99–104, 115–116
    due to abnormal forms of haemoglobin 101–2
    due to abnormal amount of reduced haemoglobin 102–4
    signs and symptoms 98–9
    treatment 126–9
Heart lesions, congenital, non-cyanotic 116–7
Heart malformation, congenital, counselling 23
  and coxsackie B virus infection 10
  incidence 4
Heart syndrome, left, 106–107, 108
Hemi-larynx 144
Hermaphroditism, true 214
Hernia, diaphragmatic 239
  genito-urinary 212
  oesophageal hiatus 23–40
  treatment 240
Herpes virus associated with pachyonychia congenita 346–7
  infection during pregnancy and malformations 9
Hip joint
  abnormalities 275–9
    examination 275–6
    screening 276–7
    bilateral signs 279
    unilateral signs 277–8
  congenital dislocation 277
    aetiology 5
    birth order and maternal age effects 10
    genetics 279
    incidence 2, 3, 5
Hiroshima, malformations after 8
Hirschsprung's disease 245–8
  abdominal distension 247
  empiric risk 246
  family studies 246
  meconium plug syndrome 247
Holt Oram syndrome 375
  dominant genes 18
Homocystinuria, and ectopia lentis 166
Hormones
  during pregnancy, effect on infant 8
Hot-foot, genetic 301
Humerus varus 273
Hunter–Hurler syndrome 138, 375–8
Hurler's disease see Gargoylism
Hyaline membrane, anterior chamber 163
Hyaloid artery 184
  persistent 186
Hyaloid cyst 186
Hydramnios, and anencephaly 27
Hydranencephaly 74–6
  features and diagnosis 76
  pathology and aetiology 74–6
Hydrocele 210
Hydrocephalus 50–69
  aetiology 51, 52
  with agenesis of corpus callosum 72
  associated with myelocele 38–41
  birth order and maternal age effects 10
  clinical features 57–60
  course and prognosis 39–41
  general management 69
  incidence 2, 3, 4, 50–51
  inflammations 56–7
  intelligence 65–6
  investigations 60–2
  natural history 62–4

Hydrocephalus (cont.)
  pathology 51–2
  sequelae, neurological and psychological 65–6
  treatment 66–8
  tumours causing 57
Hydrocolpos 211
Hydromyeloceles, in spina bifida 30
Hydronephrosis due to pelvi-ureteric obstruction 224
Hygroma, cystic 92
Hyperbilirubinaemia causing deafness 139
Hypertelorism 82, 356–7
  ocular features 194
Hypertrichosis 342–3
  and spina bifida occulta 344
Hypertrophy 262
  naevoid 337
  telangiectasic 326
Hypoplasia of aortic arch 107
  treatment 107
Hypoplastic left heart syndrome 106–7, 108
Hypospadias 201–4
  correction, 203–4
Hypotrichosis 342

Ichthyosis, congenital, associated with cataract 175
  genetics 18
  simplex 293–5
    aetiology 294
    differential diagnosis 294
    genetics 294
    prognosis 294
    treatment 294–5
  X-linked 295
    aetiology 295
    differential diagnosis 295
    genetics 295
    treatment 295
Ileus, neurogenic, x-ray appearances 250
Incidence of malformations 1–24
Incontinentia pigmenti (Bloch–Sylberger anomaly) 318–19
  associated with cataract 175
Influenza, associated with haemangiomas 332

Iniencephaly 29
Intersex states 212–19
  differential diagnosis 218–19
Intestinal obstruction
  causes 244–5
  x-ray appearances 248–50
Intrahepathic atresia 242
Iridodonesis 166
Iris 163–4
  coloboma 158–9, 163
  cysts 165

Jaw-winking 154
Jejunal atresia, apple-peel variety, genetics 18
Jervell and Lange–Nielsen, cardio-auditory syndrome 138
Joint laxity, congenital 259

Karyotypes, symbolic designation 393
Keratinization, disorders 293–5
Keratitis, interstitial, with perceptive deafness 138
Keratoderma palmo-plantaris (transgrediens) 296–7
Keratoderma palmo-plantaris with periodontosis (Papillon–Lefevre syndrome) 297
Keratoderma palmo-plantaris striata 296
Keratoderma plantaris et palmaris 296
Keratodermas, localized or regional 295–300
Keratosis follicularis (Darier's disease) 299
Keratosis follicularis bullosa (bullous form of Darier's disease) 304
Keratosis palmo-plantares 295–6
Keratosis pilaris 297–8
Kerley's lines 113
Kidney(s)
  cystic disease 223–4
  disorders 221–4
  fused and ectropic 224
  horse-shoe 224
  polycystic, 'adult' form, dominant genes 18
    infantile form, genetics 18
  solitary 224

Klinefelter's syndrome   213, 295–7
  clinical findings   396–7
  incidence   396
Klippel–Feil syndrome   266, 366–7
  and perceptive deafness   138
Klippel–Trenaunay syndrome   326
Klumpke's paralysis   274
Knee
  anomalies   280–2
  fixed flexion   281
  ulceration   281–2
Koilonychia (spoon nails)   340
Kostmann's syndrome   370

Labia, fusion   210–11
Lacrimal apparatus, abnormalities   191–2
Lacrimal drainage channels, absence or congenital occlusion   191
Lacrimal fistula, congenital   191
Laevocardia with situs inversus   123–4
Larsen's syndrome, genetics   19
Laryngeal atresia   144
Laryngeal nerve paralysis, congenital   145
Laryngeal stridor   122, 143
  congenital   143–4
Laryngeal web   144
Laryngoceles   144
Laryngomalacia   143–4
Larynx, embryology   142–3
  infantile   143–4
Laurence–Bardet syndrome   373–4
Laurence–Moon–Biedl syndrome   181, 373–4
  genetics   19
Left heart syndrome, 106–7, 108
  see also Laevocardia
Legs, abnormalities of length   279
  amputations, congenital   280
  bowing   280
  bow (genu varum)   280, 281
  dominant genes   18
  internal rotation   280
  oedema, hereditary (Milroy's disease)   18, 336–7
Lens, abnormalities   165–7
  coloboma   165–6
  ectopia lentis   166

persistent fibrovascular sheath   180, 187
subluxations, with ectopic pupil, genetics   18
Lenticonus, anterior and posterior   167
Leprechaunism   379–80
Leucodermic macules, *see* Sclerosis, tuberose
Leucodystrophy, and perceptive deafness   138
Leuconychia   340
Leukaemia, in Down's syndrome   400
Limb, lower, anomalies   274–87
  upper, anomalies   269–74
Limp baby   259–60
Lipid histiocytosis, *see* Niemann–Pick's disease
Lipochondrodysplasia, *see* Gargoylism
Lipo-chondro-dystrophy   375–8
Lipoid degenerations, familiar, ocular features   196
Lobstein syndrome   *see* Osteogenesis imperfecta
Lobster-claw foot   282
Lowe's syndrome   371
  associated with cataract   174
Lymphangiectasis, congenital pulmonary   95
Lymphangiomas   333–4
Lymph-haemangioma, diffuse   262
Lungs, 89–90
  agenesis   89–90
  anomalous lobation   89
  congenital cystic malformations   93–7
    adenomatoid   95–6
    multiple   94–5
    treatment   97
  extralobar sequestration   96–7
  hamartoma   97–8
  hypoplasia   90
  intralobar sequestration   96

Macroglossia   347, 357
Macrostomia   347
Macula coloboma   175–6
  familiar development defect   176
Macules, albinotic   315
Madelung's deformity   272

INDEX

Mal de Meleda 297
Mandibulo dysostosis 352, 353
Mandibulo-facial dysostosis 194
Marble bones, see Albers–Schonberg's disease
Marchesani syndrome 375
  genetics 19
Marcus–Gunn phenomenon (jaw-winking) 154
Marfan's syndrome (arachnodactyly) 361
  dominant genes 18
  ocular features 194
  and perceptive deafness 138
Marinesco–Sjögren syndrome 371–3
  genetics 19
Mast cell disease, see Urticaria pigmentosa
Meatal stenosis, 201, 202
Meckel's diverticulum, 248, 251
Meconium peritonitis 249
Meconium plug syndrome 247
Mediastinum, cystic anomalies 90–3
Megalencephaly 71–2
  features and diagnosis 71
  pathology 72
Megalocornea 161–2
  genetics 19
Megalopenis 209
Mega-ureter 225
Melanin, formation 315, 316
Melanoglossia (black tongue) 348
Meningitis
  ascending, associated with myelocele, 35, 39
  associated with spinal dermal sinus 50
Meningocele, anterior 93
  cranial
    clinical features 46–48
    prognosis and treatment 48
  incidence 32
  pathology 33–4
  in spina bifida 29–31
Meningo-encephalocele 183–4
Mental retardation
  associated with cataract 175
  associated with rubella in pregnancy 9
  malformations causing 69–74

Mephentermine sulphate, in cardiac murmurs 119
Mercurials, in heart failure 127
Metabolic disorders affecting skin 321–3
Metatarsus atavicus 283
Metatarsus varus 283–4
Methaemoglobinaemia
  acquired, in congenital heart disease 101
  congenital, in congenital heart disease 101
  treatment 101–102
Microcephaly 69–71
  ante-natal causes 71
  features and diagnosis 69–70
  genetics and aetiology 70–71
  pathology 71
Microcornea 160–1
Microglossia 347
Micrognathia 354
Micronychia 339
Micropenis 208–9
Microphthalmos
  causes 156–8
  treatment 158
Micropolygyria 77–8
Microstomia 354–5
Microtia 355
Micturition, disorders 220–1
Milroy's disease, see Legs, oedema
Mitral atresia 107
Mitral stenosis 107
Möbius syndrome 381–2
  and perceptive deafness 138
Mole, hairy 308
  see also Naevus
Mongolism, see Down's syndrome
Monilethrix (beaded hair) 343
Morphine, in heart failure 128
Morquio–Brailsford syndrome 377–8
Morquio–Ullrich syndrome 376–8
Mosaicism, associated malformations 16–17
Mouth
  absence 347
  anomalies 347–8
Mucolipidosis 376–8
Mucopolysaccharide metabolic defect with perceptive deafness 138

Mucopolysaccharide metabolism, anomalies 195–6
Mucopolysaccharidosis 376–8
Murmurs, cardiac, in newborn 117–19
Muscles, abdominal, absent 228, 367–8
Muscular atrophy 260
Mustard septostomy 106
  in cyanotic congenital heart lesions 115–16
Myelocele 34–46
  appearance 34
  Arnold–Chiari malformation 53–5
  associated malformations 38
  associated with hydrocephalus 38–41
  early operation, results 42–3
  faecal incontinence 44
  general management 45–6
  limb movements 43
  neurological involvement 36–8
  orthopaedic management 45
  in spina bifida 29–31
  survival rate 40–41
  treatment of spinal lesion 42–4
  urinary incontinence 44–5
  urinary tract involvement 37–8
Myelocytoceles, in spina bifida 30
Myelomeningoceles, in spina bifida 30
Myopia
  congenital, types 192–3
  treatment, 193

Naevo-xantho-endothelioma, *see* Xanthoma, juvenile
Naevus,
  amelanotic 309–10
  arachneus (spider naevus) 326
  blue 309
  epithelial 310–11
  flammeus (port wine stain) 328–30
    treatment 328–30
  molle (cellular naevus) 308
  of Ota 310
  pigmented 304–8
    classification 305–6
    definition 304–5
    diagnosis 308
    embryology and epigenetics 306–7
    genetics 307
    histopathology 307–8
    prognosis 308
    treatment 308
  spider, *see* Naevus arachneus
  Sutton's 310
  syringocystasenomatous papilliferus (syringocystadenoma) 311
  ulotrichus capilliti 311
  Unna's 328
  woolly hair, *see* Naevus ulotrichus capilliti
  see also Mole
Nails, absence 338
  atrophy 338–9
  in clubbing of digits 340
  congenital anomalies 338–44
  gigantism 339
  onchogryphosis 339
  racket 340
  shedding 339
  spoon 340
  supernumerary 340
  thickening 339
Nasolacrimal duct, congenital occlusion 192
Neck, deformities 264–6
Neural tube, closure defects 25–50
Neuroectodermal anomalies 304–14
Neurofibromatosis 263
  aetiology 312
  associated disorders 313
  complications 313
  differential diagnosis 313
  genetics 312–13
  pathology 312
  and perceptive deafness 138
  prognosis 313
  treatment 313
  Von Recklinghausen's 93, 195, 311–13
Neurological involvement in myelocele 36–8
Niemann–Pick's disease, ocular features 196
Nipples, and breasts, absence 346
  accessory 346
Nose, embryology 140–1
Nuchal naevus flammeus (Unna's naevus) 328

Obstruction
   bladder-neck 226–7
   intestinal, *see* Intestinal obstruction
   pelvi-ureteric 224, 225
   urethral, anterior 227–8
Ocular-cerebro-renal dystrophy 371
Oesophageal atresia 236–9
   diagnosis 237
   treatment 238–9
   types 236–7
Oesophageal fistula without atresia 237–8
Onychauxis 339
Onychomadesis 339
Onychogryphosis of nails 339
Optic atrophy 182–3
   causes 182–3
   treatment 183
Optic nerve, abnormalities 181–3
Orbit, abnormalities 183–4
Oro-facio-digital syndrome, genetics 19
Orthopaedic abnormalities 256–88
Ortolani's test 276, 277
Osteochondritis of medial tibial epiphysis (Blount's disease) 281
Osler–Rendu–Weber disease, *see* Telangiectasia, hereditary haemorrhagic
Osteochondromata, knee 280–1
Osteogenesis imperfecta 257–8, 363–5
   ocular features 194
Osteopsathyrosis, *see* Osteogenesis imperfecta
Otosclerosis and conductive deafness 139
Oxycephaly 80, 357
   associated with cataract 174
   ocular features 193
Oxygen, in heart failure 126
Oxygen levels in congenital heart disease 101–4

Pachyonychia congenita 341, 346–7
Papillon–Lefevre syndrome 297
Parents, advice to 350, 351, 352
   see also Counselling
Patau's syndrome 404–8
   autopsy 407
   clinical findings 406–7
   incidence 406

Patella, congenital dislocation 281
Patent ductus arteriosus 118, 119
   cardiac failure in 120–1
Pectoralis major, absence, part or all 273
Pelvic obliquity 278
Pendred's syndrome 138, 371
   genetics 19
Penis
   anomalies 201–10
   carcinoma 201
   circumcision 199–201
   rare anomalies 208–9
   torsion 209
Peritonitis, advanced, x-ray appearances 249–50
   bacterial 248
Pes cavus 284
Peutz–Jegher's syndrome, *see* Pigmentation of the skin and mucosae with intestinal polyposis
Phimosis, and need for circumcision 200–1
Pierre Robin syndrome 352
Pigmentation
   anomalies 314–21
   ocular features 197
Pigmentation of the skin and mucosae with intestinal polyposis (Peutz–Jeghers syndrome) 319–20
Pili annulati (ringed hair) 343
Pili torti (twisted hair) 343–4
Pityriasis rubra pilaris 298
Plagiocephaly 79
Poikiloderma congenitale 336
Polycoria 164
Polydactyly 271
   associated with congenital heart disease 99
   birth order and maternal age effects 10
   incidence 5
Polymastia 346
Polyposis, intestinal, and pigmentation of the skin 319–20
Polythelia 346
Pompe's disease 122
Porencephaly
   features and diagnosis 77
   pathology 76

INDEX

Porokeratosis of Mibelli 298–9
Porphyria, congenital 321
Port wine stain, *see* Naevus flammeus
Potter's facies 370
   associated with renal agenesis 219
Potts procedure 110
Pregnancy
   hormone treatment, and malformation 8
   radium treatment causing malformation 8
   virus infections during, and malformations 9
   x-rays during causing microcephaly 71
Premature infants
   congenital myopia 192
   eyes 184
Procaine amide hydrochloride in paroxysmal tachycardia 129
Propranolol in heart failure 128
Pseudoglioma 179–80
Pseudohermaphroditism female 214–16
   male 217–18
Pseudotruncus 111
Pseudoxanthoma elasticum 335–6
Pterygium 340
Ptosis 153–4
   dominant genes 18
   treatment 154
Pulmonary atresia and severe tetrad of Fallot 109–10, 116
Pulmonary stenosis
   cardiac failure in 121
   with intact ventricular septum and reversed interatrial shunt 110–11
Pulmonary venous drainage, total anomalous 112–14
Pulse in congenital heart disease 119
Pupillary membrane, persistent 186
Pupils
   abnormal 164–5
   ectopic 164–5
   ectropion of pigment layer 165
   polycoria 164
   slit-shaped 164
Purpura 368
Pyloric stenosis

hypertrophic 240–1
   genetic and environmental factors 241
   incidence and aetiology 5
Pyuria, associated with anomalies 222–3

Quinidine in ventricular tachycardia 128–9

Rachischisis, localized, in spina bifida 30
Radiography in hydrocephalus 60
Radium treatment during pregnancy causing malformation 8
Rashkind atrial septostomy 106
Rashkind procedure in cyanotic congenital heart lesions 115–16
Rectal agenesis 254
Rectum and anus, abnormalities 251–4
Reifenstein syndrome, genetics 19
Renal agenesis 223
Renal dysplasia 223
Renal failure 221–2
Renal rickets 257
Renal tract anomalies, and Potter facies 370–1
Respiratory difficulty as presenting symptom 122
Respiratory tract, anomalies 87–98
Retina and choroid
   abnormalities 175–81
   coloboma 158
   opaque nerve-fibres 176–7
Retinal septum 176
Retinitis pigmentosa, perceptive deafness 138
Retinoblastoma 180
Retrolental fibroplasia 180
   and microphthalmos 157–8
Rickets
   renal 257
   vitamin-resistant 256–7
Rubella, maternal, causing congenital deafness 138–9
   clinical features 171
   ocular signs 171–3
   treatment 173

Rubella, (cont.)
  incidence 8
  and microphthalmos 156
  ocular features 179

Sacrum, congenital absence 367
Sanfillipo–Scheie syndrome 375–8
Scalp defects 84
Scaphocephaly 80
Schaffer's syndrome, associated with cataract 175
Schiller's syndrome, and perceptive deafness 138
Sciatic nerve palsy 282
Sclerosis
  albinotic macules 315
  tuberous 385
    and its cutaneous manifestations 313
    genetics 314
    histology 314
Scoliosis 266–7
  congenital 267
  idiopathic 267–8
Sebaceous cysts, hereditary, see Sebocystomatosis, familial
Sebocystomatosis, familial (hereditary sebaceous cysts) 311
Septostomy, atrial, Hanlon's 106
  Mustard 106
  Rashkind 106
Septum, deviated, nasal 141
Sex, diagnostic problems 212–19
Shoulder, recurrent subluxation 273
Shunt, ventriculo-auricular, in hydrocephalus 67
Silver–Russell syndrome 380
Sinus
  occipital dermal 50
    associated with dermoid 50
  spinal dermal 48–50
    incidence 49
    infection 50
    pathology 49–50
Sinuses involving the skin, and congenital fistulae 344–7
Skeletal system, abnormalities 256–9
Skeletal tissue disorders 79–84

Skin
  abnormalities 289–349
  embryology 289–92
  gross congenital defects 345–6
  pigmentation, see Pigmentation
  vascular anomalies involving 325–34
Skull defects 84
Spherophakia 166–7
Sphincter involvement in myelocele 37–8
Spina bifida 29–32
  anatomy 29–30
  birth order and maternal age effects 10
  embryology 29
  familial recurrence 27–8
  incidence 2, 3, 25, 32
  lumbo-sacral 268–9
  pathology 30–31
Spina bifida cystica
  aetiology 32
  incidence 3
Spina bifida occulta
  and hypertrichosis 344
  pathology and management 29, 31–2
Spine, anomalies 266–9
Splint
  Denis Browne abduction 277
  Frejka pillow 277
Sprengel's deformity 266
Squint 187–9
  aetiology 187
  birth trauma 188
  clinical features 187
  congenital types 188
  developmental defect 187
Staphyloma, anterior 162
Stork bites, see Haemangiomas, specific capillary
Strawberry marks, see Haemangiomas
Sturge–Kalischer–Weber syndrome 326
Sturge–Weber syndrome (encephalofacial angiomatosis) 383–4
  ocular features 195
  and port wine stain 329
Subglottic stenosis, congenital 144–5
Sulphaemoglobinaemia, in congenital heart disease 102
Sutures, premature fusion 79–81
Sweat glands embryology 291

Syndactyly 271
  associated with congenital heart disease 99
Synostosis of radius and ulna 272–3
Syphilis, congenital, and cataract 173–4
  ocular features 179
Syringocystadenoma, *see* Naevus syringocystadenomatous papilliferus
Syringomyeloceles, in spina bifida 30

Tachycardia
  paroxysmal nodal 125
  supraventricular 124
  ventricular 125
Tail, faun's or satyr's 308
Talipes
  birth order and maternal age effects 10
  incidence 2, 3
  incidence and aetiology 5
Talipes equino-varus 284–7
  genetics 286
  treatment 284, 285
Talus, congenital vertical 286–7
Tay–Sach's disease (amaurotic family idiocy) ocular features 196
Tears, congenital absence 191
Teeth, anomalies 348
Telangiectasis, hereditary haemorrhagic (Osler–Rendu–Weber disease) 142, 326–7
Telangiectasia 326–34
Testes
  anomalies 209–10
  feminization, genetics 19, 217
  torsion 210
  undescended 210
Testicular feminization syndrome 19, 217
Testosterone, in pseudohermaphroditism 216
Tetrad of Fallot 109–10
Thalidomide syndrome 385–7
Thoracic dystrophy 360
Thumb
  absence 270
  congenital adduction 271
  trigger 271
Thyroid dysfunction, causing deafness 139
Tibia
  abnormal length 279
  absence 280
Tissues, connective, and dermis, abnormalities 334–44
  supporting, general affections 259–64
Toe(s), anomalies 282
  curly 282
  fifth, absence and contracture 283
  hammer 283
  interphalangeal valgus 282
Tongue
  abnormalities 347–8, 357
  absence 347
  black 348
  cleft (bifid) 347
  in Down's syndrome 357
  geographical 348
  scrotal 347
  tie 347
Torticollis
  muscular 265
  structural 265
Toxoplasmosis
  and congenital cataract 173
  effect on retina 177
  maternal, and microphthalmos 156
Trachea
  anomalies 88–9
  compression 88
  stenosis 88
Tracheomalacia 88–9
Transposition of great arteries 104–6
  cyanosis 104
  treatment 105–6, 115
Trapesius, absence, part or all 273
Treacher–Collins syndrome 134–5, 137, 352
Trichorrhexis nodosa 344
Tricuspid atresia 110
Triploidy 411
Truncus arteriosus, persistent 111–12, 115
Tuberculosis, chorioretinitis 179
Tumours causing hydrocephalus 57
Turner's syndrome 214

Turner's syndrome (*cont.*)
  chromosome mutations 16, 17, 397–8
  incidence of congenital heart disease 99
Turricephaly 80, 357
Twins
  aetiology 6
  studies, genetic-environment influences 20
Tylosis, *see* Keratoderma plantaris et palmaris

Ureterocele, ectopic 225
Ureters
  duplication 225–6
  mega-ureter 225
Urinary fistula at umbilicus 226
Urinary infections, associated with abnormalities 222
Urinary tract involvement in myelocele 37–8, 44
Urticaria pigmentosa (mast cell disease) 323–5
  aetiology 323–4
  differential diagnosis 324–5
  genetics 324
  histopathology 324
  prognosis 325
  treatment 325
Usher's syndrome 138
Uterus, anomalies 210–12

Vagina, anomalies 210–12
Valves, urethral, posterior 227
Van de Hoeve's syndrome and conductive deafness 139
Ventricle, left, diverticulum 123
Ventricular failure, left, acyanotic lesions producing cyanosis from 114–15
Virus infections in pregnancy, association with malformations 9
Vitamin A
  in ichthyosis 295
  in tylosis 296
Von Recklinghausen's disease, *see* Neurofibromatosis
Vrolik syndrome, *see* Osteogenesis imperfecta

Waardenburg's syndrome 82–3, 138, 356–7
  dominant genes 18
Waterston–Cooley procedure 110
Webbing, congenital 263–4
Werdning–Hoffman's disease 260
Wildervanck's syndrome 138
Willi–Prader–Maurance syndrome 380–1
Wiskott–Aldrich syndrome 368–9
Wolff–Parkinson–White syndrome 124
Wrist, congenital dislocation 272
Wry neck 264–5

Xanthoma, juvenile (naevo-xantho-endothelioma) 322–3
Xanthomatosis, hypercholesterolemic 321–2
Xeroderma pigmentosum 320–1
  aetiology 320
  differential diagnosis, prognosis, treatment 321
  genetics 320